Rising to the challenges of child development

How to help them find their wings

Iñaki Pastor Pons
Jara Acín y Rivera

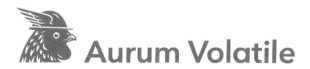
Aurum Volatile

Authors
Iñaki Pastor Pons
Jara Acín y Rivera

Layout:
Daniel Latorre

Graphic material:
Iñaki Pastor
Mathew Lee
Daniel Latorre

Translation:
Helen Williams

Edition:
Laura Ayala

Edit:
Editorial Aurum Volatile
AP. 95 - 50.080 Zaragoza

ISBN:
978-84-697-6853-2

Legal deposit:
Z-1462-2017

We would like to emphasize here that we have tried to use inclusive language throughout, although on many occasions we found the vocabulary required to represent everyone involved in caring for and raising children was lacking, or that the terms available were not politically correct, or simply did not evoke the concepts we wanted to convey. Gender-specific terms have been used with the primary aim of making the book easier to read, i.e. the masculine pronoun "he" or feminine pronoun "she" when referring to an infant, child or adolescent. This is purely a matter of style and whenever a gender-specific term is used, it should be understood to refer to both genders, unless explicitly stated otherwise.

Likewise, bearing in mind that, from a neuro-psycho-biological point of view, the mother's role is essential in many aspects of early life, some chapters contain more references to the maternal role than the paternal.

Nonetheless, it is our desire and intention to raise awareness of the important responsibility everyone involved in a child's development has, regardless of their gender or role in the care system. Moms and dads, uncles and aunts, caregivers, grandmothers and grandfathers, teachers, family friends and myriad others form part of the tribe that makes this extraordinary development possible.

We want to take this opportunity to invite you to put forward more inclusive terms that can be accepted into everyday language, so that those of us who work with families can vindicate the contribution each human being makes to the most important job in life, that of accompanying an individual's development.

"*There are two lasting bequests we can give our children: roots and wings.*"

Hodding Carter

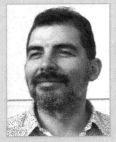

IÑAKI PASTOR PONS

Iñaki is a Pediatric Physiotherapist who specializes in child development. He is the creator and director of Pediatric Integrative Manual Therapy (PIMT) and Director of the Institute of Integrative Therapies in Zaragoza. He is the author of Manual therapy in the oculomotor system (Elsevier, 2012).

Iñaki has a master's degree in Pediatric Physiotherapy and is an International Professor of Global Postural Reeducation. He provides physiotherapy training and gives seminars and conferences in different countries around the world. He is founder of the Aragonese Institute of Health and Child Development (IASDI).

This book is dedicated to the moms and dads who dream of bringing a new life into the world and are committed to nurturing it with the greatest of love and respect. The kind of parents who are the driving force behind their children and at the same time, their refuge: who play happily with them and yet are firm in equal measure: who are testimony to the kind of love that expects nothing in return: who fight to the last in the face of adversity: indeed, whoare our hope for a better world."

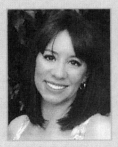

JARA ACÍN Y RIVERA

Jara has a degree in Clinical Health Psychology and she is founding partner and co-director of Elán Psicología where she is in charge of the Child and Adolescent department. She holds a Diploma in Advanced Studies in Legal and Forensic Medicine, a Master's degree in Legal and Forensic Clinical Psychology, and is an Emergency Management and Disaster Preparedness specialist. She is also a family therapist, a certified Positive Discipline trainer: a sensorimotor and clinical EMDR therapist specializing in the treatment of attachment and trauma, with special focus on early abandonment trauma.

She trains professionals, students and families in different areas relating to child care.

I want to dedicate this book to the children I have been lucky enough to meet and help. They have fueled my desire to continue learning and delving ever deeper, to cross borders and learn other languages. They have taught me that human beings have infinite power of healing and we must do everything we can to guide them on their journey, however bumpy the ride may be.

Surviving is success in itself."

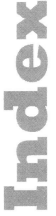

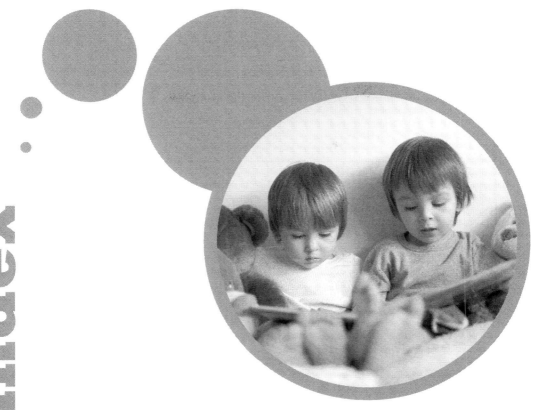

INTRODUCTION
Life has a habit of finding its own path.
How wonderful to contribute to its growth!

It wasn't our intention. Honestly, it wasn't. At least not initially!

Infants, children and adolescents have slowly but surely invaded our conscience and become the main focus of our attention and long hours of research over the years, right up to the present day.

All this time we were both moving in the same direction, from working with adults to what we consider to be the essence of the human being: development in the early stages of life.

We are both fortunate enough to work in a field we are passionate about and have the chance to gain fresh insights into each case we treat. This means we have developed our own way of working, a way that transgresses the barriers of traditional or reductionist approaches.

A fresh outlook, countless hours of research, training in different parts of the world, years of clinical practice and a holistic approach that covers all the areas involved in development are the linchpin of our work.

It is in this context that we began to share our interests, doubts, concerns, points of view, therapeutic approaches and renegade views about how certain issues were being addressed in the general framework of health care. Where the discoveries began, where new avenues of work and collaboration opened up, creating this new way of working on some of the cases we had in common. A way that takes into consideration that movement builds the brain, as does the predictability of parental care. Or that the prenatal, perinatal and first years of life are the time when much of what an individual will become in the future is programmed and therefore, this is where we should be building and repairing. Or that traumas in early childhood leave a visible and verifiable physiological imprint on brain development. Or that a lack of stimulation in infants and young children can have a greater impact on their learning than might be expected. This holistic model stems from a committed, tenacious attitude, and is underpinned by the knowledge that a baseline situation of deficient or traumatic development is reversible in most cases.

We are fortunate enough to live in an era of exceptional growth and, at the same time, deepening of the fields of both Physiotherapy and Psychology. Our curiosity about how this early programing of the nervous system takes place has been, and continues to be, satisfied thanks to scientific advances in neurological development and function.

New scientific research has caught our attention and made us determined to carry out our own investigations in search of more answers for those who come to us seeking help.

Learning disabilities, pain, attention or behavior disorders... can be approached in an inclusive, functional way, by triggering the solutions in the indivual's own organicity. More importantly, in many cases these issues can be avoided altogether by providing infants with the right stimulation and by understanding their real needs.

A new way of accompanying your child's development is possible and your role is pivotal. We want to help you in this crucial task by providing you with a clear, practical, groundbreaking guide so that, through knowledge and an awareness of all the possibilities – both your child's and your own – you can achieve your goal of helping them to find their wings.

Rising to the challenges of child development –How to help them find their wings, will give you the keys to ensure your child's development is extraordinary and to its fullest potential, so that they can adapt to the world they live in to the very best of their ability, confidently and, above all, happily.

In the chapters by Iñaki, you will learn how your child is shaped as a person and how their nervous system matures. You will clearly see the stages they have to go through to learn how to inhabit their own body and, little by little, relate to the world without you by their side. This can help you support them, lovingly stimulating their development whilst enjoying your parenting role. It is crucial you understand how they learn to control their hands, how their vision develops or how their language matures, so that you feel happy to support them and ready to enjoy every moment to the fullest as they grow and mature.

There are several chapters dedicated to learning disabilities. If your child has some kind of problem, these pages will offer you guidance and support. You will learn how medical diagnoses are made and what their limitations are and see why it is essential that a child is assessed from a functional, global perspective. The only way we can develop support programs to help these children reach their maximum potential is by using this paradigm. As you will see, there are many specialists out there qualified to help your child and your whole family.

One whole chapter is devoted to children and pain. This is a groundbreaking chapter you won't find in any other book. It will help you support your child when they are in pain, because pain is unavoidable at certain points in our lives to protect us from danger and assist our recovery. By using the recommendations in this chapter, you will be preventing your child from becoming a chronic patient in the future.

The last three chapters of the book about your child's emotional programming are fascinating. Here Jara gives advice on how to help your child develop a confident, happy personality.

These chapters are particularly valuable, because they will help you understand how to support them through those moments when life is no bed of roses. The moments of suffering they will go through, or perhaps, already have, when you have the chance to be by their side to give them vital reassurance. You will learn how to create a strong bond with your child, an experience that will make a real difference to their life, making them feel secure, worthy of love and capable of giving their best.

We really appreciate the trust placed in us when choosing this book and we are delighted it reached your hands. We know how much you love your children and are confident you will use these pages to ensure they grow up in the happiest, safest way possible.

We wrote this book in the hope and conviction that anything is possible....

Iñaki and Jara

Chapter 1

Programming
The key to a person's biologial, emotional and social make-up

Iñaki Pastor Pons

What an amazing feeling! The midwife places in your arms this helpless-looking being that awakens intense emotions you never knew existed: feelings that will stay with you throughout the rest of your life as a mother or father. Life will never be the same again. From now on, the good times will be pure heaven and the bad times, pure hell. Our children and their life-experiences dramatically increase the intensity of our emotions.

They are the greatest gift life can give you but they don't belong to you. According to Khalil Gibran, «they are the sons and daughters of Life's longing for itself. They come through you but not from you. And though they are with you, they belong not to you».

I don't know if you have just one baby or more than one; an older girl or boy, or perhaps even a great big family. Whatever the case, do you remember your children coming with instructions? Wouldn't that make life so much easier? Even though being a parent is a totally natural thing, no-one is really prepared for it. Or perhaps everyone is in some way. Being prepared is probably written in your genes and it could well be that you have the innate ability to take care of your children and raise them successfully. But in this day and age who can truly say they are in touch with their natural instincts? Western society has a significant impact on our way of being and our behaviour to the extent that hardly anyone can distinguish innate natural behaviour that has evolved over millions of years, from social behaviour acquired in the last 2-3 generations. Perhaps the huge changes in habitat and culture that humans have undergone have drowned out or blurred the voice of our natural instincts.

Human genetics are millions of years old but there is growing evidence that our first experiences in life have an enormous impact on how what is coded in our genes is triggered and develops. What happens to us early in life has a bearing on the rest of our existence, as though it were some form of programming or learning process for our brain to adapt to the life we are going to lead.

It is widely accepted that there are a large number of children with developmental, attention, behavioural and emotional disorders and learning disabilities in our society (not to mention other health-related issues such as excess weight), and it is thought that in many cases experiences early on in life played a crucial role in their future problems. This leads us to ask ourselves: which experiences determine our children's health, optimal mental development and emotional security? What determines if the child will be good at concentrating, learning, coordinating and being resilient in the future? Conversely, which factors will lead to a child developing learning disabilities, clumsiness or impulsiveness?

Join me now as I explore these issues that are so crucial to your life and that of your children.

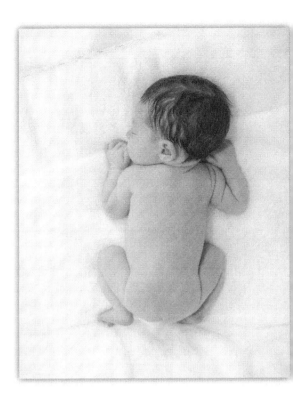

Luca is only a few days old. We can see the tuck position characteristic of the first stage after birth. Despite being fully dependent and requiring comprehensive care, he is not a blank page. His brain is already equipped with many basic survival programs and neurological programming.

What does programming mean?

To program is to provide a system with the instructions necessary for it to perform its function automatically. Normally we use the word "program" when we refer to computers or machines, but throughout this book you will discover that human beings are also full of automatisms, tasks and processes that we develop without realizing it. Spare a thought as you read this book, how many automatic functions are going on without your direct involvement? Your heartbeat, your breathing, your kidney function or the thousands of biochemical processes that are being managed right now in your liver. You may receive more information from your digestive system but that doesn't mean you control it. The automatism of the internal processes of your organs may seem straightforward, but there are other aspects that work based on programming beyond your control.

In order to read these lines, your brain carries out hundreds or thousands of tasks at full speed through very fast neuronal connections. And all this while reading the word "very fast". Position and movement of the eyes, position and movement of the head, posture control, visual input that reaches the specialised areas of the brain from the eyes, selective orientation to avoid reading "tsaf yrev" ("very fast" backwards), connections from the visual areas to the auditory areas that will determine the meaning of that word through thousands of connections called synapses. Despite being a voluntary movement, even ordering a single finger to move to turn the page is a very complex task that requires the control of hundreds of muscles in your body. The majority of these muscles are busy steadying the parts that are not supposed to move. Even as children some people suffer nervous system disorders that make the simplest of gestures very difficult, even though the voluntary order is clear.

Emotionally automatisms are even more evident when you sometimes react angrily to certain comments or situations; when you are madly in love with someone and your heart skips a beat every time you think about them; or when your emotions are running high and wreaking havoc with your body, making even the simplest of things seem complicated.

All these automatisms are forming the foundations and workings of your nature, your nervous system or your emotional world. As we will see later on, to some extent each of these processes supports your voluntary behavior and awareness, including your perception of yourself, of others and of the world at large.

The incredible thing is that each one of those automatisms has been programmed at some initial stage of our existence, although of course, they can be reset thanks to other experiences we have over the course of our lifetime.

Not everything starts at birth

A good question to start off with might be: how does the nervous system program itself or how is it programmed and when does this start?

Early programming is genetic. Every living being is created based on a genetic code that determines in a very significant way what we are and what we are like. This early programming also has a bearing on the possibility of having certain gifts or abilities, and also of developing certain diseases later in life. Science and philosophy have been debating for years which is more important, genetic inheritance or environment, genetics or epigenetics, nature or nurture. Perhaps it is just one of those classic battles between two necessarily complementary ideas. Neither can be ruled out and deciding which is more important will not get us very far. Who your children are is written in their DNA. Yet even genes need a specific environment to develop or not, to activate or remain silent. A child may have an innate ability (genetic) for music or art, but if their environment prevents them from being exposed to these kinds of experiences, they cannot possibly develop their talent to its full potential. Often, an autoimmune disease written in the genes doesn't show up until a period of severe stress or a destabilizing infection results in

hyperarousal of the immune system. Yet in other individuals, a disease programmed in certain genes will never show any symptoms.

Who your children are is written in their DNA but even genes require a specific environment to develop.

The second stage of programming occurs in the first prenatal stage up to 8 weeks after fertilization. This is known as embryogenesis, the period of human development in the womb during which the embryo is formed. At this stage the embryo is particularly sensitive to the mother's experiences. Drinking alcohol, smoking or taking drugs, different types of medicines, many chemical substances and certain types of radiation, can all have a dramatic impact on the formation of the embryo, leading to malformations or stunted growth. Women also require the correct vitamins and nutrients, which is why certain food supplements are recommended for pregnant women and those trying to get pregnant. Bear in mind that a large part of this new human being is already formed after just 8 weeks, so what happens in the first few weeks is decisive.

The fetal stage is next, lasting from the 9th week of pregnancy until birth. You could call it the third programming stage. During this stage the organs continue to form until they are fully developed and then carry on growing and maturing until birth. In this period, some sensory systems begin to function, such as the sensitivity of the skin

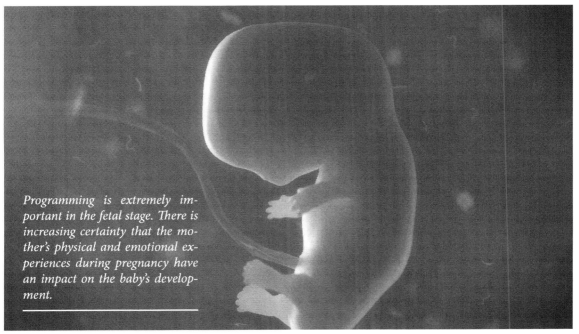

Programming is extremely important in the fetal stage. There is increasing certainty that the mother's physical and emotional experiences during pregnancy have an impact on the baby's development.

around the mouth or the perception of head movement thanks to the formation and activation of receptors within the ear, the so-called vestibular system.

The fetus is also able to perform many movements which gradually become more varied and precise. Intriguingly, in ultrasounds we see fetuses making movements newborns are incapable of, as gravity holds less sway in the aquatic environment provided by the amniotic fluid. At this stage, it is still essential to avoid toxic or damaging substances (teratogens) that may harm the fetus or cause malformations. But there are other more subtle aspects that are also important, such as the biochemical communication between the mother and child that leaves the fetus exposed to the mother's stress peaks thanks to the influx of certain hormones via the umbilical cord. The mother's nervous system is able to metabolize these substances and neutralize them quite quickly. The fetus, on the other hand, cannot deal with them or regulate them yet. We also know that some of the difficult experiences the mother has had as a result of nutritional and environmental factors, can clearly affect the way her babies are programmed for the future. The mother's well-being and her physical and emotional state, have a direct impact on the fetus.

The mother's well-being and her physical and emotional state have a direct impact on the fetus.

The first sensory system to be myelinated is the vestibular system. So, what is myelination? During the myelination process the nerves are covered in a substance called myelin which allows nerve impulses to travel faster (after all, it runs on electricity). This is one of the key processes in the maturation of the nervous system. As we will see in the chapter on movement, the vestibular system is central to orientation and balance but it is also responsible for helping to mature different areas of the brain. It is very important that pregnant women move around and keep active so that the fetus registers the movements and this system, which is so crucial to the child's neurological development, matures. If a medical condition means the mother is obliged to rest during the pregnancy, it is important to check if the baby is developing properly in the first few weeks. Did you know that by observing a baby's muscle tone and eye fixation in week 8, we can tell how he will develop in the future?

It is very important for a pregnant woman to move

around and keep fairly active so that the fetus can register her movements and its brain can mature.

Around week 16 of the fetal development stage, the first automatic motor patterns called primitive reflexes begin to appear. They will form the basis for future motor and sensory systems. Examples of primitive reflexes include; the sucking reflex when something is inserted into the infant's mouth; the palmar reflex when something brushes the palm of his hand; the rooting reflex which makes him turn his head and lips towards something stroking his cheek. There are over 100 different automatic patterns that will help the baby's survival and neurological programming. The innate movements triggered by these primitive reflexes, especially those associated with the vertebrae of the neck and the spine, help the baby to move down the birth canal more effectively and easily.

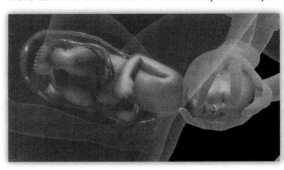

The image above shows the stage of birth where the baby's head is already out, and he needs to turn to release his body. The baby should turn by himself but sometimes he needs a little help. His primitive reflexes help him move down the birth canal. This is a defining moment in life. Do you remember your journey into the world?

As you can see, a baby is not a blank canvas at birth. He enters the world equipped with extremely basic, archaic software, which, nevertheless, is very effective! He has a series of programs and automatic applications that are responsible for contributing to his survival and helping to organize more complex, better customized programs in the future. Absolutely everything in the newborn works through automatic processes. His breathing, digestion, movements and response to the unexpected, amongst other systems, all work with primitive programs that will be updated as the child grows (just like computer updates), as he receives the appropriate stimuli and his nervous system matures. The first update begins in a part of the brain called the brainstem. The brainstem is responsible for developing the most basic survival functions, updating the first sensory and motor programs, and programming stress. As we will see in subsequent chapters, the brain is built in layers, and when the base is solid we can expect the higher functions to develop well. Which stimuli are necessary for the foundations of the nervous system to be solid? This is where the fourth program comes into play.

A child is not a blank canvas at birth.

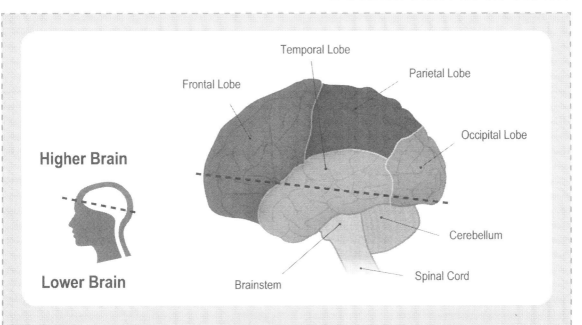

A diagram of the brain. The structure of the nervous system is quite hierarchical. The lower brain is more archaic and the higher brain more advanced, phylogenetically speaking. All vertebrate animals, even the simplest of them, have a spinal cord that conducts the nerves to the entire body. Humans have developed a very advanced higher brain called the cortex. However, early in life the embryo functions via primitive neural control from the medullary centers and then the brainstem. These two parts of the nervous system manage a human being's needs via automatic, involuntary programs. This is how, little by little as his «higher brain» develops, the infant will be capable of more intentional motor responses and in the future, of uniquely human functions such as language or math.

The first months and years have a lifelong impact

When he was first born your baby's movements were general. To move one part of his body he had to move everything. He lacked the necessary muscle control to stabilize or direct a section of his body, independently of the rest. For several days after birth a neonate is particularly lucid and attentive, perhaps in a bid to bond with his parents, and he appears to be still recovering from the major and doubtless, difficult, task of being born.

What the mother experiences is labor. What the baby experiences is birth. Sometimes a very good labor can result in a very bad birth and vice versa. A labor which goes well and leaves the mother with the feeling that «everything was easy», may coexist with a birth where the baby suffered a lot either during engagement or delivery because of pressure to his neck. Birth involves two people and yet perhaps we tend to see things more from the mother's point of view than from the baby's. On the other hand, it's hardly surprising. Can anyone remember anything about their birth other than what they've been told?

Children don't simply grow like plants, they also need to mature. In your baby's case maturing means programming, a journey that will last a lifetime. Maturing involves creating connections in the brain called synapses. The more synapses you have and the faster and more efficient they are, the better your brain will work. Let's imagine the brain is like a very advanced computer with hardware consisting of chips, cables and housing (a brain has neurons, glial cells, synapses and processing centers) and has a series of programs installed (software of varying quality), with very advanced applications that allow you to perform all the tasks you need to. Even if the programs work well, you can have several windows open at the same time, which in the case of the brain means being able to do several activities at once, such as walking and reading, or driving and talking.

What the mother experiences is labor. What the baby experiences is birth.

The development of the brain goes hand in hand with its growth. For the head to grow significantly before birth would be very limiting and dangerous as the baby must come down a rather narrow birth canal. In fact, human beings are born prematurely physiologically speaking. Really we are born ahead of time, before we are capable of adapting to the environment with a certain degree of autonomy. If we think of a foal, it can stand up and follow its parents around as soon as it is born. Comparatively speaking, a foal is much more evolved than we are. But and it's a very big «but», there is a very good reason why human beings need to be born before we are fully developed. The reason is that the rate at which we mature is dependent on the growth of our brain and if our brain were to grow any bigger, the size of our head would prevent us from traveling down the birth canal.

Children don't simply grow like plants, they also have to mature.

The truth is that it is a tight squeeze for the baby and difficult for him to come down the birth canal with any degree of comfort; birth is a very complex and dangerous process that poses many risks. The size of the baby's head is already too big for the canal which is why he has

to tuck his chin into his chest to make the diameter of the head compatible with the space in the mother's pelvis which is about 10 centimeters. The baby's position with his head tucked down is just one of the many adaptations that mother and baby make to assist the birth. In any case, even with all the help that nature offers we are still born long before we are independent, even in terms of physical movement.

The baby's maturation process and the development of his nervous system will go through different stages and processes during which new and more complex nerve connections will develop in increasingly superior and specialized centers, together with a progressive myelination that will enable the system to be faster and more efficient. At the same time the brain will grow and with it, the head.

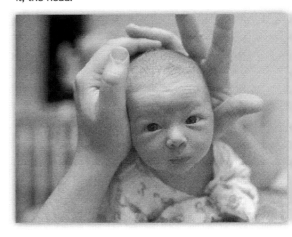

Marco's first life experiences will «program» him. Repetitive stimulation is part of his training for life.

The fourth stage of human programming occurs in the first months and years of life and includes the maturation of the sensory system, motor system, immune system, digestive system, along with emotional and social development, etc. Everything is programmed in these early stages, equipping the child to run all these different systems for the rest of his life. Even breathing is programmed. The way a newborn baby breathes, for example, is different from that of a 3 or 4 year old child because it is controlled by an archaic nervous center in the cervical spinal cord. That's why when you hear your baby sleeping, their breathing seems rapid and irregular, and you remain vigilant, checking on him several times a night. Then, a little later, his breathing becomes deeper and safer and less likely to stop suddenly. Programming affects the entire human being and will determine how different systems work during the rest of a person's life.

The brain is highly plastic, which means that its programs can be changed at any time. Encouraging news, isn't it? In fact, every time you learn something or have a physical or emotional experience, your brain changes and adapts. So, if, as you spend time on an activity, such as learning a new language or playing a musical instrument, you get better at it and it comes more naturally to you, it is because your brain is changing and improving its programs. This will always be the case; over the course of your life you will be able to learn or change things about yourself, but during the first months, maybe years of your life, programming will leave a deeper impression and will be more defined and more difficult to change than the things you learn later in life.

This is because the creation of specialized neuronal structures and synapses occurs at the same time the brain is formed, which gives the programming a structural character. That is, not only is the software programmed, but also, in some way, the hardware is created with inbuilt software. Perhaps software and hardware are better integrated in humans than they will ever be in a computer. This explains why our first experiences create physiological changes that remain throughout our lives, whether through the experience of being loved, rocked and touched, or, as we will see later on, through experiencing childhood trauma.

The brain is highly plastic, meaning you can change its programs at any point. This is very encouraging news!

So you can see why it is so difficult to learn a new language as an adult and, if you do, why you don't lose the accent of the language you learned as a child even if you spend years in another country. We know that on a psychological level, your personality and character are formed in the early years of your life and whilst in the future you will need to make changes to cope better with life, it is more than likely that these adjustments will not change the essence of who you are. This means there is a window of opportunity where experiences are decisive and assist programming.

Perhaps software and hardware are better integrated in humans than they will ever be in a computer.

The way we feel is programmed

There are different sensory systems that transmit information to your brain about the world you live in and about what is going on inside your body. Usually we talk about having five senses: sight, hearing, smell, taste and touch. However, this is a very limited approach to our ability to feel. In fact you have more senses, some of them much more important than the ones you already know as you could live without sight, but not without these other senses. For example, could you live without a sense of balance or without noticing changes in temperature?

Every single one of our senses is programmed at the beginning of our life.

EMBODIED OR SOMATIC SENSES	SPECIAL SENSES
Touch	Sight
Thermoception	Hearing
Nociception (pain)	Taste
Propioception	Smell
Balance	

A table of the different sensory systems (senses of the body), both somatic and special.

All the senses can be classified as somatic or embodied senses and special senses. The somatic or embodied senses are the sense of touch, temperature, pain, proprioception and balance. We could also include interoception or perception of our internal organs and what happens inside them. The senses of the body do not have a specific sensory organ, instead there are thousands of receptors throughout the body that inform the brain about these particular aspects, so that should some of those sensors be damaged, the brain would have access to input from the others.

The special senses are the other four you are already familiar with, minus touch which I have included here as somatic, as the whole body can feel through the skin. The special senses require very specialized organs to receive the input: the eye, the ear, the nose (or the receptors behind it) and the tongue (or the sensory organs in the mouth and behind the nose). The special senses are instrumental in your relationship with the world, to perceive what is around you, and they definitely support your chances of survival and your quality of life. It may be possible to live a very satisfactory life in any city in the civilized world without one of your senses, but this is because there is a social fabric to support you. Imagine what it would be like to be alone in the middle of the jungle or on a mountain without sight or hearing.

Every last sense, whether somatic or special, is programmed according to the type, relevance, frequency and intensity of the sensations that you have in the first few months or years of your life. The way we feel during our lives depends on the experiences we had right at the beginning. In fact it's not the sensory organs or receptors that are programmed but the brain and the processing of input from the receptors. So, for example, it is the area of the brain that handles the input from the eye that is programmed, not the eye itself.

In fact, the way you feel throughout life is not only influenced by genetics, but also by the environment you live in. The following are a few examples of sensory programming, some of which we will look at in more depth in the coming chapters.

Actually it is the brain and the processing of input from the receptors and the sensory organs that is programmed.

One of the easiest examples to understand is touch and yet, at the same time, it is one of the most complex systems. The way a child is touched during his first few months can condition his tactile sensitivity for the rest of his life. If he has not been touched, (as is the case of some adopted children), his tactile and proprioceptive sensitivity will be unbalanced and this will directly influence the way he feels about himself and others. In our opinion, given that touch is one of the pillars for building attachment, it will also affect the way the child interprets the world as a safe or, conversely, dangerous place. It is likely that these children will react in an extreme way, flinching in response to a caress or, conversely, by being clingy. In those cases where touch was a source of aggression due to inappropriate touching, abuse or neglect (which is also a form of abuse), their nervous systems could have been programmed to react in the form of fight/flight/ attachment based crying (mobilizing responses) or, worst-case scenario, in the form of submission or freezing (immobilizing responses). Some children with certain types of head or neck rigidity or nervous system conditions, can also have hypersensitivity of the skin that causes them to interpret touch as pain sometimes. This totally confuses their parents who don't understand the way their children react to certain caresses.

These experiences create deep learning for the future, affecting the way they encode and process stimuli, making them potentially threatening even in everyday situations. They leave an imprint on the memory which will influence their tactile perception and reaction to situations perceived as being dangerous in the future. As we will see later on, this can affect their perception of pain.

Touch is one of the pillars for building attachment and affects the way he interprets the world as a safe or, conversely, dangerous place.

The correct development of sensitivity in a baby's hands, which is linked to the accuracy and strength of his movements, is also dependent on the opportunities a baby has to put his hands on the floor during the first 8 months of his life and the opportunities he is given to touch new things with different textures and shapes. Even being touched on his hands by his parents can have a significant impact. Many children with developmental problems seem "clumsy" with their hands. It is difficult for them to do certain everyday things like fastening buttons or tying laces; they hold their pen in an odd way and their handwriting lacks precision or is unsteady, just as the pressure they exert on the paper is when they write. All these are signs of flaws in the way their hands are programmed in their brains.

Thermoception is the ability of the nervous system to detect temperature changes in the tissues, especially those that might affect how the body works and cause damage. Humans can operate normally within a certain temperature range, but beyond this we soon feel discomfort and pain. Again, thermoception is programmed and we can see clear examples of how people living in desert areas or very cold climates are able to adapt. When you visit these kinds of places on vacation or a day trip, you're surprised that people can stand it; but they can because they are acclimatized, they are programmed. It is interesting to note the custom of leaving infants outside in winter in extreme temperatures in some areas of northern Europe. True they are wrapped up, but nevertheless, they are outside. Or in Eastern Europe where they dip babies in ice-cold water every day in a cultural tradition designed to protect them and help them to adapt, the justification being that it protects them from diseases. These habits would be unthinkable for people living in Mediterranean or tropical climates.

Nociception is the nervous system's capacity to detect tissue damage and, incredible as it may seem, this is programmed too. Nowadays, it is widely accepted that the amount of pain a person suffers from a painful stimulus is conditioned by a series of modulators that include, among others, their own experiences or those of family members in early childhood. If the infant grew up with pain caused by neck or digestive system dysfunctions; if the child lived with relatives who were in pain and made their suffering known to all, then that person will probably have a very unique sensitivity to pain in the future, especially in these areas. This topic is both amazing and fascinating and we will look at it in more detail in a specific chapter later on. Furthermore, early experiences of exposure to life-threatening situations can affect this sensory capacity. These experiences which are perceived as «dangerous» can vary depending on the stage of development. A lack of space or nutrition in the prenatal phase could be just as life-threatening and act as a programer of pain modulation and anxiety in the future.

Proprioception is a person's ability to perceive their own body or, as Jean Pierre Roll (Professor of Neurobiology and a great expert in this field) would say, "to inhabit it, to know it, to locate it in space, to exist with and for it". This «sixth» sense is fundamental for many functions bound up with movement and thought. You control your body and your posture using this sense. It is mainly the sensitive receptors in the muscles that allow your brain to construct an internal representation. It's as though the many thousands of receptors in each muscle and tendon provide your brain with an accurate perception of the position of your limbs in relation to the others and with it a representation of your form and your position, as if it were a holographic image. In fact it is even more fascinating and it would be easy to dedicate a whole book to the subject. On the other hand, this system can suffer programming errors and we find children who drop everything, who bump into things, children who find it hard to fasten buttons or pick up a pencil; children whose movements are awkward and lack precision and coordination. Children with postural problems who lack control of their posture and movements. These difficulties show they have poor proprioception programming or a neurological pathology that affects their motor control or their way of feeling. Proprioception is programmed through movement and touch; not light touch but deep touch. Being stroked wouldn't activate it but a gentle squeeze or, better still a hug, would.

Being stroked wouldn't activate proprioception but a gentle squeeze or a hug probably would.

Balance is the ability of your nervous system to perceive changes in the position and movement of your head and body in relation to gravity and the ground and to create responses adapted to these changes to maintain your stability or your posture. Balance can adjust to an environmental influence,like when you are standing up on a bus that is slowing down or turning a bend and you steady your balance so as not to fall over; or pre-emptive, like when you get ready to go down a step or descend a ramp. You have many balance sensors and the most important ones are in the inner ear, the so-called vestibular system. However, vision, the (proprioceptive) muscle sensors of the eyes and neck muscles, or the (tactile) skin receptors of the sole of the feet also play a key role in balance. So, you perceive balance thanks to different sensory systems, but the role of the vestibular system stands out which is why we will look at it in more depth in another chapter. Poor programming of the vestibular system will affect our ability to adapt to changes in the environment and move around quickly and safely. A lack of accuracy and response in balance is one of the telltale signs in most children with learning and attention issues. Many of these children also have difficulty walking up or downstairs easily, riding a bicycle without training wheels or distinguishing left from right, which, incidentally, is the result of good vestibular programming too. Problems of balance produce anxiety and greatly affect the emotional well-being of children and adults, as we will see in subsequent chapters.

Balance is programmed right from the womb thanks to movement.

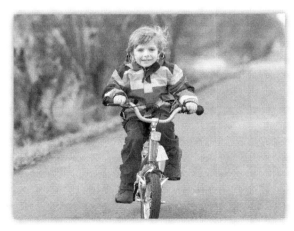

It is common for certain children with poor programming to have difficulty riding a two-wheel bicycle. John didn't find it difficult because his neurological development was good and he received sufficient stimuli.

The way you move was programmed at some point

The motor system which is responsible for planning, organizing and executing postures and movements is also programmed. The way a child develops his first patterns of movement early on in life will affect how he incorporates and benefits from more specialized gestures and movements later on. If, on the other hand, he doesn't go through the different stages of postural or motor development for some reason, it will be difficult for him to develop refined control of both hand and eye movements or global coordination. In order to learn how to control his body, a baby must go through several stages of development and use it to make increasingly finer movements. We will look at all this development in more detail in another chapter.

In the first year and a half of his life there is a paradigm shift in the child's motor skills and control of his own body. From involuntary global movements in the first few weeks to standing up and walking, the baby goes through a series of unprecedented challenges which he overcomes thanks to a strong driving force; emotional motivation. An interest in everything around him; a desire to hold his head up and look up; to follow the movements of something he is interested in, try to grab it and put it in his mouth as soon as it is within his reach and subsequently, to creep, crawl or walk when it is out of reach. All this forms part of a multifaceted process involving many milestones which a baby will reach as long as his pre- and perinatal periods were free of interferences; with no stiffness in his neck or spine, and as long as his parents provided the appropriate stimuli, including touch, movement and sufficient tummy time (when he was awake and supervised) from his very first week.

From involuntary global movements in the first weeks of life to standing up and walking, a baby goes through unprecedented challenges which he overcomes thanks to a strong driving force; emotional motivation.

It is surprising to see the general lack of knowledge about infants' needs in terms of movement and development; for example, the fact that they are left on their backs for long periods when they really need to be on their tummies to develop postural evolution and movement. The general recommendation that babies should sleep on their backs introduced in 1992 to prevent sudden infant death syndrome had a positive effect on the number of neonatal deaths and was a major breakthrough. However, there were some downsides such as the increase in the number of children with flat head syndrome (plagiocephaly) and certain sluggishness in the development of motor skills. Following confirmation of these findings, the recommendation is to use the prone position for several minutes a few times a day, always under supervision. In a nutshell «back for sleep, tummy for play».

Unfortunately, a lack of knowledge and fear means that parents daren't put their babies in this position and yet, without it, their development is hindered. There are lots of babies with minor neurodevelopmental delays, but it seems that in many countries, only a few are picked up by the health system. Medicine is very good at dealing with many life-threatening diseases, but less effective at preventing developmental problems in children. This is something that could be achieved with physiotherapists who specialize in the detection and prevention of developmental problems in healthy children (by healthy we mean those with no objectifiable neurological damage visible in an imaging test, electromyography, genetic or metabolic test). Maybe one day children will receive this level of care.

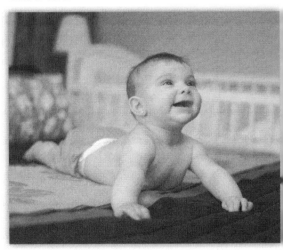

Five month old Lisa can be seen here in a position typical of this age. She is resting her weight on her abdomen and supporting herself on extended arms, with her head and upper torso upright. She is able to turn her head to both sides. Many babies who have not spent enough time on their tummies, or who suffer pain in their necks or backs, are not capable of doing this. Sadly this is more common than we realize.

The programming of motor skills is a multifaceted process involving many milestones which a baby will reach as long as his pre- and perinatal periods were free of interferences; and as long as his parents provided the appropriate stimuli, including touch, movement and sufficient tummy time from birth.

The rest of your systems are programmed too!

The immune system is included in programming. As a child comes into contact with external biological agents, bacteria or viruses in the first years of his life, so his system is trained to deal with future infections. If this trainings insufficient, we could be looking a tone of the environmental factors that lead to the appearance of autoimmune diseases. These diseases can be a sign of an insufficiently trained immune system (along with other factors such as the genetic factor obviously, and the bacterial population in the intestine, or vitamin D deficiency). Hence the danger of creating excessively clean environments for our children. It is possible that the immune systems of children who grow up in environments that are too-clean or disinfected may suffer from a lack of training which can lead to diseases or autoimmune disorders in the future; where the "confusion" caused by so-called "molecular mimicry" leads to our immune system attacking the cells of our own skin or other tissues.

Along these same lines, the role and complexity of the intestinal flora is impressive, both in terms of the assimilation of nutrients and the immune function. One of the advantages of a vaginal delivery is that bacteria from the mother's genital area migrates and populates the baby's gut (shown to be present in the gut biome). For this very reason doctors have started to insert moistened gauzes in the mother's vagina during a C-section and then use them to swab the newborn's lips. This, together with the pressure applied to the baby's chest (which empties the lungs of the liquid accumulated during birth), are thought to be factors in understanding why children born by vaginal delivery have less respiratory pathologies than those born by C-section. The colonization of intestinal flora is another example of how the immune system is programmed. You will be even more amazed to learn that the baby's intestinal flora also depends on the type of birth his mother experienced and how she was nursed as a baby. This would imply programming spanning several generations for the type of bacteria that populate the intestine. On the other hand, it's not so surprising if we think about what is perhaps the most important type of programming, genetic programming. How many generations does it take to bring about genetic programming?

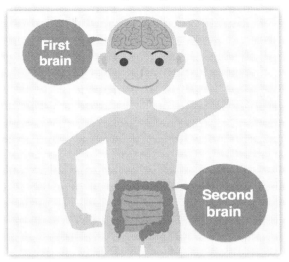

There is increasing evidence that the quality of the bacterial population in the gut has a clear bearing on human health and how the brain functions. In terms of immunity, the gut is a key hub and its role in the production of serotonin, a hormone of well-being, earns it the title of «second brain». It appears that keeping a child's gut healthy seems to be a good way of programming their happiness.

Programming also includes emotional aspects. The way in which a baby or child interacts with the adults who care for them, especially with their key attachment figure, will determine their adaptability in future relationships and the experiences they have with other people throughout their lives. Recent research in neuropsychology shows that the nature of these early bonding relationships organizes our brains, affecting our perception and relationships throughout our lives. How many of us can recount emotional trauma from our early childhood? Did you know that some of the disorders (both psychic and somatic) found in children and adults originate in these traumatic experiences? Do we really understand the extent to which this can condition a person's life journey and social relationships? Hence, it is vital we consider the need for essential training in parenting. Mothers, fathers and other key figures involved in childcare, we are all role models and «programmers», whether we are aware of it or not, and the quality and thoroughness of our care, together with our integrity, are key to shaping our children's personalities.

It goes without saying that programming includes pre-natal life, as what happens before birth determines a child's sensitivity to interpreting certain biological stimuli once born. This can affect both the metabolism and the neuroendocrine system. Pregnant women who suffer from stress give birth to children who will interpret the stimuli as being distressing and react more strongly to them. Women who are pregnant at a time or in a place where food is in short supply, will give birth to children with metabolisms designed to store food and who will be at a much higher risk of suffering from cardiovascular diseases, diabetes and obesity. The following is another study along the same lines which shows how stressful experiences during pregnancy influence the gene expression in humans; children born to pregnant mothers trapped for several days in houses without heating during a snowstorm in Quebec, had major epigenetic changes compared to the children born to mothers whose heating was repaired in just one day.

Chemicals and toxins are not the only things that can provoke changes in your body. The way your social world speaks to and treats your inner most Self, can do too. Perhaps you are not fully aware of everything that is programmed at the beginning of a human being's life and just how important it is. If you were going to build a house surely you would make sure the foundations were located in the right position and were stable and deep enough? Well, you could say that biological, neurological and emotional programming are a person's foundations.

Perhaps we are not fully aware of everything that is programmed at the beginning of a human life and just how important it is.

Everything in humans is interrelated

It is totally fascinating how some programs condition and affect others. Our sensory skills affect our motor skills and vice-versa; our sensory performance affects our immune response and this in turn has an impact on how our bowel functions, which in turn affects our energy or behavior. There are countless examples of interrelationships between the programming of all our systems. It is common knowledge that for an infant's hands to acquire sufficient dexterity and skill, he must have spent enough time on the floor supporting his weight on his hands in the prone position or crawling. This means that motor skills have a bearing on the senses. Yet, at the same time, if his proprioceptive sensory programming is poor due to a

neck problem, the baby may not develop precise movements and may even be unable to properly support his arm or hand on the floor; so, sensory performance also affects motor performance. There is a clear relationship between the sense of balance and the metabolism of the stress response, or of new and unexpected situations as a result of reflex patterns which we will discuss later on. Poor balance control causes anxiety in both children and adults alike. Auditory sensitivity affects our behavior and our interaction with others. Likewise, the way our body reacts to certain foods can determine our attention span and behavior at a given point in time. Vestibular programming may influence the development of some cognitive skills such as math.

This interaction between the different sensory systems is very obvious in children with learning and attention issues. We find clear difficulties with motor and balance control and often visual or auditory dysfunctions; glucose metabolism disorders or food intolerances. Sometimes they seem shy and other times aggressive and they are almost always anxious. This doesn't make it easy to determine which problem appeared first and which followed. When we treat children with these difficulties we often have to "reprogram" different systems and several professionals are required to do this successfully.

In children with learning and attention issues we find clear difficulties with motor and balance control and often visual or auditory dysfunctions; glucose metabolism disorders, food intolerances or anxiety.

When we see a 3 month old infant with signs of slight developmental delay (though otherwise neurologically healthy, i.e. with no diagnosed illness, neurological damage or genetic or metabolic disorders), we should be able to help him overcome it with a fairly straight forward pediatric physiotherapy procedure and by giving his parents advice on how to provide all the stimuli necessary for the maturation of his nervous system (providing there is no brain damage). As a result, the baby will learn to develop all his cognitive abilities to optimum effect. Conversely, if this same infant comes to us with learning, attention and behavioral issues when he is 7 or 8 years old, it will be much harder to correct the situation. By this age many systems have already been programmed, but in the wrong way. Now all these systems must be reprogrammed which means «erasing everything and starting over».

In this case, it probably won't be sufficient to just offer a series of pediatric physiotherapy sessions and give the parents some tips. We may need to call on the expertise of a behavioral optometrist to work on their vision or a speech therapist on their verbal or auditory skills and perhaps other professionals like a psychologist or an educational psychologist. So, as you can see, early intervention is crucial for a simpler solution and more favorable outcome.

It won't always be necessary to involve all the professionals mentioned above; in mild cases, appropriate, timely intervention on the sensory and motor systems, an eye test and a manual physiotherapy test to ensure there is no stiffness in the child's neck or tension in their head that may hinder their entire development and make the child very irritable, may suffice. Therefore, we should be working towards having all healthy children undergo a physiotherapy check-up at different times during their development, in the same way they go to the pediatrician or the dentist.

Throughout this book we will develop various aspects of programming and biological, neurological and emotional development in children and, of course, show you how to help them find their wings for unlimited development.

SUMMARY

There is growing evidence that our early experiences have a significant impact on the rest of our lives, almost as though they were a way of training our brain to adapt to the life we are about to lead. This training is called programming.

Both the way we perceive each of our senses and the way we move are programmed. All our other systems, such as the immunological and emotional systems are programmed too. Consequently, certain responses that are activated at the start of our life will trigger automatically in different scenarios throughout our childhood and even as adults.

The first stage of programming is genetic. Every living being is created thanks to a genetic code which makes a major contribution to shaping who and what we are.

The second stage of programming occurs in the first 8 weeks of the prenatal stage after fertilization. This is the period of human development in the womb during which the embryo forms and is called embryogenesis. At this stage the embryo is particularly sensitive to the mother's experiences. The next stage of programming is the fetal stage, from the 9th week of pregnancy until birth.

The fourth stage of human programming occurs during the first months and years and addresses maturation of the sensory system, the motor system, the immune system, the digestive system, emotional and social development, etc. Everything is programmed in these early stages, equipping the child to run all these different systems for the rest of his life.

It is widely accepted that a large number of children in our society have developmental, behavioral and emotional disorders and learning disabilities (not to mention other health factors such as excess weight) and that for many of them, their early life experiences proved crucial in determining the problems they were to face later on. Most of the time parents are able to provide the right support. However, there are variables beyond their control that can cause a child to suffer from developmental, neurological or emotional difficulties.

What can you do?

INFANTS

- The most important thing is to be aware that your baby is using the information he receives to develop the programs his body and mind will run on throughout the rest of his life. I advise you to sit down for a few moments and ask yourself the following questions: Am I giving him the stimuli he needs to develop to his full potential? Physically, emotionally, sentimentally, socially, in terms of diet, transcendency, spirituality, etc. What is the best you can do for his development?

- Thinking up stimuli for your baby can be a good way of avoiding the kind of restrictive helicopter parenting some people practice with their children. Their intentions are good, they want to protect them but in fact, they hinder their development. This is a major problem in today's society as people are often confused about their parenting goals, or just lack goals of any kind. What does being a parent really mean in strict biological terms? What is the ultimate meaning of this life experience? Should our aim be to ensure that our children never suffer, never face any difficulties in life and ultimately are incapable of being self-sufficient? In the absence of any real road-map, many parents focus on protecting their children and making things as safe and easy for them as possible with all the corresponding risks for their development. Perhaps our main goal as parents is to guide our children to the maximum level of self-sufficiency in the shortest possible time and in the safest possible way and, especially in the case of humans, with a good degree of social integration. Offering children stimuli throughout their development and education makes them more able and motivated. It makes them believe in themselves and teaches them to take conscious risks. After all, life is all about having experiences and taking risks. How to give them the maximum number of experiences with the minimum number of risks? This is the million dollar question for all parents.

- As we will see later on, the most important sensory stimuli for babies are movement (particularly the head) and touch. These two stimuli truly build the foundations of the nervous system. Make sure that you get your baby to move, that you carry him with you and touch him sufficiently in a conscious, mindful way.

- Offer him different, age-appropriate light and sound stimuli. And, of course, children also need to taste and smell different flavors and aromas. These senses are programmed or trained, too. Offer your children varied experiences that can be great fun when done blindfolded: like guessing aromas or flavors without seeing them. Being in touch with nature can provide an endless source of stimuli. You don't have to go to a three-star Michelin restaurant to experience flavors and aromas; far from it, with a bit of creativity this can be organized at home or outdoors in natural settings.

- Placing your baby on his tummy for about 5 minutes at least 5 times a day from his very first week of life (always when he's awake and supervised by one of his parents), can be highly beneficial for his development. You can stimulate him with touch, sounds or songs whilst he's in this position. Gradually increase the amount of tummy time so that he is able to develop his postural skills. You will see how, by 3 months he can support his weight on his forearms and by six months, how he can lift himself onto his hands and extend his arms. He can also flip over from his back to his tummy. He will be able to achieve all this if he has been carried around and has experienced movement in a more upright position. We will look at this topic in much more detail later on.

OLDER CHILDREN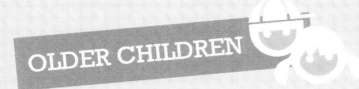

- You need to realize that you are a role model and programmer for your children and the children in your care (particularly if you are in teaching or health care.) Take a few moments to ask yourself about the core values you want to convey to them. Normally parenting styles fall into two opposing categories: too strict or too lenient. Being too lenient (a misguided form of «affection»), or being too strict (leading to emotional shut down), are the opposite ends of two complementary and necessary elements in parenting. Children can only develop their psychological structure within a framework of emotional security and integrity. So, affection is necessary when it is understood to be responding to their needs and emotions; but so too is firmness, in terms of being consistent in our emotional presence and the actions we take. This way we won't be raising little tyrants or useless "snowflakes". We will be helping them to become independent and building their emotional intelligence. It is sad to see how children become tyrants at home, making decisions that affect not only their lives but those of others, when the best thing for them would be to take up a recognized, respected place in the family, without being in the driving seat. There is a lack of respect for the most senior members and the children decide everything about family life, from what everyone eats to the things they buy. Despite the fact that psychologists and educational psychologists are constantly warning us about the dangers of a lack of parental authority and of the high levels of anxiety the lack of a reference figure causes in children who are allowed to make choices they are not ready for, many societies nowadays have trouble rectifying this situation. Perhaps it would help to consider what place a 7 or 8 year child occupies in a tribe in the middle of the Amazon, an Eskimo community or a remote Polynesian island. What is their social role? Their decision-making capacity? What jobs do they do for the community? Do you think the whole family goes hunting, or fishing or tends to the land, whilst they stay in bed deciding what everyone is going to eat for dinner tonight or what the group is going to do today? In these cultures, a child has a particular place in the family group and they help out with the jobs as soon as they are able to. They also have a tremendous amount of respect for their elders.

- After breastfeeding, food should be introduced to children in the right way and in the correct order. The fact is that there are several different theories on this subject and this means that no-one is really clear. Food is usually the best example. How should food be introduced early in life after breastfeeding? An evolutionary approach might be the sensible option. Start with the foods that humans have eaten for thousands of years; root vegetables, fruit, white meat, white fish...., then slowly build up to relatively newer foods. We don't deal with this subject here but I am sure you will be able to obtain more detailed information from pediatricians and nutritionists who are specialists in this field.

- If you were unable to accompany your child in his early stages of development because you weren't aware of the need for it, or because of other difficulties in his early years (illnesses, hospitalizations, etc.), don't panic, it can all be programmed later. The brain is an amazing thing and it can sometimes find alternative ways to build or repair itself. If you consider your child's difficulties correspond to less than optimal motor, sensory or postural development in the early years of his life, you can ask a developmental physiotherapist (at the end of this book you will discover how to find one), for an overall assessment of the current situation and for advice on how to reprogram his nervous system. It is never too late to help your child progress. Help him find his wings!

BIBLIOGRAPHY

Regarding the effect of pre and post natal stress on the development of a child's personality:

> Cyrulnik B. De cuerpo y alma. Neuronas y afectos: la conquista del bienestar. Editorial Gedisa; 2007.

Regarding how certain difficulties experienced by the mother affect the programming of her future children:

> Mitchell C, Schneper LM, Notterman DA. DNA methylation, early life environment, and health outcomes.Pediatr Res. 2016 Jan;79(1-2):212-9.

> Ravelli AC, Van der Meulen JH, Michels RP, Osmond C, Barker DJ, Hales CN, et al. Glucose tolerance in adults after prenatal exposure to famine. Lancet. 1998 Jan 17;351(9097):173-7.

Regarding prenatal factors in programming development:

> Goddard Blythe S. What babies and children really need. Hawthorn Press; 2008

Regarding the birth process:

> Arsuaga JL. El primer viaje de nuestra vida. Ediciones Planeta; 2012.

Regarding the different sensory systems:

> Blakeslee S, Blakeslee M. El mandala del cuerpo. El cuerpo tiene su propia mente. La Liebre de Marzo; 2009.

Regarding proprioception:

> Roll JP. Les muscles, organes de la perception. Pour la Science. 1998;248:92-9.

Regarding balance and anxiety or learning:

> De Quiros JB, Schrager OL. Fundamentos neuropsicológicos en las discapacidades de aprendizaje. Editorial Médica Panamericana; 1996.

> Erez O, Gordon CR, Sever J, Sadeh A, Mintz M. Balance dysfunction in childhood anxiety: findings and theoretical approach. Journal of Anxiety Disorders. 2004;18(3):341-56.

> Goddard S. Assessing Neuromotor Readiness for Learning. Wiley-Blackwell; 2012.

> Goddard S. Attention, Balance and Coordination. The ABC of Learning Success. Wiley-Blackwell; 2009.

> Smith, PF. Dyscalculia and vestibular function.Medical Hypotheses. 2012;79(4):493-6.

Smith PF, Zheng Y, Horii A, Darlington CL. Does vestibular damage cause cognitive dysfunction in humans? Journal of Vestibular Research: Equilibrium & Orientation. 2005;15(1):1-9.

Regarding the Hierarchical Theory and Programming Theory:

ShumwayCook A, Woollacott MH. Motor Control. Translating Research into Clinical Practice. 4th ed. Wolters Kluwer. Lippincott Williams & Wilkins; 2010.

Regarding the relationship between sleeping in the supine position and flat head syndrome in infants:

Argenta LC, David LR, Wilson JA, Bell WO. An increase in infant cranialdeformity with supine sleeping position. J Craniofac Surg. 1996 Jan;7(1):5-11.

Robinson S, Proctor M. Diagnosis and management of deformational plagiocephaly. J Neurosurg Pediatr. 2009;3(4):284-95.

Regarding the importance and programming of intestinal flora:

Cañellas X, Sanchís J. Niños sanos, adultos sanos. La salud empieza a programarse en el embarazo. Plataforma Editorial; 2016.

Sánchez B, Hevia A, González S, Margolles A.Interaction of Intestinal Microorganisms with the Human Host in the Framework of Autoimmune Diseases.Front Immunol. 2015 Nov 20;6:594.

Vieira SM, Pagovich OE, Kriegel MA. Diet, microbiota and autoimmune diseases. Lupus. 2014 May;23(6):518-26.

Regarding early life experiences, brain development and health:

Kundakovic M, Champagne FA. Early-life experience, epigenetics, and the developing brain.Neuropsychopharmacology. 2015 Jan;40(1):141-53.

Szyf M, Tang YY, Hill KG, Musci R. The dynamic epigenome and its implications for behavioral interventions: a role for epigenetics to inform disorder prevention and health promotion. Transl Behav Med. 2016 Mar;6(1):55-62.

Regarding secure attachment in infant mental health:

Schore A. Effects of a secure attachment relationship on right brain development and infant mental health.Infant Mental Health Journal. 2001;22:1-2, 7-66.

Regarding sensory programming and its importance in child development:

Ayres AJ. La integración sensorial en los niños. Desafíos sensoriales ocultos. TEA Ediciones; 2008.

Chapter 2

Bonding through touch
Our skin as an extension of our mind and soul

Iñaki Pastor Pons

No-one is in any doubt that infants need love and affection; but, from a biological perspective, what does showing them affection really mean? Caressing them, using a soft, sing-song voice, spending time with them, cuddling them, feeding them..?

In his now classic study of newborn monkeys, Harry Harlow left a newborn baby monkey with two surrogate "mothers". One of the "mothers" was made of wire mesh with a crudely drawn face and a bottle of milk. The other "mother" was milk-free but the wire mesh was covered in terry cloth which was soft to the touch. Which one do you think the baby monkey chose to spend his time with? Contrary to what you would expect, the monkey did not prefer the mother who dispensed milk, it chose the mother who was soft to the touch and proceeded to "attach" itself to her, snuggling up against her for long periods of time. This experiment shows that it may actually be the contact and not the act of being fed that comforts the monkey and creates the bond with its mother.

From a biological perspective, for a newborn human affection means skin contact. To be touched and more importantly, touched appropriately is to be loved. It is probably much more important than being spoken to and possibly more necessary than food itself, (within limits, of course). The everyday reality of many children brought up in orphanages in certain countries with limited care resources is shocking. Other countries take good care of their orphans but even so, many of those who are adopted have serious developmental problems when they arrive in our country. Were they fed correctly? Yes, they did not go hungry. Was their temperature kept under control? Yes, that was all taken care of. Were they clean? Yes, their diapers were changed regularly to avoid infections that could lead to potentially fatal health problems. Were they abused? The likelihood is they weren't, but did anyone touch them? Probably a lot less than they really needed. Alongside this we find there was also a lack of movement and emotional attachment. These three areas could be the pillars which ensure stable psychological and biological development. Maybe, instead of talking about "pillars" we should refer to the "roots" of a correct biological, psychological and social development.

In this chapter we discover that the skin truly is an extension of our nervous system, so that by touching our skin we are touching our brain. An infant's emotional and physical development depends on the quantity and quality of this touch. But just how important is it? What kind of physical contact does your baby really need?

Join me over the next few pages as we discover amazing things about the miracle of touch.

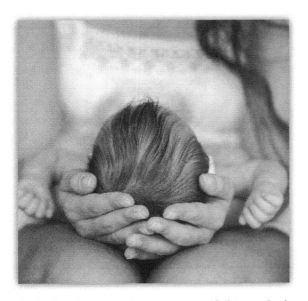

Each time he comes into contact with his mother's skin George feels loved.

For a newborn infant, affection means skin contact. To be touched and, more importantly, to be touched properly, is therefore to be loved.

Thanks mainly to the fascinating effect it has on the way the immune system works, these days no-one is in any doubt that contact is key to sensorimotor development or that is has repercussions on a child's physical growth, emotional well-being, cognitive potential and general health.

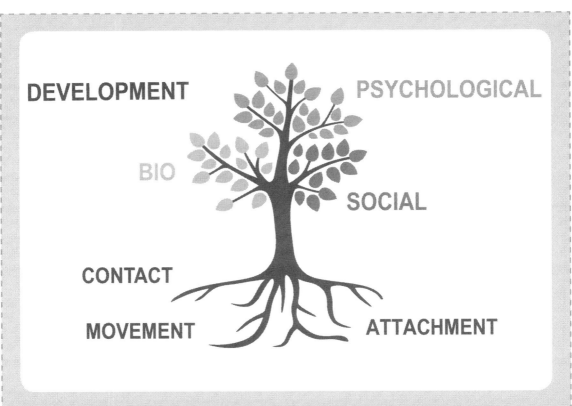

What we see here is a diagram of the three branches of biological, psychological and social development. Although they are different in adulthood, in newborns they share the same trunk and roots. Biologically and anthropologically speaking, a baby that is loved is one that is touched and cradled with affection in a safe and calm manner, thus creating a strong bond.

How and when do we start to sense touch?

When you see a newborn baby, can you resist touching his tiny hands and feet or stroking his lips? Not only are adults drawn to protecting infants and young children, but, irrespective of their family bond, they also feel the urge to stroke certain areas of their body almost as though it were some sort of genetic programming for the survival of our species. But what about the baby? When does he start to sense touch on his skin?

An ultrasound image showing Noa's nose and lips at 7 months. This entire area of her face has been sensitive to stimuli on the skin for some time now. In fact at just 7 weeks she was already responding to stimuli in this area.

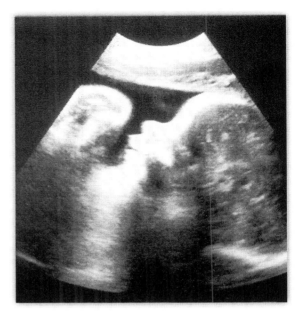

Touch is undoubtedly the first sense to develop. Barely 7 weeks after conception the embryo can already sense touch on its lips and nose; at 9 weeks on its chin, eyelids and arms, and around 12 weeks, on practically the entire surface of its body. However, although the fetus feels touch on its skin, it does not experience the sensation of being touched in the same way an adult would because the area responsible for processing these sensations is the spinal cord which is the most primitive part of the nervous system.

The spinal cord is a major part of the nervous system, but it works more as a communicator between what is "above" and "below", resolving the simplest of issues without the ability to provide complex answers or global patterns of movement (except walking which can be activated through a central pattern generator in the bone marrow). Hence the first reaction to a tactile stimulus felt by a fetus is very simple, it withdraws. This is called a "withdrawal reflex" or "response" and is mediated in the spinal cord. These reactions are pure reflexes, which means that the same stimulus always results in the same automatic response.

As tactile stimuli reach "higher" areas of an increasingly mature brain, like the brainstem, the responses become more sophisticated. For example, the rooting reflex where touching a fetus around the lips makes it turn its head and lips in the direction the contact came from. Unlike spinal mediation reflexes, brain stem reflex responses are more global and involve more parts of the body. For example, the rooting reflex is more complex than the withdrawal reflex; moving closer to seek out and find the stimulus is

much more advanced than moving away for safety. As other senses and more superior brain structures develop, the stimuli can reach more "modern" areas of the nervous system allowing a perception of oneself being touched to be developed. The neurological structures that will allow the fetus to construct this future map of itself do not develop until the third trimester of pregnancy.

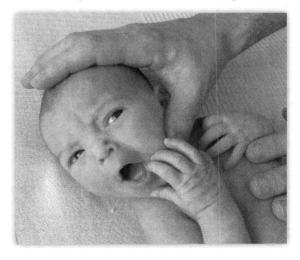

Three day-old Asher demonstrating the rooting reflex. You can see how his lower lip is moving towards the thumb stroking his left cheek.

In the first year of life, information about touch is processed 4 times faster than it is at birth. By the age of 6 it has doubled in speed again, reaching a level similar to that of an adult.

The baby develops tactile sensitivity from the top down, from its head to its toes. The mouth is the first area that becomes sensitive and this is what the baby uses to explore everything, no matter how dangerous it may be. Babies' mouths are well-developed and offer the brain very reliable information about what they touch. In fact babies are able to recognize the shape of objects they have sucked (but not seen) when they see them later, suggesting they are capable of abstract perception. This is not the case with their hands as neonates cannot visually recognize unseen objects they have touched.

This means that even though they grab things and are developing sensitivity in their hands and a significant number of connections in their brain, babies actually investigate with their mouths. They won't begin to use their hands to intentionally reach for objects until they are 16 weeks old and at first can only grasp objects that are by their side using a rather primitive pincer grip. It won't be until much later that their hands get a true feeling for what they are touching. Until they are 18 months old their sensitivity to recognizing objects is still not sufficiently developed to allow them to distinguish objects that are slightly different.

In any case, babies have a long way to go before they can differentiate any type of touch or pinpoint where they have been touched on their body. This will depend on the evolution of their somatosensory system in certain areas of the brain where we have accurate maps of our body. It also depends on the myelination of the nerve pathways. Even when this process has still to develop further, the newborn can feel with its skin better than it can see, hear or taste.

> Babies actually investigate with their mouths. Even at the age of 3, their sensitivity to recognizing objects with their mouths is still greater than with their hands.

One brain, many maps

There are many, varied maps in your brain. There are numerous maps of your body and countless maps of your exterior self. If you were to close your eyes, would you know which position each part of your body was in or where it was in space? If someone were to touch your body would you be able to tell where? Could you direct your left hand to your right ear in a single movement? Could you visualize the route to follow to get to your place of work or guide someone there who had never been before? All of the above is only possible if you have created maps in your brain.

Despite all our scientific advances, we still don't know exactly how the brain works. The only thing experts agree on is that the brain represents things. It represents things that are external to you in the form of a map, from what your house is like, to the shape of different objects. Likewise, it represents your entire body in an area of the cortex called the somatosensory area and the topography of every inch of your skin in that area of the brain is known as cortical representation. In fact, this part represents the tactile sensitivity of your body because there are other representations of your body distributed throughout the brain.

When a baby is born, she doesn't have a cortical (cerebral) representation of her body. The initial projections to the somatosensory cortex are diffuse, with many overlaps between different areas of the body and undefined edges. The limits of her body are not well defined because the primary sensory areas in the brain and the somatosensory cortex have yet to develop, as do many other areas in the brain.

So, how does the baby draw this perfect map of her body? She can create a clear map from being touched by the adults who look after her. The more a baby's skin is touched, the better the maps she builds will be. Another

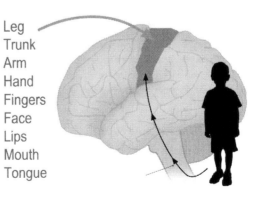

Leg
Trunk
Arm
Hand
Fingers
Face
Lips
Mouth
Tongue

We all have a virtual representation of the different parts of our body in our brain. This occurs in the primary somatosensory area of the cortex, shown here in pink. Every inch of our skin is represented somewhere in this area. It truly is a map of our body in our brain.

way she builds maps is by putting parts of her body into her mouth which, as we have seen, is the most developed part of the tactile system early on in life. Last but not least, she can create maps each time she combines information from the skin with other new information which is developing at a slower rate. This is known as proprioception. Proprioception is the information you have about the position and movement of each part of your body and we looked at it briefly in the chapter on programming. The receptors of this proprioceptive information are found primarily in your muscles, tissues and skin. They allow you to build a very accurate map of yourself, as well as influencing your posture, muscle tone and cognition.

The more a baby's skin is touched, the better and more accurately she builds the map of her body in her brain and the better her movements will be later on.

Over time and once she becomes familiar with her own body, a child will have a more accurate sense of where she is being touched. Providing of course, that as a baby she was touched often enough and in the right way, with firmness and affection and that her tactile sensitivity hasn't been affected by illness or disorders. If these maps form correctly, in the future the child will be able to perceive and control her body more accurately as she will feel each part of her body, her position in space and the amount of tension in that area, with great precision and will be able to develop movements that are well-coordinated and suitable for her environment. It is safe to say that we move our body with the same accuracy with which we feel it. This has a direct impact on learning and attention.

We move our body with the same accuracy with which we feel it.

Sometimes it reminds me of those old-fashioned switchboards where an operator would connect the telephone wires:

– *I'd like to speak to the CEO's office please.*
– *Putting you through.*

At this point the operator would connect the line and communication was possible. When we assess children who have learning and attention issues we often find that, during a test involving fast, high precision finger movements, the child takes a while to find the finger that must touch the hands right in front of her face. Some children even have to use their other hand to move one of their fingers without the other fingers on that hand moving too. As if the switchboard operator couldn't find the exact connection for the call to reach the right person.

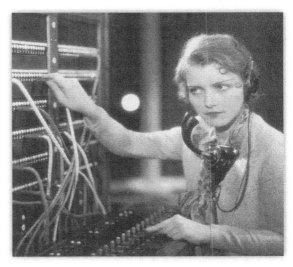

In some ways the nervous system is like an old-fashioned switchboard. Inside the brain there are millions of wires that must interconnect for everything to work properly.

There are millions of wires that must interconnect in your nervous system for everything to work properly. There are wires leading to the central control systems (management) with sensory information about what's going on both outside (the one that tells you about the temperature or pressure outside) and inside (about your muscles, tissues, joints, etc.). These wires carry sensory or afferent information.

There are also wires that originate in your central computer (your brain) and lead to your muscles to enable you to move or position yourself in the environment, (there are also wires that contract your arteries and secrete hormones... let's face it, you're not short of wires!). These wires carry the outgoing or efferent information. Last but not least, there are wires in your central control computer that organize the information you receive.

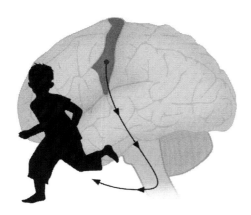

There is also an area (a map) in the brain for controlling our movements: the so-called primary motor area. It is right next to the sensory area that you saw before to enable communication to get through quickly. So that, the better you feel your body, the better you will move it.

When you were born you had no control over your own body. Or maybe in an unconscious, non-voluntary way, you did have some control over essential basics like your heartbeat which began several months ago, or over other biochemical and neuroendocrine control systems. However, the map to control the different parts of your body had not developed.

For this reason, a baby's first movements are general and involuntary, also known as holokinetic: when she moves one part of her body, everything else moves too. In fact, voluntary control and the possibility of maintaining the position of a body part is a process that takes some time. During this process she will gradually discover her hands, look at them and take them to her mouth; her feet come next. In any case, a baby will recognize and control the parts of the body that her caregivers have touched much sooner.

During the first stages of life, a main sensory map and a main motor map develop in the brain. This occurs in the so-called primary somatosensory and motor areas. These areas are next to each other since to move properly you need to feel properly. Have you tried eating or drinking when your mouth is still numb after a visit to the dentist? Hard isn't it?

The process of discovering the hands is interesting because it gives us an idea of how the brain works in these motor and sensory maps. At some point between the second and third months, infants begin to put their hands to their mouths and then clasp them together. At this point, the hands do not have a clear place in the brain's body map but thanks to oral stimulation, skin contact between their hands, and, in large part, to the loving touch of their parents on each of their fingers through games and caresses, babies begin to develop an accurate map of their hands in the primary sensory area. The better they can feel their hands in these maps, the better their voluntary grasp of objects will develop. This connection is important for them to be able to fasten buttons or hold a pen properly in the future.

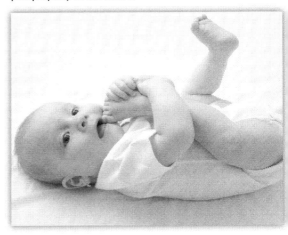

Edward needs to raise his hands and feet to his mouth and besides, he loves doing it. This way his brain becomes familiar with his body and starts to build an accurate map that will enable him to use his hands in a skilful, agile way and his feet with stability and balance.

At the same time that this hand to mouth, hand to hand and third-party touching of baby's hands is happening, the baby looks at her hands and incorporates them through visualization into other areas of her brain associating the fact that the small movements she feels correspond to visual changes. The connection of multiple stimuli contributes to the development of a map or body scheme of the hands in the brain. This is how the brain works. Everything that reaches the brain does so through at least two different simultaneous paths. This duplication of information provides certainty and depth to perception. Certainty, because if one of the sensory pathways doesn't work (if, for example, the baby has a vision problem) the map will still be created. Depth, because it gives us a much more complete and multidimensional perception.

Visual information from both eyes is combined so that if one eye is inoperative, it is still possible to perceive the environment. But this isn't the only reason. The simultaneous perception of two eyes separated horizontally makes three-dimensional visual perception possible, this is called stereopsis. Stereopsis is far more than simply the sum of the visual information from both eyes. It is the perception of depth which would not be possible if the two eyes did not supply the correct information from the retina and muscles (proprioceptive information about the length and the state of stress of the muscles). This is how the brain works: not only does it combine different information from the same phenomenon, but it sublimates this information into a deeper, more complex, "three-dimensional" or even "four-dimensional" perception which better represents the environment.

The existence of more than one sensory pathway for the same phenomenon gives our perception certainty and depth.

This is how the brain works. Not only does it combine different information from the same phenomenon, but it also sublimates this information into a deeper, more complex, "three-di-mensional" or even "four-dimensional" perception which better represents the environment.

It is essential you touch your baby as much as possible because the information she receives about her skin and tissues helps her create a much more complete and accurate brain map of her body. This means that the switchboard will be able to connect the different parts of her body more accurately when she needs to use them for increasingly precise movements in the future. Children with learning and attention issues have difficulty coordinating their body to carry out certain tasks, as if they were unfamiliar with it or unable to control it properly. The thinking is that the cortical maps in these children were not programmed correctly.

It is essential to touch your baby as much as possible because she can use this information about her skin and tissues to create a much more comprehensive, accurate brain map.

It is important you touch her hands, tiny fingers, feet, back, face, lips..., basically for you to follow your natural instincts when you see a baby. Which parts of a baby's body are adults naturally attracted to? On the whole, their little hands, tiny feet and mouths, right? This is what draws us to babies and where we want to touch them.

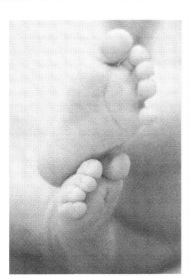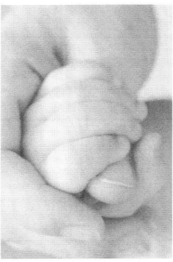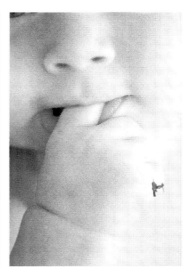

The feet, hands and mouth are the body parts with the highest representation on the maps in the brain. This is where touching in the early stages of life can be particularly important.

Could this be genetic programming for adults, designed to stimulate the area the baby needs to develop? Mouth, hands and feet are the parts of the body that interact most with the outside: for feeding, moving around and of course, for communicating with others. This is why these body parts take up more space in the brain than others as represented by Penfield's Homunculus.

Penfield's Homunculus is that distorted cartoon-like representation of the human body showing the actual amount of space each body part occupies in our sensory cortex. This is why his hands, feet and mouth are disproportionately large with respect to other parts of his body. During the brain surgeries he performed to treat epilepsy, Canadian neurosurgeon, Wilder Penfield (1891-1976), discovered that when different parts of the brain are stimulated the patient experiences sensations in specific parts of his body. Over the years he came to the conclusion that there was a neurological or "virtual" map of our body located in the sensory cortex and another map in the motor cortex.

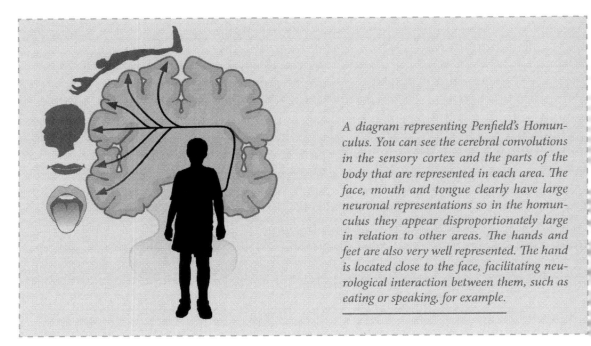

A diagram representing Penfield's Homunculus. You can see the cerebral convolutions in the sensory cortex and the parts of the body that are represented in each area. The face, mouth and tongue clearly have large neuronal representations so in the homunculus they appear disproportionately large in relation to other areas. The hands and feet are also very well represented. The hand is located close to the face, facilitating neurological interaction between them, such as eating or speaking, for example.

The reason your body map is disproportionate is something that has long fascinated neuroscientists because it raises the question once again of whether your genes or the environment play a more important role. It is a combination of your genes and your experiences that shapes your brain. The foundation of this map is undoubtedly genetic. You are genetically programmed to develop more sensors on the pads of your fingers or on your lips, places where the functions require greater precision. The more sensors there are and the better they are connected to the brain, the better the map of these areas will be, or rather, the better these areas will be represented in your brain. But genes are just one part of building these maps. It is a well-known fact that body maps in the somatosensory cortex depend on the electrical activity of the sensory fibers which carry the information from each part of your body. And this can vary according to individual circumstances. I am sure you are familiar with the quality

and beauty of some of the foot paintings produced by physically handicapped people. Clearly, for them to be able to produce these paintings, the area of the brain which represents their feet and toes is more highly developed.

So, the body maps in your brain can vary depending on the stimuli and this plasticity may not be always a good thing. If you regularly offer an infant or child the right stimuli, they will be able to build a better representation of themselves in their brain and that will have a direct impact on their coordination skills, how precise their movements are and their ability to learn in the future. If, on the other hand, they are given few tactile stimuli or receive negative stimuli such as constant or chronic pain, these experiences may also modify their brain maps, blurring them or associating the tactile experience with something dangerous. This is why modern physiotherapy doesn't just address the body when treating problems of chronic pain but also tries to improve the patient's cortical maps by using images or perception exercises to combat chronification issues. What is more, it does so very successfully.

Additionally, our earliest experiences of touch are known to determine our tactile sensitivity in the future and they play a fundamental role in the development of a child's brain. Even the sensations of touch experienced by a fetus in the womb are thought to be important in establishing their subsequent sense of perception of their own body and this prenatal programming is believed to last at least half the pregnancy. Evidently, an enriched environment postpartum develops the brain even further. The following experiment with rats gives us food for thought. When young rats are given new toys, they touch them and climb on top of them. This increases their brain activity and the size of their somatosensory cortex. If the toy is left in the same place for days on end, the little rats get bored and their cortex starts to shrink. But if the position of the toys is changed at least twice a week, the increase continues. This has tremendous implications for our children's lives as tactile sensitivity in humans is known to impact on cognitive development..

If you regularly offer an infant or child the right stimuli they will be able to build a better representation of themselves in their brain. This will have a direct impact on their coordination skills, how precise their movements are and their ability to learn in the future.

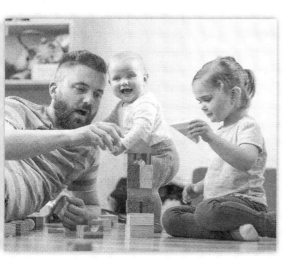

Aiden and Sophia are in a nurturing environment. Not just because of the number of toys they have but because they are playing on the floor accompanied by an adult. Playing, moving around and interacting really are brain food.

So, what do your children need? As you can imagine, a 5 month old baby sitting with a toy in her hand, propped up by a pillow to stop her from falling over, is not the best form of stimulation. Maybe because the child should spend more time on her tummy with someone by her side or exploring the environment; maybe because you should not leave a baby who has still not learned how to sit up by herself from the lying position, sitting up; maybe because she should try to reach out for the toys with her hands or by making little movements with her body or maybe because we should be touching her and playing with her at that time. Maybe because we need to ask ourselves what a nurturing environment really means.

Playing, moving around and interacting really are brain food.

The incredible benefits of contact

Contact is vital for the growth and development of almost all mammals. We know that many animal offspring need to be licked as soon as they are born to prevent them dying of kidney or intestinal failure. Human babies also need contact but it is remarkable how we have evolved from licking to touching and kissing. As many parents of newborn babies will tell you, the urge to sniff their infants remains strong.

What happens with children's bodies is similar to what happens with their minds. For a human being to recognize itself and feel comfortable and safe in its own skin, it must first have been touched and recognized physically by other human beings when she was small. In a wonderful parallel, for a human being to recognize and feel safe and secure in their own mind, they must first have been accepted and recognized by other human beings early on in life. Deliberate contact and stroking are pivotal to building her identity from the outset, just as much as responding to the sounds she makes or her emotions.

Touching therefore increases body awareness and "prevents" mental and physical dissociation because it helps to integrate the body into the Self. These body-mind connections which become permanent when established this early on, encourage the body to constitute a real part of the Self. This can be a way of healing, of regulating and channeling emotions and experiences. In addition, to feel touched, seen and heard is also a form of protection against potentially traumatic situations in the future (we perceive fewer situations as traumatic and cope better with them because we are more resilient). It is even possible that there is no difference between physical, psychological and social identity early in life and instead there is a common path that then branches off and evolves in a more complex way.

In some experiments, newborn rats that are handled are less easily scared and possess more brain receptors for benzodiazepines (tranquilizers). They also suffer less degeneration in the hippocampus (a key area of the brain for memory and spatial orientation) and their response to stress is much better. This only works if it happens during the first 10 days of their life, after that it doesn't produce the same lasting benefits.

If we human beings experience anything like these kinds of neuroendocrine responses when we have skin to skin contact with our parents, then the implication is that we need to take a long hard look at the way we manage the first months of children's lives. This is when the amount of real touching (skin-to-skin contact time on large areas of the body) and real movement (not the sort she gets from the baby carriage, but the type where the baby's head perceives slight vertical movements) are essential for development. Ironically, these are precisely the stimuli that are lacking in many households. When viewed from this perspective it is easier to understand some of the serious development problems we find in so many children adopted from institutions in different countries. Unfortunately we find them in many children born to families here too and not always due to a lack of love and care. Occasionally, it is possible that the child has been unable to integrate the contact with her mother or attachment figures correctly due to different nervous system disorders. In our clinical practice with these children and others with developmental immaturity, we regularly see how daily intervention through touch and movement noticeably improves their stress response and reduces their anxiety. Something can always be done to help them find their wings!

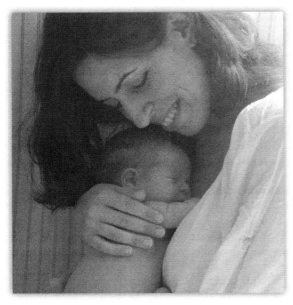

Finn loves being in full contact with his mum; he feels relaxed and loved. Skin-to-skin contact is one of the best gifts you can give yourself and your baby.

In our clinical practice with such a lot of children who have developmental immaturity, we see regularly how daily intervention through touch and movement noticeably improves their stress response and reduces their anxiety.

The fact that touch is a basic need for newborns was fully borne out by the skin-to-skin program developed in Columbia in the eighties which came about as the result of insufficient incubators for the number of premature infants being born. In this program they observed that, by leaving a naked premature infant (in poor health because of her immaturity), in skin-to-skin contact with her mother's body 24 hours a day, she regulated her temperature better than the infants in the incubators and even her weight gain and vital signs improved much faster than the infants in artificial "caregivers". Some years later research would establish that one of the development pathways of an infant's immune system is skin-to-skin contact. Over time this has led to the program being applied in hospitals that do have sufficient incubators. These days this "kangaroo care" is widely recommended across the globe and is supported by a body of evidence, particularly in premature infants.

"Kangaroo care" is thus named because of its resemblance to the early life of marsupials where the young are carried around in a bag in constant contact with the mother. Some of the benefits seen in babies are: they sleep better, cry less, breathe more regularly, breastfeed for longer, gain weight faster and are discharged before babies who have not had skin-to-skin contact with their parents.

Skin-to-skin contact has proven effective in reducing pain in infants. In a very recent study, it was found that the heel prick test carried out on all infants as part of the protocol tests in Western health systems is less painful when the mother and child have skin-to-skin contact during the test. It was also observed that there were fewer changes in heart rate, an improvement in the blood oxygen saturation and enhanced emotional communication between the mother and child.

From an immunological perspective, there is growing evidence of the beneficial effect of skin-to-skin contact on children. Another recent study shows how skin-to-skin contact between infants and their mothers in intensive care units is clearly effective in the treatment of infections of certain types of staphylococci resistant to antibiotic treatment and this contact is contemplated as part of the protocols in neonatology units.

Some of the benefits of skin-to-skin contact are babies sleep better, cry less, breathe more regularly, breastfeed for longer, gain weight faster.

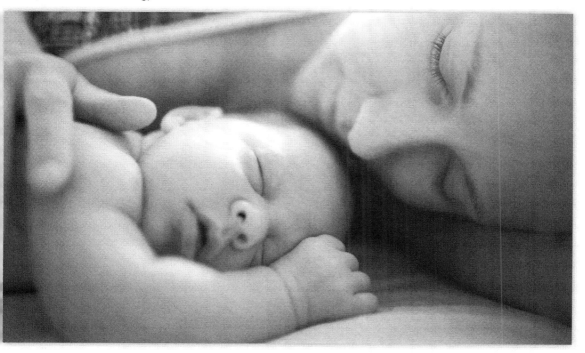

Amelia loves her mother being close and touching her. So much so that she relaxes to the point of sometimes falling asleep. Massages are fantastic for your baby but they are no substitute for hours of skin-to-skin contact.

Do our babies get enough skin-to-skin time?

If we consider the number of children who have development problems in our society (around 20%) and some of the advice like "don't pick her up, she'll get used to it", you might be forgiven for wondering if, on the whole, our babies get all the contact they need.

There are numerous social dilemmas surrounding parenting infants and children. Should I do this or that? Do I let her cry, or do I pick her up? When faced by one of these dilemmas just ask yourself: if you were on a lost island in Polynesia, part of a tribe deep in the Amazon or in a town in far-off Lapland, none of which are westernized, what would you do? Perhaps we have forgotten that human beings are equipped with genetic programming spanning millions of years that hasn't evolved as quickly as society has in our developed countries. Our biological needs are a consequence of our genetic make-up rather than a result of changing and often contradictory socio-cultural norms. Attempts to go against human nature inevitably lead to physical, psychological or social dysfunction.

If you don't know what to do with your baby, just ask yourself: if you were somewhere else in the world, totally in tune with nature, what would you do?

Babies need constant contact. Sometimes we are more preoccupied with buying them clothing that is soft and pretty, instead of giving them the most important thing of all and what they need most: something altogether simpler. We look for the softest, highest quality fabrics but fail to understand that what they need most is our own skin.

SUMMARY

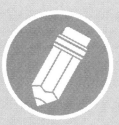

From a biological point of view, in the case of a newborn human being, affection means skin contact. To be touched and, more importantly, to be touched properly is therefore, to be loved.

The skin really is an extension of the nervous system, so touching the skin equates to connecting with the brain. The emotional, mental and physical development of the baby depends on the quantity and quality of that touch in the first years of his life.

There are many, varied maps in your brain. There are numerous maps of your body and countless maps of your exterior self. In the first stages of life a main sensory map and a main motor map develop in the brain. The better these maps are, the more accurate and efficient the child or adult's movements will be. However, for these maps to be made properly, their skin must be touched from birth.

Fortunately, even if some children do not receive enough contact or the contact they have with their parents cannot be integrated properly due to some health issue, it is never too late to touch them and help their brain to create those maps.

Children with development, learning and behavioral problems often lack precision in the perception and control of their bodies, as if their body maps had not been formed properly. In our clinical experience we see how many children improve their neurodevelopment by daily stimuli to the skin and movement protocols.

Skin-to-skin contact with their parents or attachment figures has incredible advantages for infants. Some of the benefits we see are that they sleep better, cry less, breathe more regularly, breastfeed for longer, gain weight faster and are discharged from hospital before infants who did not have skin-to-skin contact with their parents. In addition, they experience less pain during situations such as medical tests and, the icing on the cake is that they respond better to infections. For these and many other reasons, you would be wise to question if expressions like "don't pick her up, she'll get used to it" actually contribute to better parenting and individual human development.

What can you do?
HELPFUL PRACTICAL ADVICE

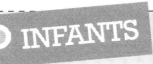

INFANTS

- Spend at least an hour a day in skin-to-skin contact with your baby with no clothing in the way. If it's cold cover yourselves up but make sure direct contact is maintained. You'll find you feel good too. There is evidence that adults secrete endorphins when they are in contact with babies, but let's face it, it doesn't take much science to prove it: all you have to do is let a baby fall asleep on top of you. You will notice how your heart rate lowers, your breathing slows down and you go into a semi-hypnotic state. Where possible, stay like this as long as you can. This advice is not just aimed at mothers it applies to fathers and other carers too. The longer the baby spends skin-to-skin, the better he will develop overall. If skin-to-skin contact is so clearly beneficial for the most fragile infants, how come it is not a standard part of child care? It's like saying that drinking water has proven effective in the recovery of dehydrated people. Surely you would recommend it to everyone else?

- Touch your baby's little hands as often as you can, pausing at each tiny finger. The same with her feet. Stroke her around the mouth, on her cheeks and face. Do it regularly. I'm sure you already do; we are programmed to. But now that you know how important it is, you mustn't forget to do it. You can enjoy doing it too. It's wonderful to feel a baby's skin.

- If you breastfeed your baby, let her try to find your nipple. Do the same with the bottle if this is her main or combined source of food. Don't just "plug" the bottle into her mouth straight away. Tap it gently on your baby's face to activate her search reflexes. This can be very beneficial for the correct integration of primitive reflexes and have a positive impact on her capacity for speech in the future. It can also prevent lingual parafunctions later on (such as sticking out one's tongue while writing), excessive salivation or behaviors where the older child is always uncontrollably biting or sucking things (such as jacket sleeves).

- Massage your baby. This can help both of you as well as creating a beautiful bond. It has extraordinary effects for the child and for the relationship. Remember to touch every part of her body firmly but don't forget this does not substitute skin-to-skin time. There are some indications that this ancient practice of massage, which is more common in certain Asian cultures, is beneficial to the physical and mental development of children, although the studies are not as clear-cut as those on skin-to-skin or "kangaroo care".

OLDER CHILDREN

- If you have an older child who has trouble with her coordination, is somewhat clumsy with their hands and whose movements, even the more global ones, lack precision, spend 5 or 10 minutes a day touching them. Not just their hands, their whole body. A pediatric physiotherapist specializing in Pediatric Integrative Manual Therapy (PIMT) can teach you the best way to touch them to "wire" their brain. Don't use a light touch, it should feel more like kneading bread. Try it! Start at the center and move out to the extremities: arms, forearms, hands and even fingers, pausing on each finger. Do the same with their feet. This isn't something that can be done mechanically it has to be done in a conscious, mindful way, connecting with them in the moment. By doing this, over the course of 30 to 40 days they will probably start to move in a more coordinated way, though you have to realize there are no magic remedies and if they have learning and attention issues it should be combined with other therapies. As we will see later on, what is needed in these cases is a comprehensive evaluation of the child's neurodevelopment and an overall treatment proposal.

- If you were unable to accompany your child in her early stages of development because you weren't aware of the need for it, or because of other difficulties in her early years (illnesses, hospitalizations, etc.), don't panic, it can all be programmed later. The brain is an amazing thing and it can sometimes find alternative ways to build or repair itself. If you consider your child's difficulties correspond to less than optimal motor, sensory or postural development in the early years of her life, you can ask a developmental physiotherapist (at the end of this book you will discover how to find one), for an over all assessment of the current situation and for advice on to how to reprogram her nervous system. It is never too late to help your child progress. Help her find her wings!

BIBLIOGRAPHY

Regarding the experiment with mothers made of terry cloth and wire:

Harlow HF, Zimmerman RR. Affectional responses in the infant monkey. Science. 1959;130:421-32.

Regarding the onset of the sense of touch, its development and significance:

Barnard KE, Brazelton TB. Touch: The Foundation of Experience. MW Books; 1990.

Bushnell EW, Boudreau JP. The development of haptic perception during infancy. En: Heller MA, Schiff W, eds. The psychology of touch. Hillsdale, NJ: Lawrence Erlbaum; 1991.

Eliot L. What's going on in there? How the brain and mind develop in the first five years of life. Bantam Books; 2000.

Regarding brain maps:

Blakeslee S, Blakeslee M. The body has a mind of its own. Random House; 2008.

Killackey HP, Rhoades RW, Bennett-Clarke CA. The formation of a cortical somatotopic map. Trends Neurosci. 1995 Sep;18(9):402-7.

On how pain stimuli can modify cortical maps and how to treat it:

Moseley GL, Butler DS, Beames TB, Giles TJ. The graded Motor Imagery Handbook. Noigroup Publications; 2012.

Moseley GL, Flor H. Targeting cortical representations in the treatment of chronic pain: a review. Neurorehabil Neural Repair. 2012 Jul-Aug;26(6):646-52.

Regarding the benefits of skin-to-skin contact:

Diamond MC. Evidence for tactile stimulation improving CNS function. En: Barnard KE, Brazelton TB, eds. Touch: The Foundations of Experience. International University Press; 1990.

Lamy Filho F, De Sousa SH, Freitas IJ, Lamy ZC, Simões VM, Da Silva AA, et al. Effect of maternal skin-to-skin contact on decolonization of Methicillin-Oxacillin-Resistant Staphylococcus in neonatal intensive-care units: a randomized controlled trial.BMC Pregnancy Childbirth. 2015 Mar 19;15:63.

Lassi ZS, Middleton PF, Crowther C, Bhutta ZA. Interventions to Improve Neonatal Health and Later Survival: An Overview of Systematic Reviews. EBioMedicine. 2015 May 31;2(8):983-98.

Liu M, Zhao L, Li XF. Effect of skin contact between mother and child in pain relief of full-term newborns during heel blood collection. Clin Exp Obstet Gynecol. 2015;42(3):304-8.

Moore ER, Anderson GC, Bergman N, Dowswell T. Early skin-to-skin contact for mothers and their healthy newborn infants. Cochrane Database Syst Rev. 2012 May 16;5:CD003519.

Sapolsky RM. The importance of a well-groomed child. Science. 1997;277:1620-1.

Vincent S. Skin-to-skin contact. Part one: just an hour of your time. Pract Midwife. 2011 May;14(5):40-1.

Vincent S. Skin-to-skin contact. Part two: the evidence. Pract Midwife. 2011 Jun;14(6):44-6.

Yoshida S, Martines J, Lawn JE, Wall S. Setting research priorities to improve global newborn health and prevent stillbirths by 2025. J Glob Health. 2016 Jun;6(1):010508.

Regarding the early initiation of maternal breastfeeding:

Lassi ZS, Middleton PF, Crowther C, Bhutta ZA. Interventions to Improve Neonatal Health and Later Survival: An Overview of Systematic Reviews. EBioMedicine. 2015 May 31;2(8):983-98.

Regarding the benefits of massage in infants:

Badr LK, Abdallah B, Kahale L. A Meta-Analysis of Preterm Infant Massage: An Ancient Practice With Contemporary Applications. MCN Am J Matern Child Nurs. 2015 Nov-Dec;40(6):344-58.

Vickers A, Ohlsson A, Lacy JB, Horsley A. Massage for promoting growth and development of preterm and/or low birth-weight infants. Cochrane Database Syst Rev. 2000;(2):CD000390.

Chapter 3

Movement, the most powerful stimulus of all
Learning how to live in this world

Iñaki Pastor Pons

Contact and movement are the two fundamental needs of any newborn infant. Children love the feeling of movement. They find it relaxing when they are babies and fascinating and great fun when they are older. As a parent no doubt you have been party to both. Do you remember how long you spent rocking the baby-carriage to get your baby to sleep? Then, just when you thought he had fallen asleep and you could finish your glass of wine with your friends, the moment you stopped and turned to go, he would let you know he wanted more movement! It's not unusual for parents to drive their babies round and round the block in the car to get them to sleep, dreading the moment they return home. Let's not dwell on the advisability or otherwise of these practices here. The fact is that movement relaxes babies. It calms them down, reduces their irritability, stimulates them and they find it fun. In fact, they actively seek it out.

When children are a bit older there is nothing they like more and there is nothing quite so easy. They ask you to spin them round like a merry-go-round, turn them upside down, flip them over… and if you don't do it, don't worry, they will find a way to do it themselves. Have you ever seen a 4 or 5 year-old spinning round at top speed, waiting for that drunken, dizzy feeling when he stops? You look on, hoping in vain that the horror on your face will prevent him from carrying on. «You're going to get dizzy» you tell him as you see his eyes gyrating rapidly as soon as he stops, swaying from side to side to regain his balance before once again hurtling full throttle into spin after spin.

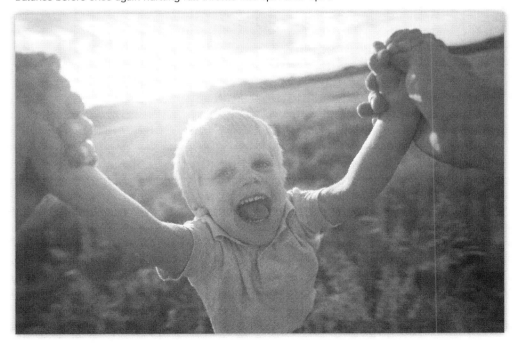

Michael loves being spun around. It's a favorite game for many children and something they never get tired of.

Why so much movement? Why is it so desirable, sought after and instinctive? How does it contribute to a child's nervous system and how can it be used to maximize your child's development?

The vestibular system is the biological system which manages and regulates our sense of balance, spatial orientation and the control of eye movements. It is thanks to this system, if it is programmed correctly, that you learn how to live in this world.

Join me now as we explore this topic which is so fascinating and so essential for your child's development.

What makes us feel movement?

In order to feel something, you have to have a sensor, a receiver or an organ in your body which is sensitive to this kind of stimulus and capable of perceiving it. You have a so-called vestibular system which enables you to feel your head movements and interpret them correctly. It is called vestibular because the organs of the vestibular system are located in a space inside the ear, (vestibule: space or set of large rooms), together with the organ of hearing. The vestibular apparatus is a set of capsules and canals which include the hearing organ (cochlea) and two types of vestibulary organs: semi-circular canals that are sensitive to head rotations, and the otolith organs, (utricle and saccule), that are sensitive to linear head movements and the position of the head with regard to gravity, for example, when you are standing up or lying down.

There are three semicircular canals each filled with liquid in all three-dimensional planes of the vestibule so they can perceive any movement of your head. Inside there are hairs called cilia which are in contact with the fluid in the canals. When the liquid moves in the canals or otolith organs through movement or the position of the head, the cilia detect it, converting the movement (balance) or hearing into an electric signal which is carried to the brain by a nerve.

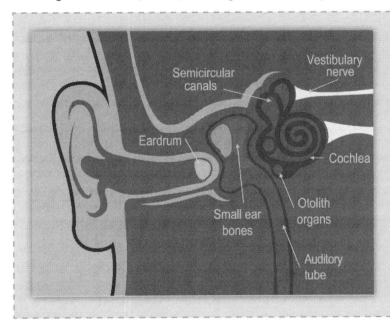

The vestibular and auditory organs are found inside the ear. The eardrum is shown in light blue, the small bones of the ear which transmit the vibrations of the eardrum to the cochlea (the snail-like shape in violet), in orange and pink. The rings above the cochlea are the semicircular canals responsible for detecting head movements. The organs of hearing and balance are very close to each other.

The information from this nerve reaches an area of the brain called the vestibular nucleus, inside the brainstem. The sensation does not reach the cortex at first, so the sense of balance is subconscious. When you read whilst you are walking you are not aware of the sensation of your head movements. It is only when things go wrong that you get a feeling something unpleasant is happening. For example, when you lose your balance through unsteadiness or when you feel motion sickness on a boat. Children with developmental or learning issues do not describe dizziness in everyday life (some of them are very sensitive to means of transport), but their balance is usually very poor.

There are pathways from the vestibular nuclei for controlling the eyes, the head, the muscles of the spine and the legs and other nerve centers. What does this mean? It means that, when you move your head, your eyes must move to stabilize the images, your neck to stabilize your head and your back and leg muscles to ensure that you don't fall over. You can imagine what would happen if this information wasn't managed properly: whenever you moved your head it would feel like the world was moving, that the walls or the floor were moving, that you were going to fall over or at the very least, it would make you feel totally disoriented. Anyone who has suffered from it knows all too well: vertigo is worse than any pain imaginable!

There are pathways from the vestibular nuclei for controlling the eyes, the head, the muscles of the spine and the legs and other nerve centers.

Nerve fibers leading from the vestibular organs take information directly to the cerebellum, where it is processed together with other information from your vision, touch and proprioception, so that, overall it helps you to control your balance. The cerebellum is one of the main keys to balance, although it also plays a role in the fluidity of movement and in language. Assessing the function of the cerebellum is an important part of evaluating children with learning and attention issues.

The information from the vestibular system reaches the cortex too. However, it does not reach a specific area, rather it is distributed in numerous areas, which gives an idea of the wide-ranging impact it has on your life.

When did you start to feel movement?

You started to feel movement very early on, somewhere around week 8 of prenatal life. The vestibular organs would have formed deep in your ear a few weeks earlier. Although the sense of touch is the first to appear in the womb, the sense of balance is the first to reach maturity. The nerve between the vestibular system and the brainstem begins to act at 12 weeks and is the first tract to mature. It is the only sensory system with significant myelination at birth, although other parts continue this process until puberty. Myelination is the process whereby an insulating substance covers the nerves enabling the speed of nerve transmission to multiply. The early myelination or maturation of the vestibular system is a great indication of the importance of balance for the development and integration of the other sensory and motor systems after birth. The vestibular system is primarily responsible for your posture, balance control and spatial and body orientation.

Even though the sense of touch is the first to appear in the womb, the sense of balance is the first to mature.

The vestibulo-ocular reflex (VOR) starts to trigger around week 10 of prenatal life. The VOR is an automatic response that your eyes make to a change of position or a movement of the head. It is your earliest balance system.

From a phylogenetic perspective it is ancient human trait. During evolution, the first animals to have heads developed a sensor system to control the position of the head in relation to gravity. This is even true of plants. Barely has a plant seedling had time to sprout roots than it needs to know which way is up and which way is down, and this requires a system that can provide information about the direction of gravitational pull.

The appearance of this reflex in prenatal life together with another called the "Moro reflex", marks the onset of sensitivity and the processing of movement. The Moro reflex is an overall response to anything unexpected. Movement and touch, together with the response to gravity, were to become one of the great stimuli for the development of the human race. By development we mean the maturation of the nervous system in the neurosensory-motor sense. An infant's posture and ability to keep his head upright depend on the one hand on the development of the vestibular system, and, on the other, on having a healthy neck. Unfortunately, there are a lot of babies with neck problems as a result of difficult births who suffer great discomfort and whose development is held back...

It is vital that specialist physiotherapists assess and treat these disorders in order to correct any deficiencies, allowing the child to reach his full potential. Later in the book you will discover the kind of physiotherapists who are good at doing this.

An infant's posture and his ability to keep his head upright depend on the one hand on the development of the vestibular system and, on the other, on having a healthy neck.

A newborn infant needs to move. The natural, cross-cultural instinct to rock babies bears witness to this. In every culture around the globe, adults rock babies and the babies regard this stimulation from rhythmic movement as something soothing. Some children enter sleep this way and some parents can't find any other way to get their children to sleep. The most important thing to understand here is that not only does this movement have a calming, soothing effect on the infant, but it is also one of the most significant keys to the child's full development in terms of: posture control, balance, attention span, emotional security, cognitive abilities in reading, writing and arithmetic, spatial orientation, etc.

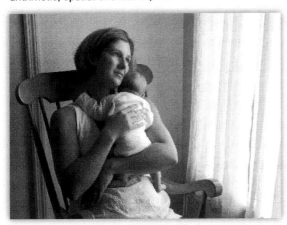

Harper loves to be with her mom and to be rocked. It soothes her and makes her feel loved. Rocking a baby not only has a soothing effect, it is also crucial for their cognitive and emotional development.

The amazing difference between a baby-carriage and a baby carrier

Imagine again if you are in that village deep in the Amazon, that island in Polynesia, or another area of the world where human beings still live in contact with nature like the tribes Salgado photographed in his book, Genesis. When a baby is born, what is the first thing his parents think of doing? Tying some sticks together to make a bed, putting the infant on top and dragging him across the floor? Sounds weird doesn't it? Well, that's exactly what we do in the western world, but using state of the art baby-carriages and wheels instead.

Baby-carriages are a great invention... for parents. They are convenient; they allow you a certain amount of freedom to do other things at the same time you look after your baby. But we should not assume they are good for the baby. Early in life human beings need to be carried in a somewhat upright position, especially after they are 4-6 weeks old. Prior to this they can nestle in a baby wrap or sling.

Baby carriers are very beneficial for infants. The vestibular stimulation they receive from the small vertical movements as the person wearing the carrier walks about is extremely important. They stimulate the muscle tone of the neck and trunk and in fact, infants that are carried have much better muscle tone. They have better head control and are more successful at meeting the developmental milestones we will see later. Secondly, contact with the parent is soothing and reassuring. As we learned earlier, contact is vitally important for developmentand has very positive neurophysiological as well as sedative, effects.

Baby carriers are very beneficial for infants. They stimulate the muscle tone of the neck and trunk and are soothing and reassuring.

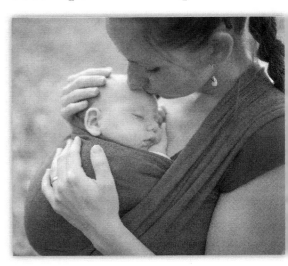

Milois delighted when they go out for a walk together but he relaxes so much that he doesn't stay awake for long.

Another benefit is the position of the hips which are spread around the parent, allowing the pelvis bones to form correctly. For this to work, it is important to make sure that the carrier system keeps the baby's legs spread out and flexed.

If your baby cries when you put him in the sling or backpack you need to check if the carrier is suitable for him. If it is, ask a specialist physiotherapist to check if he is suffering from discomfort in his back or neck.

Infants aren't afraid of movement...
well, perhaps a little,
but it is vital for them!

There is a very interesting fact which demonstrates the confusion that sometimes exists regarding the stimulus infants need and how our desire to protect them from something we haven't fully grasped, can lead to developmental issues. From birth to approximately 4 or 5 months, if an infant is moved rather quickly, he will suddenly spread his arms out. You will no doubt recall this if you have children of your own. When a baby is less than 4-6 weeks old, this reaction is accompanied by the subsequent reaction of pulling the arms in. In addition to the arms, there are other aspects we don't see: changes in peripheral circulation, an increase in the heart and respiratory rates and the secretion of stress hormones. It is an adaptive response to an unexpected movement of his head, although it can also be triggered by a loud sound or bright light. The child's automatic, overall response to an unexpected stimulus is known as the Moro reflex.

The parents' first reaction is to think that the baby "got scared" and, with the clear aim of protecting their child, (no one wants their baby to be frightened), the amount and intensity of the movements are reduced to avoid triggering this response. Far from being helpful for the infant, this can cause a serious developmental problem for him in the future. Let me explain.

Primitive reflexes such as the Moro reflex are «programmers». This means that their responses provide the nervous system with the possibility of «training» itself in the different adaptive responses necessary for our environment. As a result, brain connections relating to movement and the senses, along with immunological and neuroendocrine responses, are established. Primitive reflexes are extremely helpful for development. However, primitive reflexes which do not manifest themselves, are unused or non-integrated, create gaps in the maturation of the nervous system.

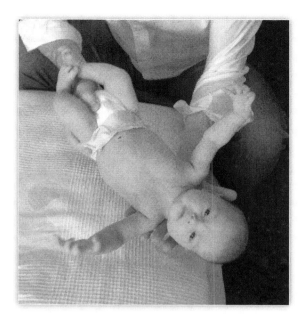

William, who is 4 weeks old, reacts to a change in position with the Moro reflex triggered by a backward head movement. The Moro reflex plays one of the most influential roles in a person's future in terms of their attention and behavior.

Primitive reflexes such as the Moro reflex are «programmers». This means that their reactions provide the nervous system with the possibility of «training» itself in the different adaptive responses necessary for our environment.

The Moro reflex in particular is great at programming a person's global response to stress, to the unforeseen and the unknown, whatever the type of stimulus may be. The Moro reflex plays a part in programming many key aspects of a person: oculomotricity, equilibrium responses, spinal righting reflexes, auditory sensitivity, tactile sensitivity, the level of immune response and many other processes. Nature's ability to economize is impressive. A single response is used to program multiple things for example; integration of the Moro reflex reduces hearing sensitivity by 20 or 30 decibels. Failure to integrate this reflex can leave auditory hypersensitivity and result in the child having difficulties with language maturation as well as unusual reactions of fear and rejection to certain loud or noisy environments. The relationship between the Moro reflex and the unexpected, frequently results in children with poor integration having difficulty entering new environments and feeling comfortable. Sometimes teachers say to parents: "He never speaks in class. What's he like at home?" The surprised parents reply: "He never stops talking at home!" These kinds of odd reactions are typical in children who have not successfully integrated the Moro reflex or who were not treated by experts in development.

The Moro reflex, which is also known as the startle reflex, has another unusual function: in conjunction with the visible response of the arms, the heart and respiratory rates also increase, and stress hormones are secreted. This prepares the infant's metabolism to react to new or unexpected situations. These responses program how he will react to stress in the future. Many children who have poor stress programming have great difficulties adapting to new situations or live in a permanent state of anxiety. Both the physical and emotional experiences encountered in the first months and years program the way a person will function for the rest of their life.

Many children who have poor stress programming have great difficulties adapting to new situations or live in a permanent state of anxiety.

For learning and attention to take place, the child must be able to inhibit any stimuli and sensations that are not a priority for the task. Whilst you are reading this book your brain is constantly receiving stimuli. Some are external; sounds from the street, the people next to you moving around, the ambient temperature, etc. There are also the sensations in your body: you may feel hungry or have an ache or pain somewhere; perhaps you can feel your clothes rubbing against a part of your body, or the chair touching your back, as well as hundreds of other sensations. With so many stimuli how do you manage to read and understand what is going on? Because your brain inhibits this information in order to focus your attention on the task of reading. Many children with poor startle reflex programming struggle to prevent their attention from wandering with every new stimulus that reaches them. Everything attracts their attention: a sound from the floor above, a classmate moving, the contact of the chair on their back, etc. Consequently, cognitive performance decreases drastically. The ability to stay on task depends, among other things, on the programming of this reflex which is linked to a large extent to movement.

In addition, other reflexes both primitive (present in babies) and postural (present throughout life), also have an impact on the quality of our learning and attention. Now you can see why «protecting» infants from feeling movement can have lasting repercussions for the child and future adult.

John has trouble concentrating. Everything he hears and any slight movement near to him manages to break his concentration so he can address this new stimulus. Many children with poor integration of the Moro reflex are unable to inhibit their responses when confronted by noise or movement. Everything attracts their attention, greatly reducing their performance.

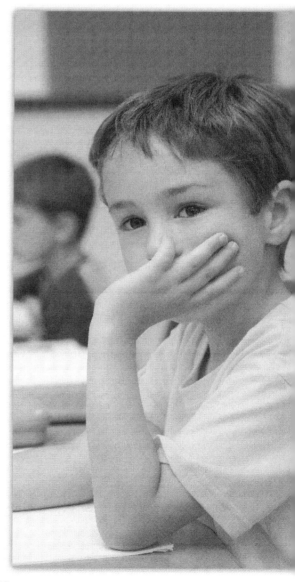

What do balance and learning have to do with each other?

Thanks to the rhythmic head movements that began during fetal life when the mother moved or walked around and which continue into the first phases of postnatal life, the brain develops connections between different areas by means of the aforementioned reflexes, and these will be important for how the systems controlling balance and eye movement function. All of this is triggered by stimulation of the vestibular system.

Even without you realizing it, the vestibular system plays an amazing role in neurological and mental development. For example, one study found a large number of children who had a poor post-rotatory nystagmus response (one of the ways of detecting if the vestibular system reacts after turning or spinning) also had clear delays in motor development. Almost half could not walk by the 18-month milestone and upper age limit

Even without you realizing it, the vestibular system plays a vital role in neurological and mental development.

It is relatively easy to understand how the sense of balance can affect the development of motor skills, but vestibular deficits are also often found in children with emotional problems, attention deficit, problems with perception, learning disabilities, language disorders and autism. Although vestibular dysfunction is probably not solely responsible for these disorders, the findings suggest that a sense of balance and movement is much more important than previously believed.

Could it be that the lack of a correctly functioning vestibular system causes cognitive dysfunctions in people? Could it even lead to problems in processing mental arithmetic and math? Research in this area would suggest so. This would explain why so many children with learning, attention, and behavioral issues have poor balance control. In fact, it seems that the lack of proper vestibular and proprioceptive programming is one of the key factors in learning disabilities. Additionally, as we have already seen, when the vestibular system is not working properly it can cause insecurity, anxiety and various other difficulties in both children and adults.

Mental development requires the development of other more basic aspects in the brain. As one of the first systems to mature, the vestibular system offers some of the earliest relevant experiences for the maturation and organization of the nervous system. These experiences are likely to play a fundamental role in the organization of other sensory and motor skills and therefore form the basis for the development of emotional and cognitive skills.

In fact, it seems that the lack of proper vestibular and proprioceptive programming is one of the key factors in learning disabilities.

A child's neurological maturity improves with movement

If vestibular problems affect brain development, some researchers wonder whether, if the situation were reversed, vestibular stimulation could improve a child's brain function, their balance, oculomotricity, head control and muscle tone. Evidence that this is the case is beginning to emerge. It is common knowledge that natural vestibular stimulation comes from being moved around and carried about, above all with an upright head. Vestibular stimulation is not as relevant in a baby-carriage. Infants who are handled and carried around, have the immediate benefit of developing muscle tone and this helps hold the head up and establish righting postures.

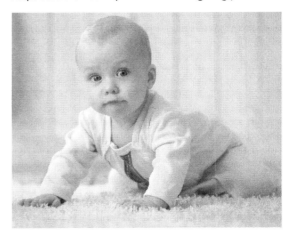

Sara, who is 8 months old is already lifting her bottom to get on all fours. Around about this age, healthy babies develop anteroposterior rocking movements which precede crawling. Through these movements they integrate spinal reflexes with regard to their limbs and strengthen their arms in readiness for crawling.

A lot of infants and children stimulate themselves through repetitive head movements. This is also true for infants between 7 and 8 months who continuously rock back and forwards, a movement that precedes crawling. Moreover, these rocking movements aid the maturation of the automatisms which are dependent on the neck and allow them to build strength in their arms. Later on, they will be able to crawl around and explore their surroundings.

Infants that are handled and carried around have the immediate benefit of developing muscle tone and this helps them to hold their head up and begin to straighten up.

In one study, infants between the ages of 3 and 13 months were subjected to 10 sessions of spinning in a chair. Twice a week, the infants were seated on an adult's lap and spun around 10 times in a swivel chair and each spin was halted abruptly. To maximize stimulation of the three channels, they were spun in different positions: sitting, sitting with their head slightly tilted forward and lying down on their right and left sides. It came as no surprise that they liked this treatment. There were two control groups, one of which did not receive treatment, and one in which the infants sat on the adult's lap but were not spun around. The results were striking.

Compared to the two control groups, the infants that were spun showed much better development, both in their reflexes and in their gross motor skills. The difference was very clear in movement skills such as sitting, crawling, standing or walking. The study involved twins; one took part in the training and the other didn't. At the end of the study when they were 4 months old, the twin who had the vestibular stimulation experience had good head control and could sit without support, whilst it took the other twin much longer to reach the same milestones.

It is even more vital that we carry infants who have developmental problems or neurological diseases.

The repercussions of this study are dramatic if we consider the quality and quantity of the vestibular stimulation that our babies receive, starting with their means of transport. When babies are pushed in a baby-carriage they suffer insufficient vestibular stimuli. Moreover, they develop better head and neck control when they are in an upright position. Babies are transported from A to B lying flat on wheel systems designed to cushion movement; therefore, it is no surprise that so many children have slightly immature development due to a lack of stimuli. Infants with neck problems or problems in prenatal development (various syndromes, diseases or some form immaturity) have more difficulty integrating the vestibular stimuli, so carrying them becomes an even more vital way, though not the only way, of helping their development.

Oddly enough, children with serious developmental issues such as brain damage or a genetic syndrome are carried less than healthy children, when their need for stimuli is much greater. It is common over-protective behavior. It's a real shame; the more movement they need, the less they get. At our clinic we see how carrying children with serious developmental problems and using vestibular stimulation alongside the usual pediatric physiotherapy on them, greatly improves their prognosis and the maturation of their nervous system.

Conversely, in the mildest cases of developmental immaturity, we see how many infants who should have been lying on their tummies weeks ago, lifting themselves up with their forearms and holding their heads up to look at the world, in fact can barely lift their heads to change position. When parents are taught to carry their babies more often, to stimulate them via movement and touch, and allow them to spend more time on their tummies whilst awake and supervised, the infant's head control improves dramatically in the space of a few days. It is a case of understanding the neurological structure of human beings and giving them what they need.

SUMMARY

Together with contact, movement is the other great basic need a new-born infant has. Children love the feeling of movement. They find it relaxing when they are babies and fascinating and great fun when they are older.

The vestibular system is the biological system which provides the leading contribution to balance, spatial orientation and eye movement control. It is thanks to this system, if it is programmed correctly, that you learn how to live in this world.

You have a so-called vestibular system which enables you to feel your head movements and interpret them correctly. Your vestibular system in conjunction with your neck and vision enable you to orient yourself in space and build your position against gravity.

Baby carriers are very beneficial for babies. The vestibular stimulation from the small vertical movements as the person wearing the carrier walks about is extremely important. They stimulate the muscle tone of the neck and trunk and in fact, babies that are carried have much better muscle tone. They have better head control and they are more successful at meeting developmental milestones.

The vestibular system plays an amazing role in neurological and mental development.

Primitive reflexes such as the Moro reflex are «programmers». This means that their responses provide the nervous system with the possibility of «training» itself in the different adaptive responses that are necessary for our environment.

The absence of proper vestibular and proprioceptive programming is one of the key factors in learning disabilities.

Moreover, when the vestibular system is not working properly it can cause insecurity, anxiety and various other problems in children and adults alike.

Children with both moderate and severe developmental issues can benefit from movement.

What can you do?
HELPFUL PRACTICAL ADVICE

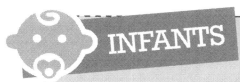

INFANTS

- Whenever possible, carry your baby in a backpack, wrap or sling or other carrying system, with the knees separated and hips spread wide against your body. This is essential to protect the correct development of his hips. By carrying your baby, his head movements will encourage maturation of the vestibular system and in turn, the correct programming of eye movements, spinal righting reflexes and the programming of stress response systems. It will also vastly improve his muscle tone.

- Hold your baby upright as long as possible when he is with you. When he is upright, he learns to respond to the pull of gravity and the vestibular system activates the spinal righting reflexes which coordinate the muscles of his neck to keep his head straight even if his body changes position. Being upright also has beneficial effects on eating since there is less chance of reflux; it prevents otitis because it helps the ear to drain into the throat; and it also encourages the action of the neck muscles on the development of the skull.

- Rock your baby a lot. Dance with him or «bounce» him in your lap. These are the sort of innate, spontaneous activities children often crave. Whilst they are playing on top of you, try to make them lose their balance by rolling them from side to side so their head is forced to react.

- Don't be afraid of picking your baby up more energetically. He needs movements that trigger balance and righting reactions. These unexpected changes of position are important so he can integrate this reflex properly. Sometimes we handle infants with excessive care. We overprotect them and, by not allowing them to fully develop their physical abilities due to lack of stimuli, we are actually harming them. Remember: when an infant is a bit scared, he is preparing his way of responding to the unexpected and stressful events he will encounter throughout his whole life.

OLDER CHILDREN

- When you play with your children, get them to roll over and over on mats on the floor or outside in the park. Perhaps you can get them to roll down a small grass slope or a man-made one using a sloping mattress. This is great for vestibular stimulation and, needless to say, great fun too!

- Allow your children to spin around if they want to. This is something we often see in healthy 5 and 6 year olds who want to experience feeling dizzy. When they stop spinning you will see their eyes are still «gyrating» until they stabilize. The medical term for this is nystagmus: rapid, rhythmic eye movements. Adults instinctively want to prevent children spinning but it is one of the ways they train their vestibular system.

- Clean mucus from the upper respiratory tract (behind the nose) with effective cleansing systems. A pediatric physiotherapist can teach you how to do this. Single doses and injections of serum are not as effective as carrying out nasal irrigation with plenty of serum which is introduced slowly and can clean the mucus lodged in the back of the nose. If he experiences mucus frequently and it is difficult to manage at home, take your child to a physiotherapist who will drain it for you. Having airways full of mucus makes it difficult to hear properly and alters the pressures that the inner ear, (where the vestibular system is located), receives.

- Limit visual stimuli from screens by restricting the use of tablets and television, replacing them with play activities: jumping, bouncing, rolling over and every other type of game that stimulates the sense of movement.

- If you were unable to accompany your child in his early stages of development and vestibular stimulation because you weren't aware it was necessary or because of other difficulties he may have had (illnesses, hospitalizations, etc.), don't panic it can all be programmed later. The brain is an amazing thing and sometimes has the ability to find alternative ways to build or repair itself. If you consider your child's difficulties correspond to less than optimal motor, sensory or postural development in the early years of his life, you can ask a developmental physiotherapist who specializes in PIMT (Pediatric Integrative Manual Therapy) to carry out a global assessment of his current situation and give you advice on how to reprogram his nervous system. Never give up hope – there is always a way to help your child progress!

BIBLIOGRAPHY

Regarding the importance of the vestibular system:

Christy JB, Payne J, Azuero A, Formby C. Reliability and diagnostic accuracy of clinical tests of vestibular function for children. Pediatr Phys Ther. 2015 Spring;27(1):102.

Eliot L. Why babies love to be bounced: the precocious sense of balance and motion. En: Eliot L. What's going on in there? How the brain and Mind develop in the first five years of life. Bantam Books; 2000. p. 145-56.

Nandi R, Luxon LM. Development and assessment of the vestibular system. Int J Audiol. 2008 Sep;47(9):566-77.

Rine RM, Dannenbaum E, Szabo J. 2015 Section on Pediatrics Knowledge Translation Lecture: Pediatric Vestibular-Related Impairments. Pediatr Phys Ther. 2016 Spring;28(1):2-6.

Regarding the vestibular system and learning:

Braswell J, Rine RM. Evidence that vestibular hypofunction affects reading acuity in children. Int J. Pediatr Otorhinolaryngol. 2006 Nov;70(11):1957-65.

De Quiros JB, Schrager OL. Fundamentos neuropsicológicos en las discapacidades de aprendizaje. Buenos Aires:Editorial Médica Panamericana; 1980.

Smith PF. Dyscalculia and vestibular function. Medical Hypothesis. 2012 Oct;79(4):493-6.

Smith PF, Zheng Y, Horii A, Darlington CL. Does vestibular damage cause cognitive dysfunction in humans? J Vestib Res. 2005;15(1):1-9.

Regarding the vestibular system and development:

Brandt T, Schautzer F, Hamilton DA, Brüning R, Markowitsch HJ, Kalla R, et al. Vestibular loss causes hippocampal atrophy and impaired spatial memory in humans. Brain. 2005 Nov;128(Pt 11):2732-41.

Clark DL, Kreutzberg JR, Chee FK. Vestibular stimulation influence on motor development in infants. Science. 1977 Jun 10;196(4295):1228-9.

MacLean WE Jr, Baumeister AA. Effects of vestibular stimulation on motor development and stereotyped behavior of developmentally delayed children. J Abnorm Child Psychol. 1982 Jun;10(2):229-45.

Rapin I. Hypoactive labyrinths and motor development. Clin Pediatr (Phila). 1974 Nov;13(11):922-3, 926-9, 934-7.

Regarding the primitive reflexes, development and learning:

Goddard Blythe S. Movement instinct. En: Goddard Blythe S. What babies and children really need. Hawthorn Press; 2008. p. 139-78.

Goddard Blythe S. Attention, Balance and Coordination. The ABC of Learning Success. Wiley-Blackwell; 2009.

McPhillips M, Jordan-Black J-A. Primary reflex persistence in children with reading difficulties (dyslexia): A cross-sectional study. Neuropsychologia. 2007 Jan;45(4):748-54.

Regarding the Moro reflex and its involvement in neurological development:

Goddard Blythe S. Attention, Balance and Coordination. The ABC of Learning Success. Wiley-Blackwell; 2009.

Regarding the vestibular system and anxiety:

Erez O, Gordon CR, Sever J, Sadeh A, Mintz M. Balance dysfunction in childhood anxiety: findings and theoretical approach. J Anxiety Disord. 2004;18(3):341-56.

Chapter 4

Don't run until you can walk
Taking things one step at a time

Iñaki Pastor Pons

It has take us an exceedingly long time to evolve into what we are today... It wasn't that long ago that we left the sea to populate the earth, became mammals and evolved into primates making the evolutionary leaps that led to the species we are today. We didn't become the variety of Homo sapiens we are now without some unsuccessful versions of homo falling by the wayside.

Evolution is not a straight line but a path with many ramifications and nature has certain obsessions; one of these is that it repeatedly uses things that work well. As a result, humans evolve in the womb from a simple cell division in an aquatic environment to the being we are at birth. Similar to how it was in the beginning; through cell division we evolved from single cell beings into more complex beings in an aquatic environment. Only in this case, because the exercise has been repeated so often, nature is able to do it in just 9 months whereas the evolution of our species took millions of years; from the cell division of a fertilized egg, to an increasingly complex organism, to what we are today. Quite a feat, isn't it?

In the early stages, the path seems common to different species. In fact, in the first weeks of life you wouldn't be able to clearly differentiate a dog, a mouse or an elephant from a human being.

It's only subsequently, at a later stage of development that we establish ourselves as humans thanks to our genetic programming. We know that at a certain stage of our embryological development we even get membranes between our fingers and toes which disappear later on.

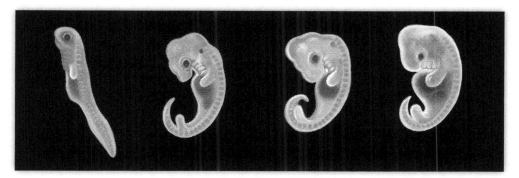

Here are reptile, bird, fish and human embryos. But ... which is which?

As you will see in this chapter, amazingly, nature mimics the evolutionary path yet again, this time outside the womb. The fascinating thing is that the time it takes to complete the full evolution of the species, i.e. to standing upright and saying our first words, is about 9 months. However, it takes much longer for us to fine-tune our abilities such as posture and balance control, or language and manual skills.

It is just as important to go through these evolutionary stages inside the womb as it is outside. Evidently, any deviation in this evolutionary path prior to birth can have dramatic consequences for the formation of the body and the brain. Yet skipping stages can also have consequences after birth, eminently on a functional level, but it is possible there could be more subtle alterations at a structural level too as a child's bones change according to the muscle tensions reaching them. If the muscle action is weak and asymmetrical, it is likely bone development will be too.

As a parent it is vital that you have basic knowledge of the stages your baby will go through. Firstly, so that you can quickly detect any delay in the acquisition of motor milestones (holding the head upright, rolling over, etc.). Secondly, so that you can help your baby through each stage through play and stimulation and by creating the best, warm, environment for her development. Some infants have minor difficulties which could be successfully overcome at each stage with parental awareness and just a little help in the form of stimulus. This would also allow her to integrate everything her nervous system needs to develop during this period. It would prevent many developmental problems in the future. Did you know that an assessment carried out on infants at specific times during their first year of life can predict their IQ and language skills at age 5–6 years? Surprising, isn't it?

Let's take a look at the stages of an infant's motor and postural development by drawing a parallel with the evolutionary process. This is purely for didactic purposes and should not be taken literally, but there are similarities which provide some interesting insight into understanding what happens to a person as they are forming.

The amphibian stage from 0 – 6 weeks old

Around week 40 of the pregnancy the baby is getting ready to leave the womb. Meanwhile, she is protected in an aquatic environment which allows her to move but at the same time cushions her from the enormous pressures that can be put on the mother's abdomen. Before we start breathing air, we are capable of living and developing in a water environment with food reaching us via the umbilical cord.

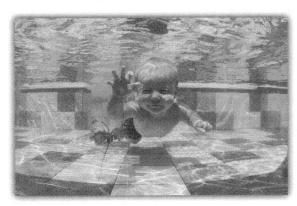 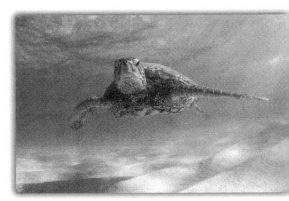

Mason is a great diver and can move skilfully around underwater just like a turtle.

It is possible to give birth in water and some mothers choose this option, although there is no real justification from an anthropological perspective. The fact is that when we are first born a reflex allows us to submerge ourselves in water without drowning. It is incredible to see how, thanks to a primitive survival reflex, an infant is able to hold its breath under water. She will lose this reflex a little later on along with the ability to submerge herself so easily and safely, although it is something that she can be re-trained to do. It is odd that this automatism does not disappear during childbirth and the reason it persists is still unclear.

We should not underestimate the difficulty of the situation human beings face when they leave their aquatic environment behind at birth. The infant moves quite well in her mother's womb, but her weight multiplies when she enters a world of air. She is trapped by gravity, without the necessary strength or muscle control to enable her to use her motor skills in this new environment.

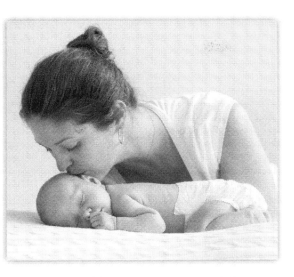

At just 10 days old Justin remains in a curled up position. He is still recovering from birth which is always an intense experience. His head is slightly tilted and turned to one side, his hips are at a 90° angle and his pelvis flexed slightly forwards. His elbows and knees are close together and he is displaying the classic neonate position.

A neonate is trapped by gravity without the necessary strength or muscle control to enable her to use her motor skills in this new environment.

This stage which lasts about 6 weeks is called the phylogenetic stage due to the presence of very archaic reflexes called primitive reflexes and it is characterized by a lack of body control. The infant has contact surface but no support surface in order to straighten herself up. Her muscles aren't sufficiently developed for her to lift her head up and her nervous system does not permit muscle coordination, so she can't steady one part of her body to move another. Her movements are global and holokinetic. When one part moves, everything moves.

When she is lying on her back her preferred head position is to one side and she has trouble fixing her gaze, something that will develop very quickly in the coming weeks and will serve as an indicator of the health of the central nervous system. It is not the only indicator, but it is a particularly significant one. Her head is slightly tilted backwards and, when she turns it, her torso makes a hollow arch in the direction of the turn. She moves her arms and legs, but in a global, non-segmented way keeping her torso, head and limbs in an asymmetric position almost all the time.

When she is lying face down a neonate is only able to lift her head in extreme circumstances. For example, if she has difficulty breathing or something blocks her light, in which cases she would be able to turn her head slightly. The hips are open at 90 degrees and the position is clearly flexed. If we see a newborn raising her head when she is lying on her stomach, far from being a positive sign of control, she probably has a neck problem involving increased tone of the extensor muscles in the neck (neck extensor hypertonia) and a concomitant contracture. Infants who suffer a lot of tension in their necks are usually irritable and have difficulty sleeping. They tend to have the worst colics because of the discomfort they are in and the impact of the vagus nerve (which branches from the back of the neck) on the digestive system.

When she is lying face down a newborn is only able to lift her head in extreme circumstances. For example, if she has difficulty breathing or something blocks her light, in which case she would be able to turn her head slightly.

If we see a newborn lifting her head up when she is lying on her stomach, far from being a positive sign of control, she probably has a neck problem.

From a neurological perspective, it is imperative she spends as much time as possible in skin-to-skin contact with her mother at this early stage. The most essential stimuli for her neurological and emotional development are being touched and carried around with skin contact.

The reptile stage: from 7 weeks to 6 months

After about 6 weeks adapting to the new environment, the nervous system can develop new skills. Initially it is able to activate muscles in a coordinated way to stabilize a body area. This means the infant can straighten its head a little and make more segmental movements without the rest of its body "wobbling".

During what could be called the reptilian stage, the infant's movements are slow, and she still cannot explore her surroundings. What she will develop first and foremost is the possibility of straightening up against gravity, using her arms and hands for support. This is a key stage and one in which she must spend long periods on her stomach whilst awake and supervised and receiving stimulation from her parents or carers. Some theories erroneously recommend infants should only lie on their backs because they cannot roll over on their own. This is a misguided view. The question is: if an infant is incapable of rolling over onto her back from her tummy, does this mean she should always be left on her tummy? Does this mean therefore, that if she is incapable of climbing into her mother's arms on her own, she should never be picked up?

An infant will stay in the same position you leave her in because she is maturing but that doesn't mean she can't be left in other positions. There is clear evidence (and evidence is far more than just a theory) that infants who spend more time on their tummies whilst awake and supervised, develop much better than infants who always lie on their backs. Not to mention the high proportion of flattened heads we find in infants who spend their first months on their backs. It is true that you should not make infants sit up or walk until they are ready to do so by themselves, but we are talking about a stage where the baby can move by herself and it is better she follows her own path to sitting up and walking. However, in early life she needs to mature whilst lying on her back, her stomach and whilst being carried or held.

Some theories erroneously recommend infants should only lie on their backs because they cannot roll over on their own. This is a misguided view.

During this period certain fundamental aspects of the brainstem mature, such as the ability to straighten the head, to move the eyes and to lift parts of the body using the strength of the diaphragm and torso. On a different level, both thermoregulation and bonding with adults continue to evolve. The primitive reflexes of survival and neurological programming are still present, but

little by little they will be integrated in a process which will «silence» them, although they will still be present «inside», helping the nervous system with its enhanced functions in the future.

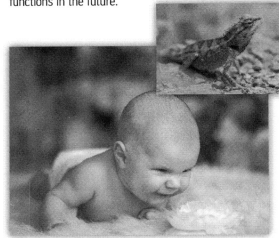

Sophia, who is 5 and a half months old is mastering the prone position and is almost able to prop herself up fully on her extended elbows which is the six-month stage. We see her feet «flying» in postural behavior known as the «swimmer» or «sky-diver» whereby she supports herself with her belly as the only point of contact.

There is clear evidence that infants who spend more time lying on their tummies whilst awake and supervised, develop much better than infants who always lie on their backs.

At 8 weeks visual fixation should make it possible for her to keep her gaze steady for about 3 seconds if you put your face up close to her or show her an interesting object close-up.

When she is on her back, she can start to lift her legs up and turn her head more easily without moving her body quite so much. You can see her body and head are closer to the midline and she is much more symmetrical than before.

Sometimes we will find her staring at something in a position which is typical of this stage: the fencer position. In the fencer's position the head is turned to the side, drawn by the sight of something interesting. The arm on that same side is stretched out while the arm on the opposite side is flexed. She should adopt this position sometimes on one side and sometimes on the other.

When she is on her tummy, she can hold her head by

propping herself up on her forearms and throwing her weight onto the lower half of her thorax. Her elbows are slightly further back than her shoulders, but the position allows her to look up and check out what is in front of her. It is absolutely essential for their development that infants spend time on their tummies whilst they are awake and supervised. The benefits have also been observed in children with Down syndrome, reducing their developmental delay.

Spending time on their tummies whilst they are awake and supervised is absolutely essential for development.

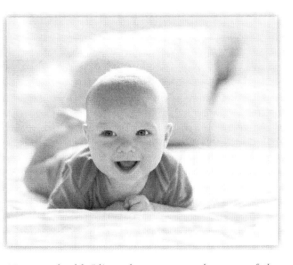

Nine week old Oliver demonstrates the start of the straightening process, in a position where his elbows are slightly behind compared to his shoulders. His eyes are also capable of fixation which is a sign of good cognitive development.

The 12 week stage is an important milestone in an infant's motor and sensory development. When she is on her back, she can keep her legs bent at an angle of 90 degrees to the hip and also raise her arms off the ground slightly which will enable her to try to reach objects later on. This ability to lift her limbs off the floor is only possible if the diaphragm and the muscles of the abdomen can stabilize the center of the body. Hypotonic infants have difficulty lifting their legs off the floor but so too

do hypertonic infants who have tension in their necks or lower backs. The former's legs are stretched and relaxed, whilst the latter's are stretched but tense; nonetheless, babies must be able to gradually raise their legs and, little by little, keep them elevated for longer and longer.

Twelve week old William demonstrates his ability to keep his legs in hip and knee flexion, touching his thighs with his hands. He will gradually be able to touch his knees, shins and feet, the latter around 6 months.

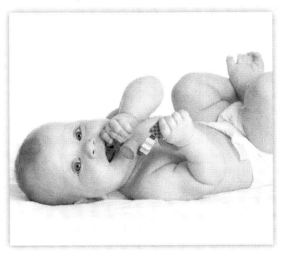

George, 12 weeks old, shows his ability to keep the legs in hip flexion and knee flexion, being able to touch the thighs with his hands. You can progressively touch your knees, shins and feet. The latter around 6 months.

Hypertonic infants have difficulty lifting their legs off the floor but so too do hypertonic infants who have tension in their necks or lower backs.

Around the 3-month mark, a baby will begin to bring her hands together. This is a key moment in the communication between the two cerebral hemispheres. At 4 months she may try to reach an object that is by her side. At 5 months she is able to reach for an object on the midline with both hands. It is important to give her objects at her sides so that she has to turn her head, move her eyes and stretch her arms out to the sides. This will develop her oculomotricity, spinal control and spatial perception.

It is important to give her objects at her sides so that she has to turn her head, move her eyes and stretch her arms out to the sides.

When she is lying on her tummy, she can lift her head and chest for the very first time, supporting her weight with her arms. From here she can move her head from side to side and explore the world. This is the first time her eyes can move independently of her head and it is a momentous occasion.

For the first time her eyes can move independently of her head as she explores the world and it is a momentous occasion.

Unfortunately, not all infants achieve these motor milestones at this stage. Infants who have spent too much time on their backs and very little on their tummies are not able to straighten up or do so inappropriately with their arms in the wrong position. Infants with neck problems that do not receive treatment from specialized physiotherapists suffer discomfort and their stages of development are hampered too. These «delays» in motor development often go unnoticed and become more significant later on. In other cases they are a missed opportunity to recognize that there is something wrong with the child and to remedy it.

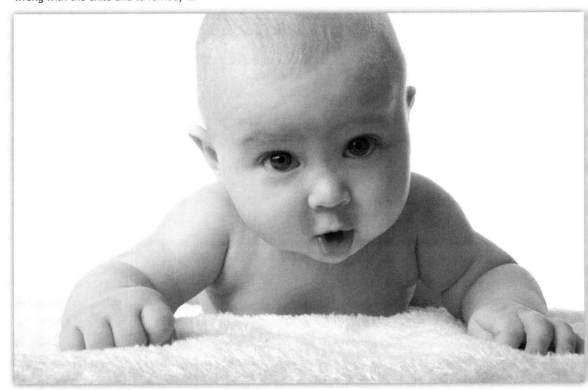

At 12 weeks Ethan is able to support himself on his forearms and remain upright and curious. From here he can turn his head or move his eyes to look to the sides. He is safe and steady and the weight of his head doesn't cause him to lose his balance because he is fully stabilized. Many 12-week old infants fall onto their side from this position due to a lack of control over their arms and end up lying on their backs again or protesting.

Gradually, between 3 and 6 months they are able to raise their legs higher and reach htheir knees and feet with their hands, until, at 6 months shthey can lift them to htheir mouth.

After 5 months their favorite position is no longer lying on their backs. They discover the wonder of rolling over, playing and lying on their side. By 6 months they are able to turn over by themselves, if they have had sufficient «tummy time» on the floor and so long as there are no joint or muscular dysfunctions in the lumbar spine or the hips that impede coordinated, functional movements. They must also have sufficient muscle tone. Infants that have too much tone due to stiffness in their backs often roll over prematurely, but they do it in a strange way. These infants arch themselves from head to foot in order to propel themselves into a roll. The correct way to do it is to flip from a raised leg position in an easier and more harmonious way.

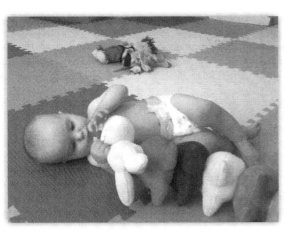

At 5 months Jacob is able to roll over onto his side and stay there as he plays. This allows him to spend some time concentrating on playing.

Infants that have too much tone due to stiffness in their backs often learn to roll over ahead of time, but they do it in a strange way.

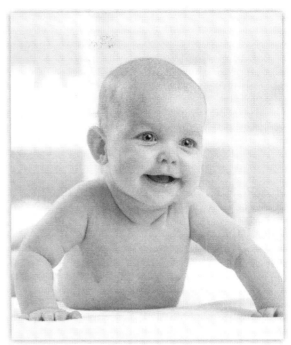

Logan demonstrates the position typical of the 6-month mark as he straightens himself up on extended forearms. His ability to fix his gaze reflects his maturity. It won't be long before he tries to go in search of whatever object has caught his attention, by creeping or crawling.

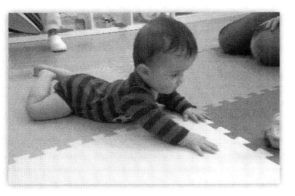

Isabella demonstrates a skill which is typical at 4 and a half months: contralateral support. We see how she rests her weight on her left forearm and the inner part of her right knee which is slightly flexed, in order to stretch her right hand out. This skill is essential for her to be able to crawl later on as it requires contralateral limb movements. Many babies with mild lower back disorders are unable to change the position of their hips each time they choose to reach for a toy with one hand or the other.

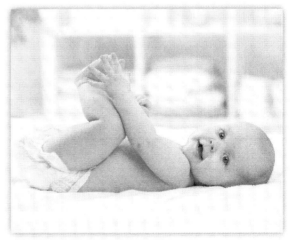

Infants start to grab their feet at around 6 months, and it is a wonderful phase. By doing so, Logan is getting to know himself and stimulating development of the sensory areas which represent his hands and feet in his brain. He only needs to do one more thing to make it perfect... get them into his mouth!

During this stage it is important that they spend time on their stomachs with stimulation and supervision so that they develop strength in their arms and torso. Give them safe objects to reach out for and play with. If they lack a little strength in their arms, help them to straighten their torso whilst lying on their stomachs. Keep touching them and carrying them around. Infants that are carried develop better than infants who are pushed in strollers. If they don't hit the milestones for this stage give or take a week or two, I would recommend you speak to your pediatrician and ask a specialist physiotherapist to evaluate their development.

The mammalian stage: from six to 9 months

After sixth months an infant's brain begins to mature in key areas of her social and emotional being. Her limbic brain takes a step towards maturity and her face is noticeably better at expressing emotions. She shows how she feels through an amazing range of mimicry. At the same time, she sees herself as part of the group and demands to be recognized as such. This is typical of many mammals.

In terms of posture and motor skills, once her elbows are fully extended, she can support herself by spreading her hands and has the ability to flex her hips, she is just one step away from crawling on all fours. The early stages of being on all fours can be seen in her attempts to get her stomach off the ground. At first infants often propel themselves backwards until they gain strength in their arms and control over their hips.

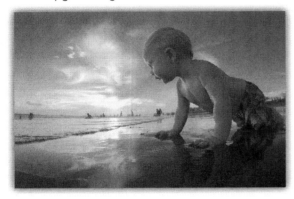 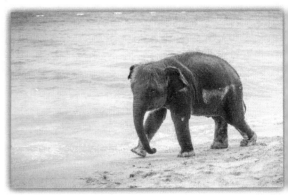

Liam is crawling along the beach like a four-legged animal. He is able to move around, explore his surroundings and enjoy new experiences. For a few moments he can be independent, although he will always maintain visual contact with his Mom to make sure he can return to his safe place at any given time. It's exciting exploring the world isn't it?

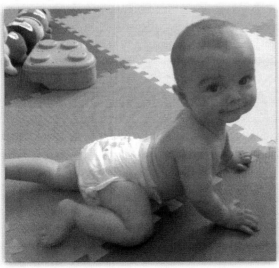

Jacob, who is almost 7 months old, looks over the moon. He has mastered the floor and can move around it. All he needs to do now is find a way of exploring the world more quickly and one that allows him to reach a higher level in the future. Could crawling be the answer?

At 7 months an infant must be able to support her weight on extended arms and bend one leg. This position indicates the infant's ability to get on all fours and it is something she begins to practice with dogged determination. Infants who experienced difficulties alternating leg flexions when they were on their stomachs at the 4 and a half months milestone will find it difficult to bend their hip now. This will probably lead them to skip the quadruped position and proceed almost directly to standing. If an infant had difficulty with only one of their hips because of tension in their lower back, we will see asymmetrical crawling with one leg in the correct position and the other twisted inwards or outwards. This situation requires attention and guidance from a pediatric physiotherapist to help her develop more graceful movements at home.

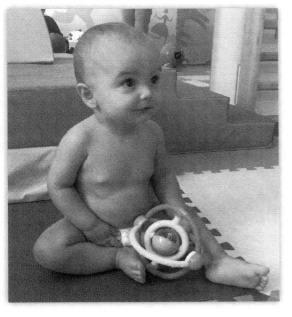

At 8 months, Jacob can sit upright without any support and with a totally straight back which, by the way, looks very elegant. A common error is to sit infants up prematurely, at a time when they aren't able to get into, or out of, that position on their own. The sitting position where babies are supported by a throw or support pillow and left with a toy in their hands, is a prison for them and can lead to sensory and motor development delays. You only need to look at the backs of children who are made to sit upright ahead of time to see that they are curved and slouched. A baby who sits up on his own a bit later on has a straight back which is capable of steadying his shoulders should he want to look for something above head level.

A common error is to sit infants up prematurely, at a time when they aren't able to get into or out of that position on their own.

The 9-month milestone is a particularly important one as it is when we develop many of the characteristics so typical of our species. This is when infants acquire the pincer grip; the ability to sit up from lying down without any help or support; the urge to be upright and their first words. These four motor milestones are a fundamental step in neurodevelopment and are essentially human milestones. Isn't it strange that pregnancy lasts 9 months and then it takes us another 9 months to acquire these very human abilities?

The 9-month milestone is a particularly important one as it is when we develop many of the characteristics so typical of our species.

At 9 months, attempts at standing up coexist with crawling. Crawling is a feature that shapes the motor and neurological development of the human being, and has become a source of controversy amongst those who think it is essential and those who do not consider it to be important, in view of the fact that children function more or less normally later. It must be added here that everything nature provides in terms of motor and sensory development is important, regardless of whether we fully understand why. There are obvious benefits to crawling: it awakens sensitivity in the hands, integrating the extension reflexes; allows contralateral coordination between arms and legs in preparation for walking in the future; allows the baby to explore the environment; allows spatial vision and orientation to develop; allows the infant to leave her mother's side and have a taste of independence before returning to her, and maybe other areas we don't know about. After millions of years of evolution, everything nature does is for a reason.

There are obvious benefits to crawling. It shapes the neuromotor development of the human being.

Even more important than the fact that an infant doesn't crawl is to know why she doesn't. What happened to prevent her from developing that control over her body? The most frequent causes are either hypotonia in children who have some kind of developmental disorder or who lacked stimulation and movement, or hypertonic extension of the legs in infants who suffered neck problems following a difficult birth and couldn't be assessed or treated by specialist PIMT physiotherapists.

It would be a different matter altogether to suggest that the absence of crawling causes obvious developmental difficulties. This is far from the case. There are infants who start crawling later on, even after they have learned to walk and they are still able to integrate the benefits of doing this. This why it is advisable for parents to join in any games and activities on the floor with their children throughout their childhood.

For experts in development, crawling is a more human stage than creeping. It is possible that creeping may have been present before the arms could be extended forwards and there was hip flexion in the prone position. In any case, both creeping and crawling enable the baby to get to know her environment, discover new worlds, new things to touch and suck, new places that are at different heights and that she is determined to reach. At the same time, all this exploring takes a baby away from her mother which causes separation anxiety. With separation comes the comforting possibility of returning to the safe arms of mom. This separation and return also programs the child's inner sense of security. It is not a good thing to stop infants from experiencing even the slightest separation anxiety as it prevents them from developing their own resources in terms of self-sufficiency and trust in the world. As Boris Cyrulnik says: «When we are not afraid of our environment, we are no longer surrounded by our family... we are imprisoned by it!»

Even more important than the fact that an infant doesn't crawl is to know why she doesn't. What happened to prevent her developing that control over her body?

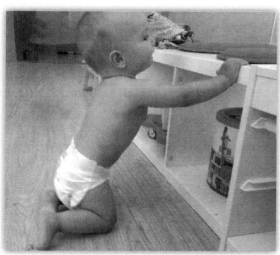 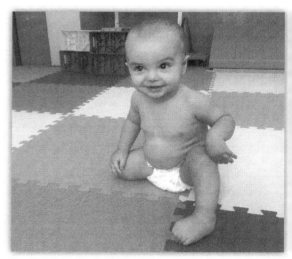

Jacob, who is 10 months old shows us that he is just one step away from standing up, if he hasn't done so already. He is in the tripod position where one foot is planted on the floor and the opposite knee is resting on the ground.

The primate stage: from 11 to 17 months

12-month-old Sophia taking her first steps in the swimming pool. She is amazed by the feeling of her feet on the floor and the cool water on her legs. This is an amazing experience for her as she feels how she is able to move. However, her legs are very bent, as are her upper limbs, a reminder of our ancestors. She waddles from side to side and her back is still not fully unfurled which is why she doesn't yet have lumbar curvature or lordosis which is indicative of the maximum upright posture in humans

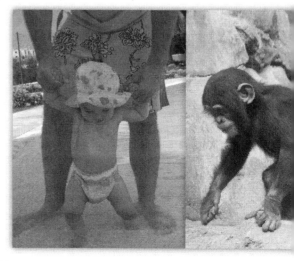

As discussed earlier, the distinction between the amphibian, reptile, mammal or primate stages is purely didactic and non-linear. Moreover, the stages of development actually overlap. For example, the pincer grip is a feature close to primates, but it only starts around the 9 month mark; the emotional aspects and group relations which we associate with the mammalian stage, continue to develop throughout life. However it is important to understand that we are the product of millions of years of evolution with nature finding the best path for us as individuals and for our species. So we can help our baby live through each stage of their development safe in the knowledge that it is serving their neurological and psychological maturation process.

After launching into conquering what is above floor level around the 9-month mark, an infant slowly starts to explore this space in a new way, vertically. Her first attempts at walking are pretty unsteady. Once she has managed to stand up with the help of her arms, she is only capable of walking sideways holding on to the surface that helped her to get upright. It is common to see an infant circle an entire coffee table in front of the sofa without letting go. This is her first attempt at walking, and it is essential for developing certain aspects of coordination between arm and leg movements.

Her parents can help her to walk sideways in both directions by encouraging her (with toys, keys, and nowadays, mobile phones). This stage of walking before she starts walking «independently» should be developed slowly. Speeding processes up -walking too soon for example- means skipping stages that nature needs to mature the nervous system and to improve coordination and balance. It is not advisable to use a baby-walker or to hold the child's hands so they can walk in open spaces, before they have walked sideways. An infant shouldn't do anything she hasn't yet been able to do by herself if all she needs to achieve it are the right resources, i.e. a little time and some stimulation. This applies to sitting up and walking as there are many experiences our baby can have with us that she would not manage on his own that are just as wonderful, such as being upside down, being carried, dancing or playing in our arms.

Once she has mastered walking sideways, the child must move on to walking "between islands" where she will leave one surface and pass on to another a certain distance away, for example, switching the support of one chair for another. This is how she gains confidence and coordination.

The next step is walking independently, only this time the child won't be able to stop. She toddles from Mom to Dad without being able to stop on the way, hoping to make it to her destination and fall into her parent's arms. It is a cute stage, but she walks unsteadily. Only later, around 15 months, will she develop the ability to walk and stop; she will be able to stop, bend down, pick something up off the floor and then stand up

> Speeding processes up -walking too soon for example- means skipping stages that nature needs to mature the nervous system.

and continue walking. Statistically it is often considered normal for a child to start walking before the age of 18 months. However, the reality is that children who start walking after they are 16 months old often have other developmental immaturity issues. It is important to check their development by carrying out a specific physiotherapy examination using tests or objective scales of development to verify, not only their gross motor control (gait), but other aspects of their development: fine motor skills, language or autonomy.

As she starts to stretch her legs and develop a lumbar curve, it could be said she has reached the upright stage of human motor development. From here on the bones of her legs, femurs and tibias will begin to change shape slightly and this will continue gradually until she is 7 or 8 years old. If this rotation does not develop correctly, especially in the case of children who did not crawl or who crawled asymmetrically, or sat in the W position, they will end up pigeon toed or with flatter feet and prone to tripping up more frequently. This is easy to fix with the help of a physiotherapist who specializes in development.

At 14 months Jacob is able to do a small «squat». It is a clear sign of balance control. Not only can he walk, but he also controls his center of gravity to get up and down off the floor without help.

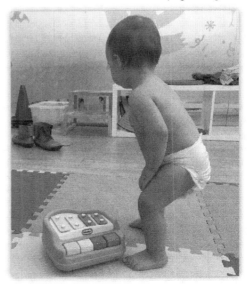

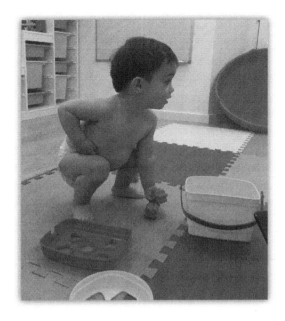

At 15 months, Isabella has mastered different heights. She is stable and this enables her to stop and handle objects without having to return to the floor.

It is important to allow children more time in open spaces, to give them the opportunity to experience movement in different ways and come into contact with nature as much as possible. All of these things further enhance a child's motor skills.

The human stage. From 18 months to 7 years... 70 years... or the rest of our lives

Without doubt this is the longest stage. In fact, it could be said it lasts a lifetime. It is the stage of maximum development of purely human qualities. Of course, there is improvement of balance, coordination, gross and fine motor skills but what truly sets this stage apart is the development of the skills unique to humans: language, math, literacy and abstract thinking.

Two year olds are good at walking, although stairs can be a bit tricky. They simply enjoy moving, running and climbing independently. The best part is jumping off the bottom step.

By two and half they should be able to put some of their clothes on. Sometimes we just don't know what they are capable of until we give them the chance. At this age they can toss a ball to you.

At three they should be able to alternate their feet easily when climbing stairs; they really enjoy riding a tricycle and can control speed. They can also run as if they were jumping or riding a horse and they should be able to jump forwards. In terms of clothes, they can put their pants, socks and shoes on, although fastening buttons can still prove tricky.

At this age they can more or less stay dry during the day and are practicing controlling the need to urinate at the same time they are developing the habit of going to the bathroom.

What truly sets this stage apart is the development of the skills unique to humans: language, math, literacy and abstract thinking.

When they are four years old they can go downstairs one step at a time. This is where we can pick up on children with inadequate balance, the ones who feel insecure on the stairs and always require some support. It is a sign of inadequate programming of balance and movement control. They can fasten large buttons, feed themselves (with the exception of using a knife) and eat and talk at the same time. Most are responsible enough to wash their hands and face, or brush their teeth.

*In the following pages:
The summary table shows the different stages of development and their characteristics, as well as the kind of support that can be provided. It is merely an overview of what is in fact a very detailed process.*

Stage	Characteristics	Parental involvement
0-6 weeks newborn	**Prone position:** The infant is in a «fetal tuck» position. She has a hard time controlling her head and can hardly lift it up. **Supine position:** She lacks control and makes unintentional movements; primitive reflexes. She seems unsteady and sways to the sides when she moves.	Start to put her in the prone position for 5 minutes, 5 times a day when she is awake and supervised. Provide plenty of skin-to-skin contact and carrying. Touch her hands, face and around her mouth a lot. Put your face close to her so that she follows you with her gaze.
7 weeks to 6 months	**Prone position:** She gradually straightens out until she can stretch her arms out with her hands open. **Supine position:** She gradually lifts her legs up until she can grab her feet and put them into her mouth. From 4 months onwards she is able to grasp objects with her hands. First on one side and then with both hands on her midline. At 5 months she can roll on to her side to play. **Language:** At 6 months there is considerable mimicry. She wants to be part of the group and blows raspberries.	Leave her in the prone position for longer periods. Provide plenty of skin-to-skin contact and carrying. Put your face close to her so that she follows you with her gaze. Offer her objects first at the side and then gradually, more in the middle. Talk to her a lot. Tell her everything that's happening around her using your normal language and vibrant tone.
6-10 months	**Prone position:** She starts to lift her bottom up until she gets on all fours. She sometimes seems to crawl backwards when she pushes with her arms. She will gradually progress from this position to sitting up on her own. She has a taste for exploring her surroundings. At 9 months she stands up for the first time relying on objects or her parents for support. **Prone position:** She rolls over much faster so she can go explore her surroundings. Sometimes she will lie on her back so she can suck things she finds interesting. **Social:** She bangs her toys. **Language:** She combines syllables and may even say her first words.	Provide a safe environment so she can move around and explore freely. Continue with skin-to-skin contact and massages too. Play with her on the floor. Continue to talk to her a lot and tell her everything that is going on. At the start of this stage, use stimuli to help her roll to both sides. Gradually help her to get onto all fours if she finds it difficult.
11-17 months	**Prone position:** At the beginning she crawls at top speed. It's her best way of getting around, although she increasingly fancies walking so she can reach everything above her. **Standing up:** First she learns to walk sideways. Then she walks between support areas. Later on, she walks around freely without being able to stop. Finally, she is able to walk around freely, stop, bend down to pick an object up from the floor, stand up again and continue on her way. **Language:** The number of words she uses increases. She can identify objects and point to them or name them with sounds. She says «Mom-Dad».	Help her go through all the stages of walking. Don't use a baby-walker. Let her learn to walk by holding on to things. Gradually help her to walk more. Allow her to go barefoot at home. At most put socks on her but leave her feet free. Continue to play on the floor with her. Continue crawling. Allow her to be in contact with nature.

Stage	Characteristics	Parental involvement
18 months to 7 years	**Fine motor skills:** Between 2 and 4 she becomes able to build towers using more and more bricks. At 3 she can draw a vertical line. At 4 she can draw a circle. At 5 she can draw a child made up of at least 3 parts. At 6 she can draw a child with 6 parts and copy a square. **Gross motor skills:** At 2 she enjoys moving, running or climbing. At 3 she can walk up and downstairs and jump forwards. At 4 she can balance on one foot for 2 seconds. At 5 she can balance on one foot for 5 seconds. At 6 she can walk along a line. **Language:** At 2 she can combine words and is able to point to and recognize several animals. At 3 she can name 6 parts of her body and some friends. At 4 she can name some colors and is able to explain what an object is used for. At 5 she can define at least 5 words. At 6 she is able to say opposites. **Social-independence:** At 2 she can put some of her clothes on and throw a ball to another person. At 3 she is able to wash and dry her hands. At 4 she gets dressed unaided. By 5 she is completely independent.	Allow her to be on the floor. There are some great craft books for all ages. Get into the habit of making things at home. Play with her time and again. Don't leave her in front of a Tablet or TV indefinitely. Set a time limit from the very first day and make sure it is always met. Provide lots of contact with nature. Encourage her and allow her to become independent. Little by little encourage her to help around the house. First with her own things and then with other people's. It's a good idea to always get her to leave her shoes together when she takes them off. Never, ever do it for her. Give her independence in even the simplest things. Gradually she will be able to clear her plate and glass up from the table or pick up her clothes... Don't do anything for her that she can do for herself (except of course, in an emergency or if there are difficulties...). Sport is great but a variety of games – like the games and activities organized at summer camp– promote a greater variety of skills. Play with her time and time again.

At five years old children know how to dodge obstacles; they can jump very well and even do long jumps with two feet; they can climb safely; skip rope and do acrobatic movements. Their laterality should be well established by now: it started to develop some time ago but will still require a few more years to fully mature. At this age they like to help with housework, although this should be introduced as part of normal everyday life. They play with toy blocks and like to build houses or dens with cardboard, towels or anything else they find. They eat independently, even using a knife. They can dress themselves very well, although they still ask for more help than they really need.

By the time they are six all their skills have clearly been refined, but children face profound changes on very different levels, physically, mentally and emotionally. Between the ages of six and seven we find the following changes, amongst many others:

• The cerebellum begins to take clear responsibility for controlling posture and movements which become smoother.

• They lose their baby teeth.

• The facial sinuses develop more clearly and the face takes on the features it will have in the future.

• Abstract thinking appears. The child begins to develop the ability to understand generalizations and, in terms of language, double-entendres.

• Literacy can be fully achieved.

• The leg bones are about to finish maturing into what will be the future adult bone.

From here on they never stop changing and evolving. The brain shows a fascinating ability to adapt throughout life. Children continue to learn from their experiences, perfecting their abilities and building and improving their relationships with others.

SUMMARY

The human being replicates the evolution of species up to 3 times. The first time over millions of years, the second for 9 months in the maternal womb and the third time during its first year of life when the stages we go through are reminiscent of phylogenetic evolution, allowing the brain to develop certain skills.

The stage up to 6 weeks of life, (known as the phylogenetic stage due to the presence of very archaic reflexes called primitive reflexes), is defined by a lack of control over the body. The infant's musculature is not developed enough for her to lift her head and her nervous system does not allow muscle coordination, so she can't steady one part of her body to move another. Her movements are global, holokinetic. When one part moves, everything else moves too.

During what could be called the reptilian stage, the infant's movements are slow, and she still cannot explore her surroundings. What she will develop first and foremost is the possibility of straightening up against gravity, using her arms and hands for support. Whilst lying on her back a, baby will start to lift her arms and have control over them until at 6 months she is able to pick objects up with two hands with a certain amount of accuracy. She can also put her feet into her mouth.

From the sixth month mark, an infant's brain begins to mature in important areas of her social and emotional being. Her limbic brain takes a step towards maturity and her face is noticeably better at expressing emotions.

At 9 months, attempts at standing up coexist with crawling. Crawling is a feature that shapes the neuromotor development of the human being and has become a source of controversy amongst those who think it is essential and those who do not consider it to be important, in view of the fact that children function more or less normally later on. Actually, crawling is important for the development of many aspects of the nervous system, but it does not shape an individual's life.

After launching into conquering what is above floor level around the 9 month mark, an infant slowly starts to explore this space in a new way, vertically. Her first attempts at walking are pretty unsteady. Once she has managed to stand up with the help of her arms, she is only capable of walking sideways holding on to the surface that helped her get upright.

What can you do?
HELPFUL PRACTICAL ADVICE

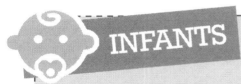

INFANTS

- Enjoy each stage of your baby. Every moment is unique and will only come around once. I'm sure you've heard it all before but, sometimes, even when we know it to be true we don't change our ways. Spend time with her as there really is no better way of spending your time. Every human life is a miracle, but the early stages of life are even more beautiful.

- Don't think about what's coming next. We say things like; «Let's see when she's able to hold her head up» without valuing the importance of the here and now; or «Let's see when she starts to crawl» without appreciating the fact that she is learning to control her head; «Let's see when she starts to walk?» we say, without enjoying crawling with her. The difficulty we have living entirely in the present not only affects our lives but we run the risk of transferring it to our children's lives too as we miss precious moments with them.

- Try to fully understand what your baby needs at each stage in order to help her, to experience it with her, to encourage her if she has any difficulty. Try to ensure she does everything on each side: head position, rolling over, reaching for objects, etc.

- If you find that your baby is slow in acquiring the motor and postural patterns she should have at her age, try touching her and carrying her more and providing more tummy time (when she is awake and supervised). These three things will help to stimulate her development.

- When she is a few months old if you find that her legs are always stretched and tense, try to help her into bending positions. If she keeps complaining seek help from a good developmental physiotherapist who specializes in PIMT. He will fully understand the situation and the possible causes.

- In the same way that it is important for a pediatrician to examine your baby regularly a pediatric physiotherapist should assess her neurological development at key times during her first year of life. Ideally, checkups on how your baby is acquiring all of her skills should be carried out at 8 weeks, 3 months, 4.5 months, 6 months, 9 months and 12 months. Pediatric physiotherapists who specialize in child development use tests and target ranges to determine if your baby is meeting the expected developmental milestones for her age. They can guide you in terms of stimulation, carrying methods and games.

OLDER CHILDREN

- If your child is no longer a baby, try to get her to spend time playing on the floor too. Every time she is on the floor, she inevitably adopts positions associated with the history of development. This way she can complete any stages she may have missed. When she is on the floor you will see her on her stomach, crawling and changing position from sitting to all fours. Parents sometimes find it hard to let their children play on the floor, but it is simply a question of understanding its importance and adapting the space by laying a good area rug.

- If you were unable to accompany your child in her early stages of development because you weren't aware of the need for it or because of other difficulties in her early years (illnesses, hospitalizations, etc.), don't panic, everything can be programmed later. The brain is an amazing thing and it can sometimes find alternative ways to build or repair itself. If you consider your child's difficulties correspond to less than optimal motor, sensory or postural development in the early years of her life, you can ask a developmental physiotherapist who specializes in PIMT for an overall assessment of the current situation and advice as to how to reprogram her nervous system. Never give up hope – there is always a way to help your child progress!

BIBLIOGRAPHY

Regarding how an assessment of an infant's development can predict their IQ and language skills at the age of 5-6:

Peyre H, Charkaluk ML, Forhan A, Heude B, Ramus F; EDEN Mother-Child Cohort Study Group. Do developmental milestones at 4, 8, 12 and 24 months predict IQ at 5-6 years old? Results of the EDEN Mother-Child Cohort. Eur J Paediatr Neurol.2017 Mar;21(2):272-9.

Regarding the importance of skin-to-skin contact:

Kristoffersen L, Støen R, Rygh H, Sognnæs M, Follestad T, Mohn HS, et al. Early skin-to-skin contact or incubator for very preterm infants: study protocol for a randomized controlled trial. Trials. 2016 Dec 12;17(1):593.

Regarding the importance of tummy time:

Wentz EE. Importance of Initiating a «Tummy Time» Intervention Early in Infants With Down Syndrome. Pediatr Phys Ther. 2017 Jan;29(1):68-75.

Zachry AH, Nolan VG, Hand SB, Klemm SA. Infant Positioning, Baby Gear Use, and Cranial Asymmetry. Matern Child Health J. 2017 Jul 19.

Regarding the importance of emotional development in children:

Cyrulnik B. De cuerpo y alma. Neuronas y afectos: la conquista del bienestar. Editorial Gedisa; 2007.

Regarding the optimal development of infants based on in-depth knowledge:

Vojta V, Schweizer E. El descubrimiento de la motricidad ideal. Ediciones Morata; 2011.

Regarding the benefits of crawling:

McEwan MH, Dihoff RE, Brosvic GM. *Early infant crawling experience is reflected in later motor skill development. Percept Mot Skills. 1991 Feb;72(1):75-9.*

Regarding development from birth to age 3

Gross D. *Infancy. Development from Birth to Age 3. 2nd ed. Allyn & Bacon; 2011.*

Regarding the stages of development on the Alberta Infant Motor Scale:

Morales-Monforte E, Bagur-Calafat C, Suc-Lerin N, Fornaguera-Martí M, Cazorla-Sánchez E, Girabent-Farrés M. *The Spanish version of the Alberta Infant Motor Scale: Validity and reliability analysis. Dev Neurorehabil. 2017 Feb;20(2):76-82.*

Piper MC, Darrah J. *Motor Assessment of the Developing Infant. WB Saunders Company; 1994.*

Regarding how physiotherapy can help infants:

Campbell SK. *The Child's Development of Functional Movement. En: Campbell SK, Palisano RJ, Orlin MN. Physical Therapy for Children. 4th ed. Elsevier-Saunders; 2012.*

Håkstad RB, Obstfelder A, Øberg GK. *Let's play! An observational study of primary care physical therapy with preterm infants aged 3-14 months. Infant Behav Dev. 2017 Jan 21;46:115-23.*

Regarding the need for open spaces and movement:

Adolph KE, Franchak JM. *The development of motor behavior. Wiley Interdiscip Rev Cogn Sci. 2017 Jan;8(1-2).*

True L, Pfeiffer KA, Dowda M, Williams HG, Brown WH, O'Neill JR, et al. *Motor competence and characteristics within the preschool environment. J Sci Med Sport. 2017 Aug;20(8):751-5.*

Regarding neurological development and the development of laterality:

Ferré J, Aribau E. *El desarrollo neurofuncional del niño y sus trastornos. Visión, aprendizaje y otras funciones cognitivas. 2 edición. Editoral Lebón; 2006.*

Chapter 5

We see the world with our brain not our eyes

Iñaki Pastor Pons

Vision is possibly the sensory system which has evolved the most. We have lost some senses along the way due to phylogenetic evolutionand there are others which, whilst not technically lost, have at least stopped improving. This is true of the sense of smell which is much more highly developed in other species. In humans it may have a greater impact at an unconscious rather than a conscious level. Did you know that odors are a great marketing tool? A particular odor can make you feel a certain way without you even realizing. Everything in your unconscious mind affects the most primitive part of the brain which is why smell is a key sense in the first weeks of life when everything archaic is particularly active.

Vision works the opposite way round to other senses; in humans it is barely developed at birth but it evolves over time into a particularly relevant one. In fact, a whole host of vision-based technologies have been developed even ones that create non-existent worlds of virtual reality which can be accessed through vision.

Your visual skills may be a true reflection of how your nervous system is programmed and they rely on the development of other systems such as the vestibular or proprioceptive systems. Without them, vision would just be a super-sense with no internal references or foundations and would cease to be effective.

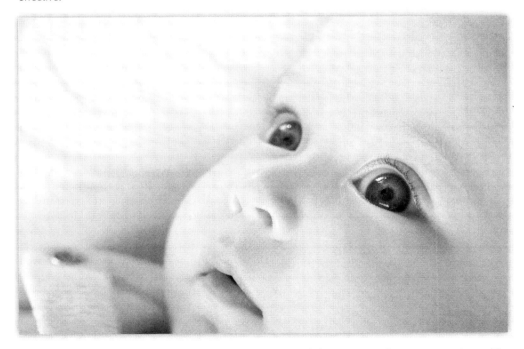

Susan doesn't see the world with her eyes, she sees it with her amazing brain. Vision is not like simply using a camera to take photos or videos, it is a much more complex process.

The way you see is a reflection of who you are. Vision is so important that it sometimes reveals aspects of your behavior too. Often the ability to see close up rather than faraway and vice versa corresponds to a particular way of viewing life; in a concrete or abstract way. Your ability to see the bigger picture in life or focus on one thing can also say a lot about the way you deal with the micro or macro global reality you live in.

Going to school requires the ability to see, listen and do things all at the same time, although visual and auditory aspects become increasingly relevant as students get older, with movement taking something of a back seat. Leaving aside the merits or otherwise of this approach to education, it is important to realize that the state of our vision, our visual skills– which are numerous and not confined just to "sight" (the ability to recognize a character at a distance with each eye)– are vital for success in our school days. By academic success we mean that a child is able to fully develop on a cognitive, physical and emotional level and acquire as much knowledge and skills as he can with a big smile on his face and the feeling that he is flowing, learning and making progress.

How can you ensure that your child's vision develops correctly? How can you tell if his visual system is well equipped for schooling and literacy? Might the visually demanding technological reality we live in full of televisions and tablets, be too much for our children?

Join me now as we delve into the fascinating world of the sensory system.

By academic success we mean that a child is able to fully develop on a cognitive, physical and emotional level and acquire as much knowledge and skills as he can with a big smile on his face and the feeling that he is flowing, learning and making progress.

How vision develops early in life

Compared to our other senses, vision has yet to fully develop at the beginning of life. A newborn's sense of touch, hearing, smell, taste and perception of head movement (vestibular movement) are developed to some extent during prenatal life. Vision on the other hand is very primitive at birth. It is possibly the least stimulated sense of all during pregnancy.

Vision is very primitive at birth.

A newborn can barely see objects 8 to 12 inches in front of him and, although it appears he can recognize his mother's face, the finer details (focal vision) are blurred: his ability to process ambient vision which detects movement, is somewhat more advanced and is associated neurologically with many structures in the brainstem, motor and sensory nerve fibers in the neck, trunk, arms and legs. This is why motor development, posture and vision are so closely related.

The ability to process fine detail (focal vision) develops in several stages, allowing interest and curiosity to stimulate the development of more advanced cognitive and perceptual functions. The infant can now get a sense of the shape and volume of things, not just through his vision, but also through touch, especially with his mouth. Remember, it will be several months before the tactile sensitivity in his hands will be able to provide his brain with spatial recognition, while with his mouth he can get an idea of the shape of the object he is sucking and use spatial recognition later. Despite relying on his mouth to interact with the environment, the activation of groups of neurons in his brain will enable his vision to develop quickly over the space of just a few months.

Motor development, posture and vision are closely related.

One of the characteristics of the neurological immaturity of a newborn is his inability to fix his gaze. If you put your face up close at a distance at which the infant can see, he will scarcely be able to hold his gaze for 1 or 2 seconds.

Gaze fixation is a major neurological milestone which occurs around the 4-week mark; 50% of infants will develop gaze fixation by this stage. By 8 weeks all infants should have developed visual fixation and be able to stare at an object or at their mother's face for more than 3 seconds. At the same time, he can start to piece together an image of the object he is seeing in his mind's eye.

By 8 weeks all infants should have visual fixation and be able to stare at an object or their mother's face for more than 3 seconds.

Until he is one month old and in the earliest stage of his postnatal neurological function, a newborn is only able to fix his gaze if his head is held still. If you support his head your baby is able to fixate even before 4 weeks. This gives an idea of just how important head control is for vision, something that no vision expert should overlook. We will look at this in more detail later on.

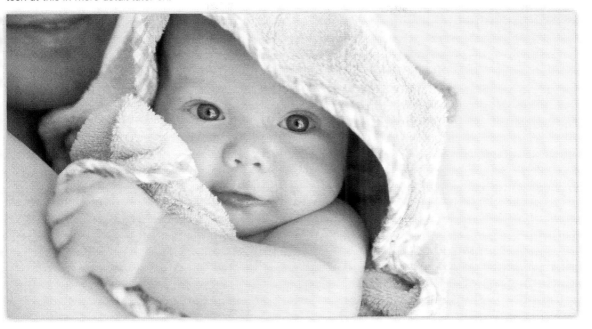

Ryan can focus better when his head is held. It is a sign of just how important the neck and vestibular system are for developing proper vision.

Eye movement or oculomotricity, improves in parallel with the visual system. Although it is a totally separate system from vision, the two systems have such a close relationship that if one of them fails, it is impossible for the other to function correctly. Let me give you an example. Imagine you had a video camera, how could you record a clear, crisp image if the camera wouldn't stop moving? You need to stabilize and control eye movement in order to develop your vision. At the same time vision helps to keep the eyes well focused. This is a good example of significant interaction between two very different systems.

An infant is unable to move his eyes even slightly to the sides without moving his head until he is 3 months old. Up until then it is impossible to distinguish his eye movements from his head movements and the movements of his head from those of his body. In fact, a newborn makes whole body movements because he cannot steady one part of his body to move another.

Apparently, by 6 months many of the fundamental visual skills such as depth perception, color vision or eye movement, have developed. An infant's visual skills and sensory-motor development are interdependent. In fact, postural development and the development of the visual system go hand in hand.

An infant's visual skills and sensory-motor development are interdependent.

How vision works

Were we to compare the eye to a reflex camera or video camera, vision might seem a very simple process. However, the reality is very different. Vision is a highly complex process and, in fact, the area in the brain dedicated to vision is much bigger than the area of all the other special senses put together. A large number of brain structures are required for visual processing as it also entails other sub-processes.

The starting point is light. As light enters the eye through the pupil it activates different receptors in the retina which convert this stimulus into an electrical signal that travels to the brain through the optic nerve. Some of the input from the retina of one eye will remain in the same hemisphere and some will cross over to the optic chiasm in the other hemisphere (one of the places where pathways in the nervous system cross). This way each cerebral hemisphere has a perception of the other's field of vision. This means that your left hemisphere sees everything to the right of what you are seeing.

From an embryological perspective, the retina derives from the same tissue used to form the nervous system or the skin, called the ectoderm. So it could be argued that the retina is actually an extension of the brain. From here the retinal input is redirected in three directions comprising the three functions of the visual system. On the one hand, a certain amount of the nerve cells from the retina reach a center responsible for coordinating eye, head and torso movements in space. This center is called the superior colliculus. This first visual pathway is possibly one of the most primitive and it allows you to move your eyes, head or torso (or all three combined) to track moving objects in your field of vision. We are not made to look out of the corners of our eyes. In less than a minute it causes us fatigue and discomfort so we move our eyes and head to keep our eyes in a comfortable centered position.

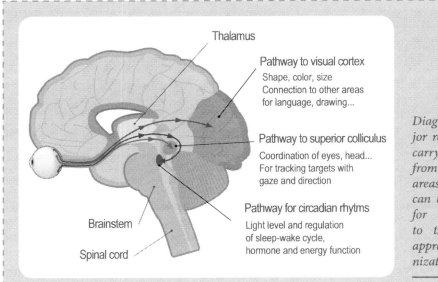

Diagram of the three major retinal pathways which carry the necessary input from the eye to different areas of the brain so that it can be processed and used for enhanced adaptation to the environment and appropriate internal organization.

It could be argued that the retina is actually an extension of the brain.

A significant proportion of the nerve cells that come from the retina reach the thalamus. The thalamus is a hub that receives everything that needs to reach the cortex, ordering and distributing the incoming input so that it can be redirected to the areas of the brain that are most involved. Visual input reaches the thalamus and then continues to the visual area located in the occipital cortex or visual cortex, at the very back of the brain.

Put your hand on the back of your head: that's where the visual cortex is. This is the area of your brain you use to see details of things; their shape, color, depth, etc. So, the fact that you are reading this book means that this part of your brain is receiving signals from your eye and is able to organize and decode them. Just think, if you were reading this book in Korean (for example: 당신이 한국에서 이 책을 읽고 하는 경우: 'if you are reading this book in Korean'), you would see the straight lines, circles and signs clearly, right? Of course you would. But it isn't enough to simply see the details. In order to read, not only must you be able to see, you also have to be able to decode the written signs. This happens in another area of the brain: the temporal cortex. For this to be possible, the input has to pass from the visual area in the occipital cortex to other areas. In many children who have issues with learning or literacy, even though they see the text well, they are unable to move their eyes precisely or have difficulty connecting visual areas with language.

A third of the input from the retina plays a very unique role. Allow me to explain. As you read this book, a certain amount of environmental light is entering your eyes without you even noticing. Perhaps it's daytime and light is coming in through the window. This light stimulates the retina and this unconscious pathway triggers the production of certain hormones linked to your circadian rhythm. Light in the mornings activates stress hormones such as cortisol; whereas, when it gets dark your body secretes melatonin, which promotes sleep and rest. The circadian rhythm's visual role is managed in another area of the brainstem.

This means that, not only do you use your vision to recognize the world around you, but also to coordinate the movements of your head and torso and to regulate your internal clock, as well as many other fascinating tasks. In short, your vision allows you to adapt to your environment. For example, when someone throws you a ball and you catch it on the fly; or when you walk through your house without banging into anything; or when you pick one glass up from a bunch of glasses without knocking the others over; or when you are energized in the morning and sleepy at night. Vision also enables you to develop cognitive abilities such as reading and writing; designing a tool or painting a picture that conveys perspective or your innermost feelings.

This means that, not only do you use your vision to recognize the world around you, but also to coordinate the movements of your head and torso and to regulate your internal clock, as well as many other fascinating tasks.

A global model of vision

As you are beginning to realize, vision is much more marvelous and complex than a mere camera. According Dr. A. M. Skeffington's model of vision, vision is the outcome or result of four sub-processes. Visual processing is distributed via the pathways that reach the visual cortex and involves a large part of the brain. Good development of these four sub-processes will result in visual perception that is not only correct, but also useful, enabling your child to adapt to their environment and develop their full cognitive potential. These sub-processes are:

- Identification process.
- Centering process.
- Recognition process.
- Antigravity process.

Let's take a look at a simplified version of these sub-processes.

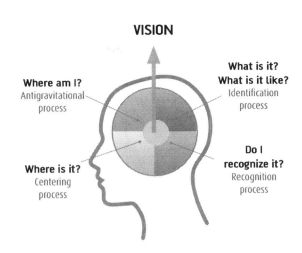

VISION

Where am I?
Antigravitational process

What is it?
What is it like?
Identification process

Where is it?
Centering process

Do I recognize it?
Recognition process

Vision is the outcome or result of four coexisting sub-processes. However, each one is managed in a different area of the brain.

The **antigravity process** attempts to answer the question: where am I? One of the visual system's responsibilities is to provide us with external references that can help us figure out what gravity and the world we live in are like, since the antigravity function is very powerful and absolutely essential. This input is key to maintaining balance. Postural instability increases significantly when our eyes are closed and we are less effective in more challenging situations, for example, standing on one leg. Depending on our neurological programming and how much we practice, we should be able to do it with our eyes open, but try doing it with them closed. Antigravity and postural control does not have a specific area in the cortex instead it is spread out like vestibular input. In contrast, more specialized nuclei do exist in the brainstem (lower part of the brain), such as the vestibular nuclei responsible for maintaining our stability.

The **centering process** attempts to answer the question: where is it? In other words, this process tries to determine where what I see, is, and this input is processed by the parietal cortex where the association areas which receive input from other senses such as the tactile or auditory senses are located. I'm sure you must have experienced a loud, unexpected noise at least once when you were walking down the street. When that happened, did you look directly at the source of the sound? Of course you did. But how did you do it? Somewhere in your brain the auditory input had to be processed to create a spatial (and therefore visual) map to guide the exact eye movement. Vision is used to create maps of space which you can use to orient yourself and find your way. These maps are created with other vestibular, tactile and proprioceptive input. This is why even blind people have activation in areas relating to vision, particularly the areas associated with spatial maps.

The **identification process** attempts to answer the question: what is it? What is it like? The brain tries to define the color, shape, texture, size and aspect of everything we see and this is handled in the visual cortex. Vision is often narrowed down to this part alone. Consequently, establishing visual acuity with one eye and then the other cannot in itself suffice to determine the health of the visual system, as this is only part of the story. The visual system is far more comprehensive and vast in its processing and functions.

The **recognition process** attempts to answer the question: do I know it? Do I recognize it? What do I know about it? Not only is it important to see the detail and features of what I see and locate it in space, but I must quickly associate it with something familiar and be able to identify it. Is it familiar? What is it called? How many times have you seen or thought about something but couldn't remember what it was called? However, you could describe its shape and position in space. This is a key part of facial recognition or language processing and perhaps requires a neurological pathology to identify more clearly that visual recognition has distinct pathways and areas to other visual processes. In the book The man who mistook his wife for a hat, neurologist Oliver Sacks describes the case of a musician who, following an illness, could describe abstract aspects of objects such as their size or shape, but had lost the ability to identify the most familiar of objects, including recognizing his wife's face. What is the point of knowing what something you can see is, if you can't associate it with something familiar or give it a name? This process is managed by the temporal lobe of the cortex, which in turn is home to the areas responsible for hearing and speech. Children with specific reading difficulties may experience problems with this sub-process. They read an exam question, but they do not understand what is being asked of them. They read a series of syllables, but they are not able to sort the sounds out according to what they see.

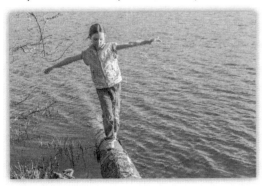

The visual system is of enormous help controlling Scarlett's balance thanks to its antigravity function. It also orients us spatially and, when it is well-developed, it can even calculate distances and times, so we can catch a ball someone throws to us, for example.

Following simultaneous processing of the four sub-processes, a perception of what I see emerges. This suggests that what I see is not input, but output. This can be hard to understand at first but it is the key to helping children with difficulties. Vision is not information input but information output, an emergent process. Vision is the outcome of your brain processing the input from the retinas plus all of its experiences and other perceptions. It may sound paradoxical, but this is the way the brain works, and not just in the case of vision. Hearing, touch and even pain undergo a complex process affected by many different factors, resulting in a perception of the world I live in. This means that there is no pure perception of the outside world. Instead there is rapid processing which takes into account various aspects such as past experience or sensory input from other sensors. At the end of this very rapid processing we have access to a perception of the world.

As Paul Harris would say: «The person incorporates elements of all the senses to build a space world». And this internal space world is never an objective copy of the outside world which is why there are dozens of optical illusions that make us realize how our brain tries to build something coherent from the retinal input. This lesson in biology could equally be applied to philosophy and it would even be a good remedy for extremism or the sterile discussions so many people have about the same issue and whose perception of it is the right one. They will never get anywhere as it is quite possible they were both right from the beginning. This is a good thing to take into account when teaching children about cooperating, not competing. Another person will always have a different, interesting perception of the same reality as you. It would be good to learn to listen to it instead of just writing it off as wrong.

Our space world is never an exact copy of the real world, no matter how sure we think we are.

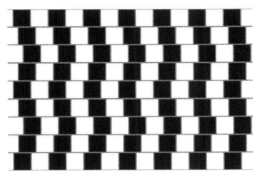

Vision is the outcome of your brain processing the input from the retinas plus all of its experiences and other perceptions.

An optical illusion of crooked lines... or are they straight and parallel? What do you see? Drawings like this can show you to what extent what you see is the mental processing of your own perception. Actually, the lines are absolutely parallel (you can check them with a ruler), but the distribution of the colors makes your brain "interpret" them as crooked.

«The person incorporates elements of all the senses to build a space world». (Paul Harris)

Therefore, you don't see the world with your eyes, but with your brain. This global approach to vision allows you to differentiate the term vision from sight. Both terms are usually confused, but there is a world of difference between them, as discussed by Pilar Vergara in her book, *Tanta inteligencia, tan poco rendimiento (Is your Child Intelligent, but Underachieving?)*. Sight is simply the ability to see something clearly. Vision goes beyond this as it is not just about gathering input from the retina, it also meets the need for what we see to have a meaning and place in the world.

Vision and movement

There are two clearly differentiated systems in the eyes controlled by their own neurological structures. Both systems are independent yet interdependent and they are vision and oculomotricity. The visual system is the one which allows us to build a perception of the world around us, locate it in space and make sense of it (this is a complex process as we saw in the last chapter). This is based on light stimulating the retina and this stimulus being converted into an electric signal.

Likewise, oculomotricity is made up of two parts; on the one hand the muscles that position and mobilize the eyes in the head and on the other; the set of proprioceptive receptors in the extraocular muscles that inform the brain of the position and movement of the eyes. In short, a motor and a sensory part in the same system. We talked briefly about vision earlier and we have already seen that there is a visual pathway to guide you in space. Now, let's look at the muscular function that moves the eyeballs and informs the brain of its position in space.

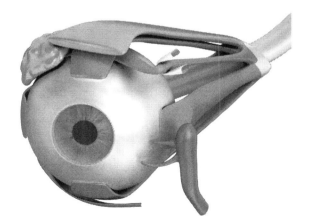

The oculomotor system has six extraocular muscles to position and move the eyes. These muscles are activated voluntarily, for example when we want to look up or to the right, or automatically when we walk or travel by car without getting motion sickness.

Oculomotricity moves and positions the eyes and has three major responsibilities: it ensures the correct location of things in space, secures steady focus and allows depth perception of a given space.

In order to appreciate your environment and locate it correctly in space, you need to know where your eyes are in their sockets and where your eye sockets are in relation to your torso (where your head is). If you don't have the correct information about the position of your eyes, the input they provide about the world, particularly in terms of «where» you are, cannot be used by the brain or will lead to confusion. There are a huge number of proprioceptive receptors in the extraocular muscles which inform the brain about the position and movement of the eyes. If this information is missing or faulty, you will have problems locating objects in space or ensuring there is a safety zone around your body.

Have you ever wondered why people sometimes bump into door frames or against tables that they had clearly seen beforehand? They collide because they miscalculated the distance, and in this case vision wasn't exactly to blame. The same thing happens when we want to pick something up from a table and knock over the glass right next to it by mistake. This is caused by a miscalculation in the location of things in our peripersonal space. Normally, the proprioceptive system is the one in charge of vision and of creating an exact map of our peripersonal space. Many children with learning and attention issues are especially clumsy in their movements or misjudge distances. This is not just about their vision it has to do with a sub-optimal perception of their body too.

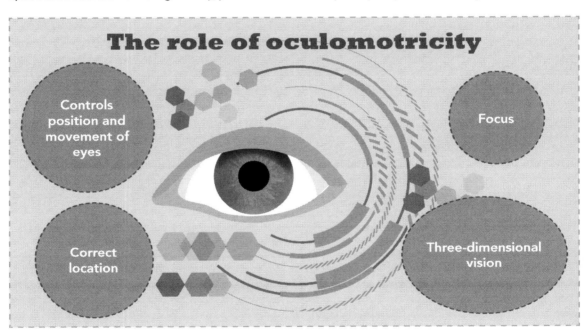

The role of oculomotricity

Controls position and movement of eyes

Focus

Correct location

Three-dimensional vision

To be able to get something clearly in focus with a camera you have to hold it still for a moment, right? What happens if you move or your hand shakes? You will end up with a blurred photo. Therefore it is vital that you are able to fix the position of your eyes to take the information about your surroundings in properly. It might sound simple but, in fact, it is very complex, because we never stop moving. Your head moves back and forth when you walk or rock back and forth, yet your vision doesn't go out of focus, does it? This is thanks to certain components of oculomotricity such as the gaze fixation reflexes. There are three types of fixation reflexes: the vestibulo-ocular, cervico-ocular and optokinetic reflex. These three reflexes are constantly at work making sure that, even if you move, you are still able to see clearly and in detail. However, fixation isn't always perfect in spite of these three reflexes, so the brain has to carry out final post-production tasks on the image, rather like the editing suite of a TV network.

The vestibulo-ocular reflex depends on the vestibular system being healthy and working properly as we saw in the chapter on movement, just as the cervico-ocular reflex depends on the neck being healthy and working properly. Therefore, when someone suffers whiplash in a car, a few days later they start to show signs of visual problems and focus, as well as unsteadiness or dizziness and other aches and pains. This is why many children with developmental problems, a lack of stimulation in their early childhood or neck problems, have visual disorders or difficulties which are noticeable in their posture, reading and writing or when they are asked to copy shapes.

Many children with neck problems have visual difficulties which are noticeable in their posture, reading and writing or when they are asked to copy shapes.

There is another function of oculomotricity for a comprehensive perception of the environment and its depth. The fact that there are two eyes and that each one is in a different position on the face (and in space) means that, although they are both looking at the same object, they don't necessarily see exactly the same perspective of the object. The brain is able to create something marvelous from this small difference between the two images; a three-dimensional vision of reality. This is the most advanced skill of visual perception and it is achieved thanks to the reciprocal position of the eyes, which in turn is secured by the muscles in the eyes and neck.

Without an effective vestibular system and good neck position, vision is like a supersense which lacks internal references and foundations, and loses its effectiveness.

There is a law of phylogenetic and ontogenetic evolution: the last thing to be achieved in evolution is the first thing to be lost. One of the first losses a child with visual difficulties suffers is the loss of stereopsis or three-dimensional vision. Stereopsis can be recovered through effective vision therapy even in people with strabismus, as described by neuroscientist Susan Barry in her fascinating book *Fixing my gaze*.

Vision for sight and balance

Now that we've seen the sub-processes involved in creating vision, let's take a look at some of the other details which are important in order for you to grasp how it

works, understand your child's difficulties and help them in their development.

If you look carefully at this book you will realize that you perceive much more than just the book.

Your peripheral vision can see the room you are in, the furniture or objects around you, part of the floor or ceiling and the corners of the room. This is a perception of your peripheral vision which picks up everything in your field of vision. We are not usually aware of peripheral vision as, normally, we are paying attention to what we are focusing on. In fact, the central part of the retina has the highest density of receptors and barely a few millimeters outside of this we lose half of our visual acuity. Therefore, if we want to see something in detail we have to use our central vision, also known as foveal vision.

However, peripheral vision makes a huge contribution to two of the sub-processes of vision we saw earlier, focusing and antigravity. In other words, peripheral vision has different roles:

- It provides field information about everything around you just like a map or radar.
- It acts as an alarm if something new moves in your field of vision. This triggers a very rapid eye movement to direct your gaze to the object that moved, identify it and, providing it doesn't pose a threat, abandon it to focus on your prime source of interest.
- It provides you with a visual «anchor» for balance, giving you a baseline for what is horizontal and what is vertical in the world around you.
- It enables you to make the necessary space and time calculations in order to cross the road or go down an escalator in a shopping mall.
- It enables you to be good at sport; as you are running someone can throw a ball to you and at the same time you can be aware by merely glancing, where your teammates and opponents are.

Peripheral vision can also be called spatial vision and it is closely involved in the prediction, preparation and control of movement. Hence it is a type of vision that people should train in for sports. But not just for sports either, children with learning and attention issues, who, unfortunately, are prone to clumsiness, frequent falls and difficulties with reading and writing should also be trained. The simultaneous action of peripheral vision and central vision is a great tool for speed reading, because with a single "swipe" of your eyes you can span different words and increase your reading speed exponentially.

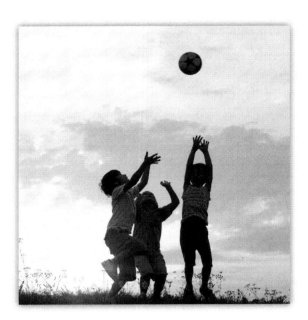

Peripheral vision is very important for sports and physical activity. It allows you to calculate the trajectory of the ball or locate the position of the players. It is also trainable.

«Spatial vision is intimately involved in the prediction, preparation and control of movement».

(Robert Sanet)

Peripheral vision develops at the beginning of life by relating your body to your peripersonal space. Each time an infant moves his arms as he plays with objects, brain connections are being created uniting the tactile with the visual, and likewise the proprioceptive. This process of building spatial perception is very important and will mature even further during his lifetime. His perception of space will be even better if his vestibular programming was optimal, if he was moved, rocked and carried as an infant.

We need to allow the child to build this map of his body in his peripheral visual space. This is why it is important to ensure that babies are not always in the same position in their crib, especially if there is a wall on one side, as the peripheral visual field on one side could develop very differently from the other. It is a good idea to change children's position in class so that they have different peripheral visual experiences.

The dilemma arises when eye patches are prescribed to treat minor strabismus, in an attempt to prevent an eye from becoming "lazy", but at the expense of stunting development of the peripheral field which is so essential for an individual's neurological organization. This treatment is being rendered obsolete by other more innovative procedures, such as occluding one of the lenses of the glasses with a translucent tape. It is worth pointing out here the revolutionary model of therapy for strabismus and amblyopia developed by Spanish optometrist Pilar Vergara in her book *Strabismus and lazy eye*.

It is important to ensure that babies are not always in the same position in their cribs, especially if there is a wall on one side, as the peripheral visual field on one side could develop differently from the other.

Visual skills for school

Now you know that vision is a comprehensive, complex process and not the simple act of recognizing a letter at a distance. Hence, vision professionals must be able to evaluate the full scope of the visual system to check that children can complete the tasks they are faced with at school age. In Spain, literacy programs start at around the age of 5 whilst, in other countries, they are deferred until the age of 6 or even 7. All children should have a full eye exam around the age they start to learn to read and write. If this test is carried out by a «behavioral» optometrist, it will be even more comprehensive and will evaluate other systems of the child's neurological development that affect vision. Ophthalmologists play a crucial role in diagnosing or ruling out diseases that can affect the visual system and it is mandatory they are involved in all cases of strabismus. However, it is essential an optometrist is involved in the case of learning difficulties, problems with processing, reading speed or fatigue. You can learn more about how to find professionals for developmental problems at the end of this book.

When children start to read and write often call it «the wall» because for many it seems like a huge wall. This is when many learning difficulties become apparent. In turn, the difficulties they have overcoming this wall have a bearing on the self-image the child develops of himself and how he compares himself with others; the pressure from parents who do not want their child to be left behind in something so important; and the exhaustion they feel, as the effort is so great for some children that they either shun the task completely or end up worn out and with little to show for their hard work.

The visual system relies on the child's neurological maturity and on the way other more primitive systems develop prior to this.

An understanding of how visual processing works and how it is developed when things are going well, presents us with a concept which should underpin the work carried out by all professionals: the visual system relies on the child's neurological maturity and on the way other more primitive systems develop prior to this. Similarly, vision subsequently becomes the linchpin for many other systems. Therefore, a good vision professional will not try to repair the visual system without first checking the foundations of the building, the substructure of the neurological development. These foundations are the vestibular and proprioceptive systems in the neck. Both offer the necessary base from which the automatic movements and reflexes can occur, which in turn underpin the visual function.

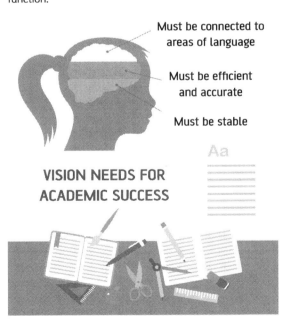

Must be connected to areas of language

Must be efficient and accurate

Must be stable

VISION NEEDS FOR ACADEMIC SUCCESS

In terms of vision, there are three basic requirements for academic success:

- **Vision must be stable.** As we saw earlier, the vestibulo-ocular and cervico-ocular reflexes are responsible for holding our gaze steady. The maturity of these reflexes depends on how the infant was moved early in life, whether he reached developmental milestones well and whether or not there was tension in the muscles or joints in his neck. When we are dealing with children who are underdeveloped, if we start reeducation or vision therapy without checking these other two systems first, it can make visual outcomes slower or mean they are not sustained over time. A child with no balance will hardly read well. There are some very interesting papers that back this up. This is why many optometrists have physiotherapists specializing in PIMT work on these systems to facilitate the outcome of vision therapy.

- **Vision must be efficient and accurate.** As we will see in the chapter on learning difficulties, higher cognitive functions must be supported by the correct functioning of the «lower brain», the ancient part of the brain that controls posture, balance and reflexes. If this «lower brain» isn't programmed properly, the higher cortical functions will step in to help stabilize it and the individual will lose their ability to concentrate, do arithmetic or speak. Keeping up this dual task causes tremendous fatigue. It is down to the correct functioning of the «lower brain» whether or not the process of seeing is tiring for the child. The «higher brain», which is fantastic for everything cognitive, is very unspecific for managing basic programs. Do you by any chance remember your first salsa class or driving lesson? Until the processes are automated, focusing all our attention on moving our feet or changing gears at the same time we are turning the steering wheel, isn't enough to ensure things go smoothly and accurately. Can you remember how exhausting it was too? Well, that's how exhausted the children who have to resort to overworking the «higher brain» to compensate for poor programming in the «lower brain». Once again a physiotherapist specializing in PIMT can help the optometrist structure and integrate the automatic functions that are supported by the proper functioning of the brainstem and the spinal cord, which together comprise the «lower» brain.

- **Vision must be able to fully connect with the cortical areas of language.** One of the visual sub-processes is recognition: Do I recognize it? What is it called? This sub-process takes place in the temporal cortex of the brain which, in turn, is responsible for language. If the language areas are not well-developed or if auditory processing is poor, the movements and fixations of the eyes whilst reading will not communicate well with the area of the brain that knows how to name the sound (phoneme), use the sound in a precise sequence or give the sound a meaning (an understanding of the text that is being read). The battle over whether the accountability for dyslexia is phonological or visual is, and always has been, a futile one, about who is right or which professional is more important in this problem that seriously affects society and concerns us all. There can be no good solution for any dysfunction that comes from the conceptual mutilation of the nervous system. Even though scan results speak of a lack of activation in the temporal areas of phonological recognition, establishing causes and consequences is a more complex issue because these findings may in turn be the consequences of failure in other circuits. It is communication between the visual and the auditory that doesn't work therefore, several professionals need to work together to connect these two wires. An optometrist and a speech and hearing specialist, or a speech therapist, must work very closely together on specific reading difficulties. As you would expect, it isn't a case of fixing just one thing, but of improving the communication between two parts of the brain. Given that brain function relies on communication and connection, by helping the brain we are helping to establish these connections. Perhaps the lack of communication between areas in the brain could be a good metaphor for the lack of communication amongst the professionals who deal with these areas.

Brain function relies on communication and connection. So, by helping the brain we are helping it to establish its connections properly, especially the ones between visual and language areas for reading.

In addition to these three optimal visual processing characteristics, the cognitive mechanisms that manage attention must be well developed as they can affect reading difficulties. This is why we need to break free of previously held convictions that have dominated research on reading difficulties.

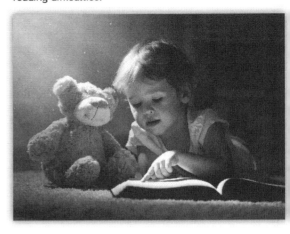

Lisa loves reading. Reading requires well-developed cognitive attention mechanisms, as well as optimal visual processing.

We must build bridges between neuroscience and education and create a new common field of natural sciencefocusing on the human being; from fetal development, development and stimulation in early life, language development and mainstream or special education. This relationship between neuroscience and education could be enriching for human development, providing that the mutual expectations of experts in each field can accommodate it.

What can you do?
HELPFUL PRACTICAL ADVICE

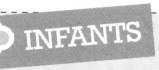

INFANTS

- Vision starts to develop in the first moments of life. Stimulate your baby's fixation systems; when he is still a newborn, bring your face up close to his, about 8 inches away, and move gently from side to side so he follows you with his gaze. He will have to turn both his head and his body to do this because he won't be able to use his eyes to look to the sides until he is 3 months old. Let him fix his gaze on you and your face whilst he is breastfeeding. Devote this time to communication between the two of you; touch his tiny hands and connect your gazes. This is a major driver of biological and emotional development. It is vital you live fully in the moment.

- When your baby is 6-8 weeks old, put him on his tummy regularly to stimulate him and stand in front of him so that he raises his gaze to look for you. Talk to him so he finds you with his gaze, this will stimulate the straightening systems in his back and neck.

- Up until he is 5 months old, offer objects from either side, not directly to him. Neurologically speaking until then he is only capable of grasping things at his sides (from 4 months he is able to reach out with his hands. In addition, turning his head and eyes to each side is very good for the maturation of the vestibular system, the neck and for oculomotricity. Lying underneath a hanging toy that he is unable to reach and that doesn't encourage eye movement, is a poor stimulation strategy and perhaps even a very subtle kind of torture. Let him look at things and grab them first on one side, then on the other and then repeat the process. This will improve his hand eye coordination and prepare the way for him to rollover from his back to his tummy as his interest in the object and his desire to grab it becomes an important incentive.

OLDER CHILDREN

- Monitor and curb screen time (television, tablets or mobile phones). It is true that your child was born in a digital age and his development should include IT systems and screens. However, a child's brain and nervous system require movement and tactile and vestibular experiences in order to develop. Moving around, jumping, rolling, touching, feeling… are all better for his development than sitting on a sofa staring at a screen. Screen time also reduces a child's interest in building his own creative, make-believe play space. If you have children yourself, you will have noticed how, after they have been playing with the tablet for a while, it is very difficult for them to give it up of their own accord; it's as though it creates addiction or anxiety. So changing activity is likely to cause a fairly heated argument followed by your child saying bitterly, «Now what am I supposed to do?» and flatly refusing to try anything you suggest. Conversely, have you ever seen how 6 and 7 year old spend a day with zero screen time? They build their own play space which is quite often make-believe, using whatever they find around the house. They develop their creativity in a much more comprehensive way and interact more often and more successfully with other people. However, it is also true that if they have no screen time, they require more attention from their parents. We need to do some soul-searching to decide what the best thing for our children is. Technology plays a key role in adapting to modern life but it cannot be a substitute for parents or physical, experiential or creative activity. Have a tech-free day from time to time. Go completely gadget free. It might be challenging but it will be awesome!

- Spot the signs your child has a problem with their vision. The most obvious signs are; refusing to read; unusual postures when reading or writing; clumsiness in certain movements and misjudging distances (walls, steps or people). There are many other signs, but these are three of the most obvious.

- Adopting odd postures when reading; getting very close to the paper; turning the paper a lot when reading or writing; over-tilting of the head or hunching of the back. These can all be signs of a vision problem and should be checked by a vision specialist.

- Clumsiness and misjudging distances is the third major sign of a vision problem. Does your child knock other glasses over when he wants to pick his glass up? Does he take undue care coming down the stairs? Does he misjudge distances with his friends and sometimes seem aggressive? Labelling a child as clumsy is unhelpful as it conceals the fact that there could be other underlying problems. The visual system locates where we are in space and allows us to calculate our safety zone so we can reach whatever we wish to touch or pick up easily and accurately. If we spot any of these signs an optometric assessment is required. Difficulty moving smoothly and easily always goes hand in hand with immaturity in the proprioceptive system which tells the child where his body is in space. Therefore, a specialist developmental physiotherapist should assess the organization of the child's sensory and motor systems and collaborate closely with the optometrist.

- All healthy, neurologically-developed children want to read, acquire knowledge, write, draw, etc. If a child doesn't like reading, it's very simple, he finds it hard work. There is no other reason. It isn't a question of personal taste. It is a clue to a vision problem which may reside in the input (a refractive problem such as hyperopia, myopia or astigmatism); or may be a visual processing problem, or a problem controlling eye position and movement. Children will refuse tasks that require effort or cause discomfort. In a way they are smarter than we are.

- Make your child's visual work easier by using visual hygiene measures. Here are some pointers for maintaining visual efficiency and reducing fatigue: take rest breaks (5-10 mins per hour); look into the distance during rest breaks (it is not enough to merely change activity); manage stress (if, on top of straining our eyes, we are nervous too, our visual system blocks, gets tired and malfunctions more quickly); use good lighting (never read with just a desk lamp); use a lectern tilted at a 20-25 degree angle (no more), even for reading; keep a visual distance of at least 40 cm. There are other aspects that can make a child's visual work easier but these are perhaps the most worthy of attention. Ask your vision specialist for more information.

- If you saw signs of a potential vision problem but didn't know how to interpret them, don't worry. You did your best and it's okay. Now that you have more information you can find the specialists who can assess and assist your child. The human brain is an amazing thing and it can sometimes find alternative ways to build or repair itself. Never give up hope there is always a way to help your child progress!

BIBLIOGRAPHY

Regarding a child's visual development:

> Eliot L. *What's going on in there? How the brain and mind develop in the first five years of life.* Bantam Books, 2000.

> Kiorpes L. *The Puzzle of Visual Development: Behavior and Neural Limits.* J Neurosci. 2016 Nov 9;36(45):11384-93.

Regarding visual fixation in babies:

> Vojta V, Schweizer E. *El descubrimiento de la motricidad ideal.* Editorial Morata; 2009.

Regarding coordination of the eyes and neck for seeing:

> Freedman EG. *Coordination of the eyes and head during visual orienting.* Experimental Brain Research, 2008;190(4):369-87.

Regarding how vision influences the circadian rhythm:

> Morin LP, Allen CN. *The circadian visual system.* Brain Research Reviews. 2005;51(1):1-60.

Regarding visual recognition as a sub-process of vision:

> Sacks O. *El hombre que confundió a su mujer con un sombrero.* Editorial Anagrama; 2009.

Regarding the difference between sight and vision:

> Vergara P. *Tanta inteligencia, tan poco rendimiento.* Pilar Vergara; 2008.

Regarding new therapies for amblyopia:

> Vergara P. *Estrabismo y ojo vago. Mitos, leyendas y verdades.* Rona Vision; 2014.

Regarding the importance of proprioceptive receptors in vision:

> Donaldson IML. *The functions of the proprioceptors of the eye muscles.* Philosophical Transactions of the Royal Society of London B: Biological Sciences. 2000;355(1404):1685-754.

> Treleaven J, Jull G, Grip H. *Head eye co-ordination and gaze stability in subjects with persistent whiplash associated disorders.* Manual Therapy. 2011;16(3):252-7.

Regarding how to restore stereopsis:

Barry SR. Fixing my gaze. A scientist's journey into seeing in three dimensions. Nueva York: Basic Books; 2009.

Regarding spatial vision:

Sanet R. Spatial vision. En: Suter PS, Harvey LH. Vision Rehabilitation: Multidisciplinary Care of the Patient Following Brain Injury. CRC Press; 2016.

Regarding dyslexia and attention:

Shaywitz SE, Shaywitz BA. Paying attention to reading: The neurobiology of reading and dyslexia. Development and Psychopathology. 2008 Fall;20(4):1329-49.

Regarding the role of phonology in dyslexia:

Hulme C, Snowlin MJ. Reading disorders and dyslexia. Curr Opin Pediatr. 2016 Dec;28(6):731-5.

McCardle P, Scarborough HS, Catts HW. Predicting, explaining and preventing children's reading difficulties. Learning Disabilities Research & Practice. 2001;16:230-9.

Regarding the role of the visual pathway in dyslexia:

Bucci MP, Mélithe D, Ajrezo L, Bui-Quoc E, Gérard C-L. The influence of oculomotor tasks on postural control in dyslexic children. Frontiers in Human Neuroscience.2014;8:981.

Gori S, Facoetti A. How the visual aspects can be crucial in reading acquisition? The intriguing case of crowding and developmental dyslexia. J Vis. 2015 Jan 14;15(1):8.

Regarding education and neuroscience:

Koizumi H. The concept of «developing the brain»: a new natural science for learning and education. Brain and Development.2004;26(7):434-41.

Willingham DT. Three problems in the marriage of neuroscience and education. Cortex.2009;45(4):544-5.

On screens and attention and learning difficulties:

Álvarez C. Las leyes naturales del niño. La revolución de la educación en la escuela y en casa. Aguilar; 2017.

Chapter 6

Hands on:
the crucial role that hands play

Iñaki Pastor Pons

They say that the hand is one of the key features that made us human; that all those years ago when humans were still crouching and covered in hair, they started to stand up to free their hands. They used their hands to pick up objects which they could make into something else and this competitive advantage has allowed our species to get to where it is today. Primitive man had no claws, no teeth; he wasn't fast-moving and couldn't blend in with his surroundings ... but using his hands he could make spears, knives, ride horses and build hideouts with branches.

The manipulation of objects also brought with it the chance to look close-up and develop visual skills which are uniquely human such as convergence (the ability to bring the eyes in to focus and locate things that are very close to) and three-dimensional vision to perceive the volume of things and the distance of objects around us.

Manipulation led to art; the possibility of using our hands to decorate our bodies, to paint or sculpt things to create a new level of self-expression.

Our hands are very skillful and can be exceedingly accomplished; playing a musical instrument, sewing, drawing, etc. The saying goes that you are not aware of how much you need something until you lose it. The same applies to your hands. If you can't use a finger or a hand because of a cut or an injury it is unbelievable just how much you struggle to do things that seemed so simple before with your other fingers or hand. Now, fastening a button or even eating, suddenly become high-precision tasks when previously you never gave them a second thought.

Children need to develop their hand function properly but not all of them do. Would you like your child to have strong manual dexterity skills? Join me now as we discover how.

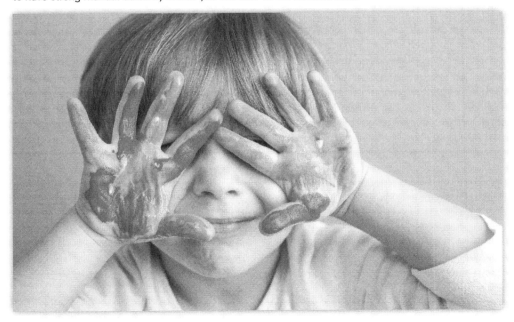

Archie hides behind his hands after using them to express his artistic side. Our hands are a beautiful expression of human development.

Manipulation led to art; the possibility of using our hands to decorate our bodies, to paint or sculpt things to create a new level of self-expression.

The history of our hands

But how did they become what they are? You weren't born with skillful hands. Human hands need to be woken up, activated and programmed to reach their full potential which will be both beautiful and quite extraordinary provided their development follows the optimal evolutionary path.

Human hands must be woken up, activated and programmed.

So, how can our hands be woken up? How can they become useful and skillful? When we are born our hands are very inexperienced and primitive. Two basic facts show us how primitive they really are. On the one hand, an infant can't hold anything of its own accord. Yes, she can grab at it, we see that in newborns. But she can't hold it, although her hand does close when something brushes against her palm. It's a bit like a carnivorous plant that closes its «jaws» in a totally involuntarily way when a stimulus touches it inside. The hand has no will power and therefore no control. This form of grasping is called the palmar grasp reflex or grasp reflex. The palmar reflex is a so-called primitive reflex, it is one of the automatisms you were born with that help you to survive and program the development of your nervous system.

The palmar reflex helps with survival as it allows the infant to be carried, or at least that is what it was used for originally. An evolutionary change has led to us losing this ability. Scarcely three days after birth a baby chimpanzee can be carried around by its parents by clinging on to their hair. Human beings are the result of a complex phylogenetic evolution. But imagine the surprise that all human newborns must feel when they see that their mother only has hair on her head. It must be a huge shock. Luckily we don't remember that moment. It turns out that we have lost the hair on our bodies, especially women, but newborns still retain this memory or legacy which allows

them to use the reflex to cling on with their hands or feet. Or maybe not? Do you think your baby would be able to hold on like this? I'm not saying you should try it, just ask yourself if she would be able to.

Actually, she would. Developmental researchers in the early twentieth century observed that a neonate was able to hang on to a rope (like a clothesline), clinging by its hands and feet thanks to palmar and plantar grasp reflexes. Nowadays we don't try that kind of thing, but we do know that the role of that first grip was for moving around.

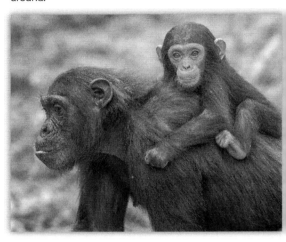

A baby chimp uses her own means to move around by clinging on to her mom's hair. This is something chimpanzees are able to do just a few days after they are born.

Of course there are more differences between chimpanzees and humans than just the amount of body hair. Human infants are far more immature when they are born as human development is linked to the size of the brain and were it to grow more during pregnancy, the infant's head would have even greater difficulty passing through the birth canal than it does already.

The first grip is automatic, a reflex. There are spectacular images of caesarean sections where an infant can be seen holding on to one of the gynecologist's fingers even before it leaves its mother's womb. Primitive reflexes are present at birth, but they develop much earlier. A fetus has a grip reflex at 4 months; as you can see, well before birth. The infant will progressively lose this grip reflex, like so many other primitive reflexes, when she develops the ability to choose what she picks up. At around 4 months a baby begins to throw her hand out to grab something that is at her side and the reflex can be integrated and inhibited.

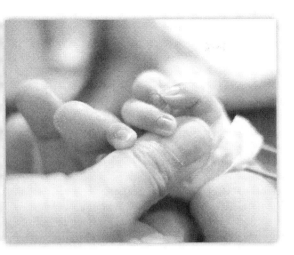

Barbara, who is still in hospital because she was premature, grasps her mom's finger with the palmar grasp reflex.

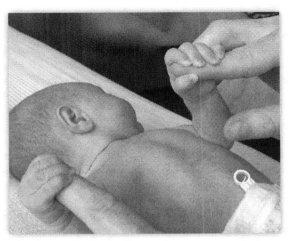

At barely three days old, Scott has a strong palmar grasp reflex. You can see how forceful his grip is. This isn't something he does voluntarily but rather because his hand has been stimulated.

The maturation of the nervous system evolves from reflex motor behaviors to voluntary motor behaviors. As more advanced brain areas are activated, the automatic ones are suppressed in order to support movement patterns in a more subtle way, yet without hindering voluntary movement. If the reflexes were to remain active when the conscious or voluntary capacity starts, instead of helping us, they would make things more difficult. Think what a problem it would be if your hand closed every time something touched it. For example, imagine your hand closed when you picked up a spoon to eat your soup and you had to hold the spoon (without dropping it) while straining to prevent your hand from clenching your fist. Just think how much energy you would use!

Well this is what it's like for so many children with major or minor developmental problems, where palmar grasp reflexes have not been integrated properly due to their immaturity and their hands have not been programmed properly. The reflex is still active and it hinders the quality and fluidity of their movements in tasks such as writing or cutting out with scissors. The problem manifests itself in a poor pincer grip which doesn't improve despite insistence from parents or teachers because the effort required to sustain the correct grasp is too great.

The other sign that the hands of a newborn human require maturation is that in the very early stages of life her thumbs remain tucked inside his hands and only emerge a few weeks later. When they do, they become increasingly active in preparation for the job they were designed for, which, by the way, is a very human characteristic; opposition to the other fingers to grip objects.

Waking the hands up. What does it take?

There is a long way to go from the grasp reflex to being able to play the guitar a few years down the line or to creating a work of art. As we saw earlier, your hands need to be stimulated and programmed.

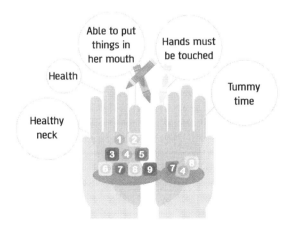

For an infant's hands to wake up she must be in good general health, have a supple, relaxed neck and receive stimuli to help them mature.

The first, most primitive stage of our development is characterized by our first automatic grip and our thumbs tucked into our fists. From here on, if everything goes to plan, we will go through different evolutionary stages.

This will require a series of conditions or circumstances:

    a. Bodily integrity and health.

    b. Correct neck function.

    c. The infant's fingers and hands must be touched (her feet too).

    d. The infant must have a lot of tummy time until she can support her weight on her hands.

    e. She must be able to put things in her mouth.

Bodily integrity and health

Manual dexterity will mature and develop if the neurological, muscular, articular and other body structures are intact and healthy. This is the first step. In addition to structural integrity, our nervous system must be healthy. The damage caused by some brain conditions can prevent us from developing our full potential in certain parts of our body. There are also different, unclassified genetic syndromes and other developmental disorders that affect the start of embryogenesis and can compromise the function and dexterity of the hands.

Correct neck function

This is the most neglected condition. The functionality and structure of the neck must work well. The nerves reaching the hand come from small spaces between the cervical vertebrae that form the neck. These nerves are responsible for transmitting the sensations of touch, pressure, temperature, etc. from the hand to the brain so that it can adapt to whatever we touch. The nerves also transmit motor commands from the brain so that the muscles of the arm and hand can make precise movements. The spinal cord at neck level has another role too; it controls the exchange of sensory and motor information and regulates the amount of muscle tone in our arm and hand. If the tone is very high, the hand will be stiff and it will be difficult to carry out precise tasks. Conversely, if the tone in the hand is too low it will drop things, lack strength and with it, fluidity and accuracy. The brain is the supreme commander of what goes on in the hand, but for everything to work properly, the neck must be in correct working order for high-precision tasks.

In order for the hand to work, the neck must function correctly with no stiffness or blocks.

The body has a rule that says automatic actions support voluntary actions. This means that in order to perform a voluntary, intentional movement, your body must develop thousands of automatic tasks that enable you to focus solely on your objective. Remember the «higher» and «lower» brain? Everything works according to this law. Need an example? How many do you want? When you reach forward to pick up a cup of coffee, the muscles of your legs mobilize automatically to stabilize your body, before your hand has moved an inch. The brain anticipates the forward displacement of its center of masses using a terrific anticipation system. Thousands of other automatic actions work in the same way too, such as torso or shoulder stabilization, goal-directed gaze shifts, visual focus shifts, new distance calculations, etc. Well, something along these lines occurs for every action.

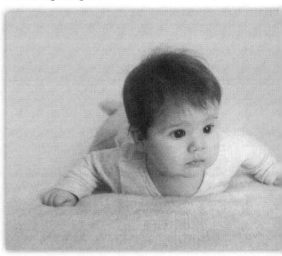

Four month old Evelyn has problems controlling her arms. Her forearms and elbows should be well supported at shoulder level. It is unlikely she will be able to straighten her torso or maintain this position without complaining if she doesn't get this support. Her parents need training to help her sort it out.

Neurodevelopmental disorders that affect learning disabilities (we will look at this later on) hinder a child's performance and education and this happens because their automatic responses are immature. The motor function (e.g. coordination), sensory function (e.g. balance), and cognitive or mental function (e.g. attention, reading, or math) are typically impaired.

The neck is often neglected in the hand function. A lot of infants (around 20%), have flattened heads associated with torticollis or ahead position preference that is non-physiological – as during the first eight weeks it is normal for infants to prefer to turn their head to one side in particular. A position that is non-physiological is where an infant clearly prefers sleeping on one side beyond these eight weeks and cries if you turn her over. This is a sign of cervical dysfunction which is usually mild and can be easily remedied by a specialist physiotherapist.

Most of these neck problems are the result of difficult births. However, many parents and experts don't consider there is a problem with the infant's neck unless they see it is completely locked. Unfortunately, there are more problems than you might think.

The majority of these problems which, whilst not serious, are quite common, can cause problems with hand function. We often see infants who don't put their arms and hands in the right place to support themselves when they are on their tummies. This makes it hard for them to hold their head up and they cry when left facing down or only use one of their hands to grab toys. Sometimes when parents see this they think their baby is showing their handedness. This isn't the case as right or left preference is chosen much later as we will see further on.

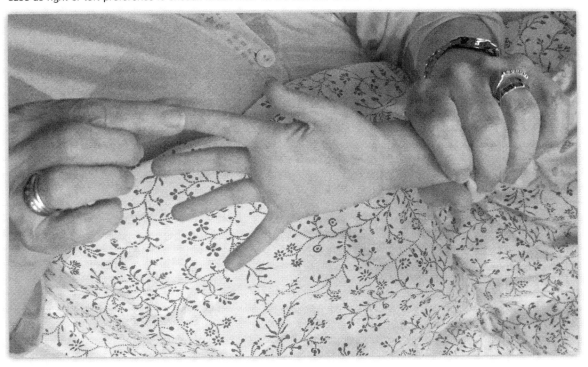

A grandmother singing to her granddaughter as she touches her hand. An elderly person's hands as they play a stimulating hand game. When you were little did they play: «This little piggy went to market, this little piggy stayed at home...» with you? Did you know that this kind of game where an adult plays with each of the child's fingers as they sing or chant a rhyme exists in many cultures? What is the biological purpose of these games?

The infant's fingers and hands must be touched (her feet too)

An infant's hands and fingers must be touched by adults. This is essential. There is a map of your whole body in your brain; a map that represents each part of your body. You have many maps, but more specifically you have sensory and motor maps. The sensory map allows you to know without looking, where you have been touched even if it was only the slightest of touches. The motor map allows you to move your fingers one by one without looking, as if you knew exactly where each one was. It also allows you to move one independently of the rest. When you were born, this map was sketchy and kind of blurred. It required stimulation to be programmed.

In every culture around the world, old people sing songs and plays games as they touch little children's hands. I have seen similar songs in many languages and it's something I love. When different cultures spontaneously develop gestures and ways of interacting with babies, it is a sign of a natural instinct and urge to enhance our species. It's the same with carrying infants; it happens in a spontaneous way in different cultures, except in ours of course. Is it because our society is more advanced than the rest? Could it be that certain sociocultural models separate us from our roots? As we saw, wearing children on our bodies stimulates the maturation of their nervous system, activates the muscles of their neck and back, trains eye movements, helps to create a bond between infants and parents or caregivers, prevents hip problems and is soothing. There is evidence to prove all this. But surely there must be many more benefits that we are not aware of? And what do we do, we push them around in a baby carriage and tell ourselves it's better for the baby... really?

In every culture around the world, old people sing songs and play games as they stroke little children's hands.

Like carrying children around on us, lap rhymes involving hand stroking are common all over the world. There is undoubtedly an evolutionary advantage to this as connections are created in the sensory and motor areas of the brain that map the hand. What happens with children's bodies is similar to what happens with their minds. For a human being to recognize itself and feel comfortable and safe in its own skin, it must first have been touched and recognized physically by other human beings when it was small. The same is probably true of the psychological side; for a human being to recognize and feel comfortable and secure in its own mind, it must first have been accepted and recognized by other human beings early on in life. Deliberate contact and stroking are pivotal to building an infant's identity from the outset, just as much as responding to the sounds she makes or to her emotions. Using touch in this way increases body awareness and "prevents" psychophysical dissociation because it helps to integrate the body into the Self. These body-mind connections, which become permanent when established this early in life, encourage the body to constitute a real part of the Self. This can be a way of healing, regulating and channeling emotions and experiences. Additionally, the feeling of being touched, seen or heard is also a form of protection against potentially traumatic situations in the future, (we find fewer situations traumatic and cope better with them because we are more resilient). It may

be that there isn't even any difference between physical, psychological and social identity early in life and instead there is a common path that then branches off and evolves in a more complex way.

It is vital that adults touch infants on their hands and feet in an affectionate, playful yet firm way so that the child's hands wake up in their brain.

The infant must spend time on her tummy. Lots of time!

Another prerequisite if her hands are to be programmed properly is that the child must spend time on her tummy. What has this got to do with her hands? The impact of tummy time on the dexterity of her hands in the future is subtle and not easy to grasp at first glance, but it is of vital importance for the way the hands function.

As we saw in the chapter on the stages of a baby's development, initially a newborn is curled-up and lacks the strength to raise her head. As she develops, she becomes stronger and has the urge to see and look ahead; the visual part is important here. When she begins to lift her head up somewhere between 6 to 8 weeks, she does so by resting on her forearms. In order to lift something, she needs a firm base to push off and the floor is ideal for this. When she starts to lift her head up, hesitantly at first, she initially gets support from her forearms but in order to spend more time upright she will gradually need higher quality support.

At 3 months an infant is able to raise her head for quite some time by propping herself up on her elbows. She is able to keep her head centered and she has the ability to turn to see the world around her. The 3-month milestone coincides with the time infants begin to hold onto objects put into their hands, although there is little incentive and the grip reflex is still quite present. This means they are able to grasp but not let go.

At 4 to 5 months her ability to maintain support and stability in the prone position improves and she is able to thrust her hands out in front to pick things up. At 4 and a half months she hits a very important milestone which will determine many of her coordination skills in the future. At this stage she is able to lean on one side and reach out with her opposite hand while flexing one hip and creating a contralateral support with her limbs. Inhibition of the palmar grasp reflex has begun already and will make way for a more intentional hand function.

At 6 months an infant should be able to sit up with her arms fully stretched out and hands completely open. As soon as she can support herself on her open palms the grasp reflex stage ends once and for all and the awakening of the hands begins in earnest. With this support, reflex movement helps to tone muscles in the arm and hand. She can open her thumb and her hand is activated in a subtle but very necessary way. From here on, if she has spent enough time on her tummy and has no problems in her neck, torso or hips, the infant will progress to all fours where her manual dexterity will continue to develop.

The next step is grasping objects by slightly flexing her wrist. And the next milestone at 9 months is using her thumb and index finger for her first pincer grip. This will allow her to pick up a raisin or a similar sized object size from the floor. Developmental synchrony is great. At the same time his first pincer grip appears, she develops other uniquely human aspects too; the ability to speak and stand up. At 9 months an infant says her first words and with support and help she

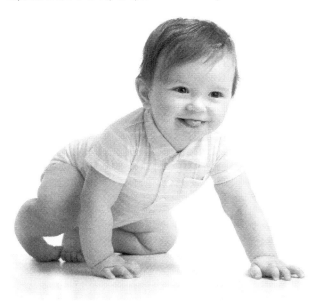

can stand up. How amazing; pincer grip, speaking and standing. Isn't nature wonderful? Our most human traits, the ones that make us different to every other species, all appear at the same stage in our development. But don't forget that these three signs are evidence of a more mature brain, of neurodevelopment that is hitting the right milestones at the right time. She still has a long way to go.

The pincer grip continues to develop into more complex pincer types, finer and more precise motor skills that will lead us to a major unprecedented developmental milestone: tying our shoe laces.

Brandon is happy on all fours. He knows he can go anywhere. By supporting himself with his hands on the floor he is stimulating deep sensitivity in his hands and activating muscle tone.

Unfortunately, too few infants spend enough time on their tummies because, due to a lack of training, their parents tend to act out of fear rooted in ignorance. Evidently this represents a failure of our social model which has not known how to guide parents or teach them about infants' needs. Other parents take their child out of the prone position as soon as she grumbles. Some infants with problems in their spine or neck are unable to get their forearms into the right position and their parents have to help them to position their arms in a way that provides support.

Unfortunately, too few infants spend enough time on their tummies.

At the age of 6 or 7 children undergo an even more significant development; their cerebellum, the part of the brain that organizes motor skills amongst other things, starts to evaluate the difference between their expectations and the results of their actions. Thanks to this increased activity of the cerebellum we learn to develop our motor control much faster. Let's look at an example: if we shoot a basketball at a basket and we're not used to doing it, we will probably miss. The ball will fall to the right or the left, the shot will be too hard or too soft, either way it won't achieve our objective of scoring a basket. We get another chance to shoot. Our cerebellum takes note of the difference between our initial intention and the final outcome and will adjust the parameters of the throwing motion so we get closer to the desired result. The visual system also plays a part in this kind of motor learning through perception and spatial projection. Sooner or later we will score a basket.

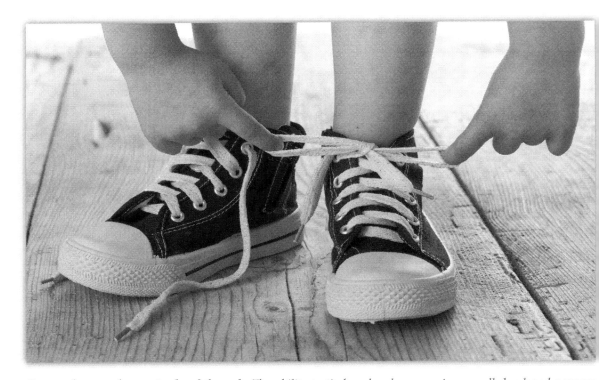

Donna shows us her major breakthrough. The ability to tie her shoe laces requires a well-developed nervous system.

She must be able to put things in her mouth

Another way the brain is able to recognize the infant's hands, create neural connections with them, fine-tune their sensitivity and improve their control and dexterity, is to bring them into contact with things like toys. More importantly, it takes the hands to an area of the body where the brain has developed prior to the hands: the mouth.

The first part of the body where sensitivity awakens is the mouth; even the mouth of an eleven-week fetus is sensitive to contact. Nature loves economy, the fact that an organ or an action has not one, but several benefits. Or, in other words, that one thing can be used to develop several others. The mouth is a good example of this. As well as being useful for feeding, breathing or communicating, it also provides one of our first sources of knowledge about the environment. It is easy to see why infants put everything in their mouths, because they learn about everything through their mouths. It is a wonderful organ for exploring the world and procuring calmness.

Because their natural instinct is one of protection, this behavior makes moms and dads nervous. They want to prevent infants from getting dirt in their mouths, but a balance must be found between making a child's environment safe and allowing her to develop. This is the eternal conflict of being a parent.

Clasping her hands together and taking them to her mouth whether on their own or with a toy, is a necessary step. Our hands and mouth are meant to be together and we are about to find out why.

The mouth and hands are biologically and neurologically designed to work together.

Our hands and mouth are designed to work together

Our hands and mouth are meant to be together. Long before they found each other, when the brain was developing, the hands and mouth formed next to each other in the primary sensory area that houses the map of our entire body.

You often find the hands and mouth close to each other even when there is no apparent physiological reason for it. Sometimes we touch our chin or mouth whilst we are thinking. How many people do you know bite their nails when they are anxious? How many little ones –and not so little ones– suck their thumbs? When you talk to someone who speaks a different language you move your hands more don't you?

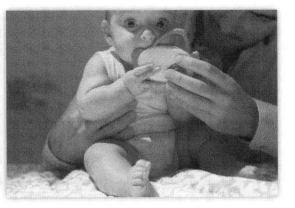

Jessica is thrilled about the opportunity to learn through sucking. The mouth is a highly developed organ of perception.

What is the purpose of the neurological connection between the hands and the mouth? It must be something very important. Well yes, it is. There are two basic functions that require the hands and mouth to work together. The first one is feeding. You won't find many functions that require coordinated motor patterns of several parts of the body more important than feeding. The second one is communication. As we will see later in the chapter on language, the hands and mouth work together as one strong, perfectly coordinated team. In fact, our mouth developed vocalization in order to improve the function of language that was previously the responsibility of the hands. This way the hands were free to take over other tasks, although they didn't entirely cast off their communication function.

There are two basic functions that require the hands and mouth to work together: the first is feeding and the second, communication.

In order to support the aim of joint programming, one of the first automatic primitive reflexes brought hand and mouth coordination even closer through the development of a sensorimotor relationship. This response is known as the Babkin reflex.

The Babkin reflex is a primitive reflex, in other words, a very archaic first movement pattern that is used for survival and to program a mature and functional nervous system for the future. If you stroke or apply pressure to a newborn's palms in her first 4 weeks of life, her mouth will automatically start to open and close as if she was sucking. It is quite remarkable. Midwives have been aware of this since ancient times, so that whenever there were any difficulties, they could help the infant suck by applying pressure to her hands. Any mother who listens to her instincts will have caressed her baby's hands while she was breastfeeding. It is common for adults to be attracted to infants' hands and feet, it's as though it was in their DNA.

Any mother who listens to her natural instincts will have caressed her baby's hands while she was breastfeeding.

In order to support the mouth-hand relationship from the neurological «subsoil», the Babkin reflex, like all primitive reflexes, must be inhibited, though it should not disappear altogether. If it is not integrated, it will hinder the function of the hands and mouth. This reflex is poorly integrated in a lot of children with developmental difficulties. Of course if you press a child's hand, her mouth doesn't open, but if you look carefully at her mouth while you caress the palm of her hand, you will see how her lips move or tighten involuntarily and, in some children, we see the tongue move or even stick out.

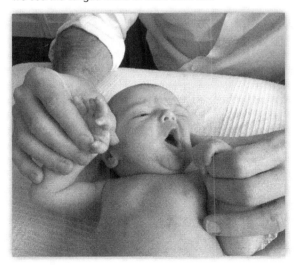

Ten day old William demonstrates the Babkin reflex. You can see how touching the palms of his hands triggers a complex mouth movement, a kind of simulation of sucking movements.

How can neurodevelopmental immaturity affect the hands?

- Poor manual function: precision, strength, coordination, etc.
- Poor pincer grip and therefore, poor, untidy handwriting.
- Poor pronunciation of different sounds.
- Involuntary movements of the tongue or the jaw when using the hands.

With appropriate intervention it is possible to integrate this relationship so that they are able to move independently. Hand movements should not trigger mouth movements and vice versa.

Laterality

We can all understand that something as complex as the nervous system needs to be well organized to function properly. There are several types of organization but two stand out in particular: one is hierarchical organization where, as areas of the higher brain are activated, the lower ones can be silenced to continue working on the more automatic body functions. Therefore, as the nervous system matures, the postures, reflexes or gestures change. A neurodevelopmental specialist can detect if certain gestures, postures or reactions are in line with the child's age or correspond to an earlier stage, suggesting delay or immaturity.

The second type of organization of the nervous system is laterality. No doubt you have heard of it. A person is right-handed or left-handed. Questions arise when we know of someone who is ambidextrous: is it an advantage or a disadvantage? We have all probably heard talk of a child having crossed laterality. But what exactly is laterality?

A neurodevelopmental specialist can detect if certain gestures, postures or reactions are in line with the child's age or correspond to an earlier stage, suggesting delay or immaturity.

There are two hemispheres in the brain, one on each side. Each one controls the opposite side of the body, in other words it receives information from the opposite side and is able to act on it. For example, the right hemisphere controls what happens in our left hand, but we manage the input from our visual field in the left hemisphere. This is because the nerves ascending to the brain cross before reaching it.

In addition to controlling the opposite side of the body, each hemisphere has specific functions, although both are involved in most activities. The left hemisphere, for example, is the so-called symbolic side which manages language and sequential information processing, while the right hemisphere is more specialized in processing input from the body, emotions and an understanding of the world we live in.

Laterality should be seen as the orderly distribution of functions between the two hemispheres. It is much more effective to use order and automation than to use the entire brain for everything. This occurs at brain level, but your body has made its own choice too.

«Laterality should be seen as the orderly distribution of functions between the two hemispheres».

Jorge Ferré y Elisa Aribau

We don't function equally with our right and left sides. Try writing your name with your opposite hand; what used to be a simple, almost automatic process becomes a task which requires your full attention. The preference for one side or another is a maturation process and has its advantages in evolutionary terms.

Many species including frogs, birds and mammals have left brain dominance for vocalization. However, right hand dominance, also known as laterality, is a specifically human characteristic. Monkeys also possess a Broca's area (the region in humans linked to speech production). However it includes so-called «mirror neurons» and besides, it is bilateral. There is some evidence that Broca's area has expanded in the left hemisphere of human brains and is involved in both speech and manual skills. Moreover, higher primates do not have hand dominance as humans do, or at least not in such a clearly defined way. Chimps tend to be slightly more right-handed than left-handed but only those in captivity and with the ratio 2:1. Humans on the other hand are right-handed with the ratio 9:1.

Right hand dominance may have come about because of the association between hand gestures and vocalization in the evolution of language, i.e. we are right-handed because we are able to speak.

Humans start to «choose» their laterality between the ages of 3 and 5 and it continues to develop and mature until the age of 12. Laterality must be well-defined at the preschool stage so that by the time reading and writing commences, the child already has solid foundations and a clear preference regarding directionality.

But children don't just have hand dominance, a natural selection by which they develop more skill and resolve with one hand than with the other. They also develop lateral preference of their eyes, ears and feet.

In order to detect a person's laterality, we must observe their spontaneous responses in different tasks. Usually it is not enough to test just one, especially if their nervous system hasn't matured sufficiently and their preference is unclear.

Which is your dominant side?

Follow the instructions below to find out:

- Which hand do you write or eat with? Which hand would you bang the table with?

- Which foot would you kick a football with, or stamp your foot with when you are angry?

- Pick up a ring or make a ring shape with your fingers. Keeping both eyes open, look through the ring and focus on a small object a few feet away, like a letter on a picture or a glass. Keep your hand still and close one of your eyes. Now close the other one. In one of the cases the object will remain inside the ring and in the other it will be completely off center.

- Put your ear against the wall as though you wanted to listen to what was being said in the other room. Which ear did you use? Place a glass over one ear to listen to the sound of the sea like you would with a shell. Which ear did you choose?

Did you only choose your right side or your left side, or was it one side for some tasks and the opposite side for others? If this is the case, you may have crossed laterality.

What is crossed laterality? To what extent is it important? For a long time, crossed laterality was one of the labels used to attempt to identify the causes of learning disabilities. But perhaps nowadays we see it as a possible sign of immaturity in the organization of the nervous system, although this is not always the case. Imagine if you will a right-handed person, who due to a health problem in one eye, has left eye preference in her vision. This person may have optimal cognitive performance; her nervous system may be organized and adapted to a particular situation. There could be additional consequences, her ear or foot preference might be distributed between the two sides as well for example or show no preference at all.

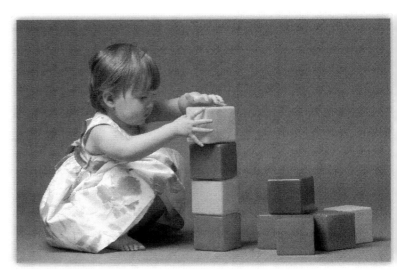

Karen displays very sound manual skills. We can see from the precision of her actions and the alertness of her fingers that her right hand is dominant. She uses her left hand as an assistant. Lateral organization allows her to be much more precise.

Imagine a company that has two buildings, one on each side of the street. The purchasing department is located in one of the buildings. Where would it make the most sense to put the economic management department for enhanced performance and communication? In the same building, right? If one of these departments was in the other building (always assuming that in the example there is no telephone or internet), a messenger would have to run across the street to transmit messages between the two departments. Crossing the street is not a problem in itself if the messenger is fast and they don't send him with pointless messages. The messenger can be trained until he is as speedy as if he were in the same building.

This is what happens to many people who have crossed laterality but good cognitive and language performance. However, in the case of children with developmental problems, not only are the departments poorly distributed (something that could be rectified), but they also have slow messengers who get lost along the way, stop for a coffee at the coffee shop, or get out at the wrong floor when they arrive at the other side and are continually searching for the right place.

Perhaps the different areas and departments don't have the right name on the door and it isn't easy for the messenger to find them. This could be a metaphor for a developmental problem associated with laterality. It could be called lateral disorganization.

Therefore, crossed laterality is a sign of a possible neurodevelopmental immaturity if disorganization is also present. However, in our opinion it is one of the many manifestations of developmental delay. It should definitely be taken into account and form part of a comprehensive neurodevelopmental assessment, but it should not be considered the root of the problem.

Crossed laterality is a sign of possible neurodevelopmental immaturity. It should definitely be taken into account and form part of a comprehensive neurodevelopmental assessment, but it should not be considered the root of the problem.

Children with «sleeping» hands

The hands and their ability to function are high on the agenda when checking for neurodevelopmental delay or immaturity. As we saw earlier, the hand is linked to cognitive function and language and certain connections are made as each person develops. The way our brain develops is linked to the way we use our hands. This is not just true because of the theory behind evolution, it can also be observed in practice in all infants.

In order to assess a child's hands and how useful they are, we need to observe several aspects:

- How does she use her hands? Does she drop things? How good is she at dressing herself, fastening buttons or tying her shoelaces?

- How does she hold a pen or pencil? What is her handwriting like? Is it small and fluid or, conversely, large, messy and irregular?

- When she crawls does she place her hands flat on the ground with her thumbs wide open? Or does she keep her fingers tucked in and her thumbs in her fist? Does she bear down just on her thumb and the tips of her other fingers without resting the palm of her hand on the floor?

- When she is inactive do her hands appear to be «asleep»?

So, as you can see, if we want to assess a child's manual skills it isn't enough to simply observe her performing a specific task such as writing. We also need to see her doing something that requires strength: or, even more interestingly, when she is doing nothing at all. In fact, this last point is a major clue.

One of the clearest examples that a neurodevelopmental problem is affecting the hands, is something I refer to as the sign of «sleeping» hands. A healthy hand should always be active, lively, with restless fingers, or at least in some degree of pre-tension. When at rest, the fingers remain outstretched with the thumb comfortably open.

«Sleeping» hands are usually always half-closed, the thumb is alongside the hand and the hand itself looks as though it has been «unplugged». The child may well be talking to you but it's as if no electricity reaches her hands.

To assess a child's manual skills, it isn't enough to simply observe her performing a specific task such as writing. We also need to see her doing something that requires strength: or, even more interestingly, when she is doing nothing at all.

«Sleeping» hands are ones that are always more or less dysfunctional. This has a significant impact on handwriting in terms of the accuracy of the strokes, the size of the letters and general tidiness. They drop things, are clumsy and appear to lack strength. Yet it is not simply a matter of strength. It is as if the brain had difficulties communicating with them. For some reason, the hands didn't wake up during the neurodevelopmental process.

It is our job to wake them up and it can be done. In fact, we do it every day with surprising results if the steps are followed correctly and parents are persistent in their approach. Interestingly there is evidence that, in order to reach for something and pick it up successfully, first you must have postural control. Our practice bears this out. Many of the children we deal with who have difficulties with their grip or manual skills also have difficulties with their balance or coordination.

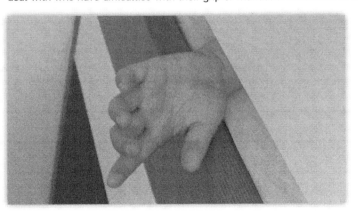

Seven year old Andrea is asleep but her hand is «awake». Her hand is active, open, and her thumb is slightly separated. This is the sign of hand that is very useful even when it is at rest.

Of course, you will have guessed by now that the hands do not miraculously wake up by filling hundreds of exercise books with writing. That would be like the paradox of the road to Santiago. Nobody would ever think that by doing the Camino de Santiago, a lame man would be walking smoothly and briskly by the end of it. However, there are people who think that if they have a knee problem, «working out», will cure it. Sometimes we think that the only way is to insist on more and more work; more hand exercises like dropping beads into a container. And it's true we do need to persevere. But at the same time, we need to be aware that these measures will not be effective on their own if the actual cause has not been addressed, or neurodevelopment rewired the way that nature would. We need to try to solve the problem and make the brain-hand connection and the maturation of the nervous system easier.

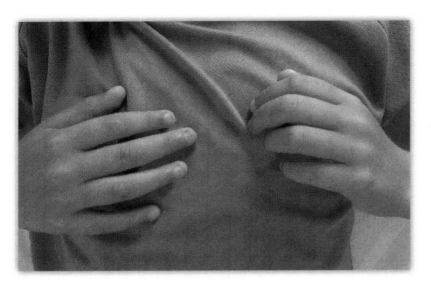

Seven year old Liam's hands are on his chest. Yet there is a difference between his hands, isn't there? This is not the result of brain damage. In this case the absence of hand functionality is linked to developmental issues, probably a neck problem at birth. Which hand do you think is affected?

SUMMARY

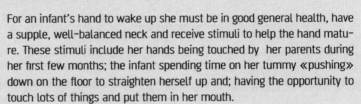

When we are born our hands are very inexperienced and lack intentionality and control. They are able to hold onto things thanks to an automatic reflex called a grasp reflex. Human hands need to be woken up, activated and programmed to reach their full, magnificent potential.

For an infant's hand to wake up she must be in good general health, have a supple, well-balanced neck and receive stimuli to help the hand mature. These stimuli include her hands being touched by her parents during her first few months; the infant spending time on her tummy «pushing» down on the floor to straighten herself up and; having the opportunity to touch lots of things and put them in her mouth.

Our hands and mouth are biologically and neurologically designed to work together. This is why infants have reflexes that integrate the hands and mouth. If you touch a neonate's palm she will start to suck. This sound combined programming will be used for feeding or for speech.

Many children with developmental and learning problems have clumsy hands to one extent or another and they also have difficulties pronouncing certain sounds.

Laterality is a specialist area in neurology. Ideally, lateralization should occur in one hemisphere of the brain so it has priority over the movement and perception of the eye, ear, hand and foot on that same side. This organization and specialization of the nervous system is lacking in many development-related problems and they require help in the form of reprogramming and maturation of the nervous system.

What can you do?

HELPFUL PRACTICAL ADVICE

INFANTS

- If you have a baby, touch her hands a lot, press and caress her palms and each tiny finger. Do it regularly, especially when she is breastfeeding or having her bottle. If you do this for the first few months you will notice she sucks much better when you gently press the palm of her hands. This will help integrate the Babkin reflex and give her better hand-mouth coordination in the brain going forward.

- Allow your baby to spend a lot of time on her tummy on a firm surface. You need to do it for 5 minutes every few hours from her first week of life whilst she is awake and supervised, gradually increasing the amount of time as she grows. If, when you place her on her tummy at 2-3 months, she isn't able to hold her arms properly and they open at the sides, you need to support her forearms and elbows more or less at shoulder level. If she has difficulty controlling her arms or you find she grumbles a lot in this position (a sign there is pain in her neck or back), seek the help of a physiotherapist specializing in PIMT. There is a section on how to find specialists who can help at the end of the book.

- Let your baby suck her hands. This key milestone occurs around the 3-month mark. By doing this she integrates the perception of her hands and can create a more accurate map of them in her brain. Let her put her feet in her mouth too, something that will happen at around 6 months. She needs to create a good representation of her feet in her brain too. This will make your child more balanced and improve her movements.

- Let her put toys in her mouth but first make sure they are safe. If she can suck a toy after holding it, she will get a much better idea of the object's shape and volume. It will help her develop. Remember that her mouth is much more effective than her hands for exploring the world, at least until she is two or three years old.

OLDER CHILDREN

- Encourage your child's autonomy. It's true that we adults do everything better and faster but learning takes time and learning to use your hands takes years. She will only develop her skills by doing things for herself. Don't dress or undress her if she is old enough to do it by herself; make sure she has enough time to do it at her own pace. Of course, in all households where there are kids schedules are very tight in the mornings and sometimes we end up shouting. Encourage her to start getting dressed earlier or, at the very least, let her dress and undress herself on her free days. But if she can do it on a daily basis, all the better. Never feed a child who is capable of feeding herself using cutlery, even if it is specially adapted. Parents sometimes secretly enjoy feeding their children it's a form of guilty pleasure. But they will learn to do it perfectly well if we just give them the chance. Even with the best will in the world, help can be highly incapacitating for children and the elderly. Sometimes our love for another person requires us to take a step back so they can occupy their rightful place in the world.

- Play with your child ont he floor regularly. This simple act will make him put her hands on the floor and this will wake them up to a certain extent. When an infant's hands make contact with the floor as she is developing it allows integration of the grasp reflex and unlocks the hand for other, more advanced tasks. If your child skipped stages such as crawling, playing on the floor can help her make up for this. Notice if her fingers are stretched out and her thumb separate when she supports herself with her hands as you play on the floor. Ideally this is how they should be.

- Play at speaking with your hands with her. There are games where you have to act out or communicate something using your hands whilst the other players attempt to guess what it is. This will build his manual skills associated with language development. You can also sing songs where the hands act out the words to a specific beat. This will be a real booster for her.

- Play clapping games with your child or encourage her to play them with her friends. Girls tend to do this more than boys but it is a very useful rhythm and coordination activity for everyone's brain.

- If you notice that your child's hands seem particularly clumsy, or see any of the other signs described above, seek help. She may be having other difficulties, with her autonomy, academic performance or language, for example. She may be really struggling to keep her head above water to avoid disappointing you and could be paying a high price for it. Get a specialist physiotherapist to carry out an overall assessment and check if there is stiffness in her neck or back. An occupational therapist can be of great help too.

- If you were unable to accompany your child in her early stages of development and provide stimulation for her hands, either because you weren't aware of the need for it or because of other difficulties in her early years (illnesses, hospitalizations, etc.), don't panic, everything can be programmed later. The brain is an amazing thing and it can sometimes find alternative ways to build or repair itself. If you consider that your child's difficulties correspond to less than optimal hand control, there are different specialists who can be of great assistance. Never give up hope – there is always a way to help your child progress!

BIBLIOGRAPHY

Regarding the grasp reflex in fetuses and neonates:

> Peiper A. Cerebral function in infancy and childhood. Consultants Bureau; 1963.

Regarding why humans are so immature at birth:

> Arsuaga JL. El primer viaje de nuestra vida. Ediciones Planeta; 2012.

Regarding how reflexes which are not fully integrated can hamper development:

> Goddard Blythe S. Attention, Balance and Coordination. The ABC of Learning Success.   Ed. Wiley-Blackwell; 2009.

Regarding the number of infants who have certain neck problems:

> Rogers GF, Oh AK, Mulliken JB. The Role of Congenital Muscular Torticollis in the Development of Deformational Plagiocephaly. Plastic and Reconstructive Surgery. 2009;123(2):643-52.

Van Vlimmeren LA, Van der Graaf Y, Boere-Boonekamp MM, L'Hoir MP, Helders PJM, Engelbert RHH. Effect of pediatric physical therapy on deformational plagiocephaly in children with positional preference: a randomized controlled trial. Archives of Pediatrics & Adolescent Medicine,. 2008;162(8):712-8.

Regarding body maps in the brain:

Blakeslee S, Blakeslee M. The body has a mind of its own. How body maps in your brain help you do (almost) everything better. Random House Trade Paperbacks; 2008.

Regarding the different stages of hand development in infants:

Vojta V, Schweizer E. El descubrimiento de la motricidad ideal. Asociación Española de Vojta. Ediciones Morata; 2011.

Regarding the Babkin reflex:

Peiper A. Cerebral function in infancy and childhood. Consultants Bureau; 1963.

Regarding the lateralization of functions in the brain:

Ferré Veneciana J, Aribau Montón E. El desarrollo neurofuncional del niño y sus trastornos. Visión, aprendizaje y otras funciones cognitivas. 2nd ed. Ediciones Lebón; 2006.

Regarding lateralization and its relationship with language:

Corballis MC.From mouth to hand: gesture, speech, and the evolution of right-handedness. Behav Brain Sci. 2003 Apr;26(2):199-208; discussion 208-60.

Hopkins WD. Chimpanzee handedness revisited: 55 years since Finch (1941). Psychon Bull Rev. 1996 Dec;3(4):449-57.

Regarding the way infants vocalize differently when touching bigger objects:

Bernardis P, Bello A, Pettenati P, Stefanini S, Gentilucci M. Manual actions affect vocalizationsof infants. Exp Brain Res. 2008 Feb;184(4):599-603.

Regarding the importance of postural control for improved manual dexterity:

Hadders-Algra M. Typical and atypical development of reaching and posturalcontrol in infancy. Dev Med Child Neurol. 2013 Nov;55 Suppl 4:5-8.

Chapter 7

The dawn of language
A paradigm shift for the brain

Iñaki Pastor Pons

Language is one of the uniquely human skills and a sign of millions of years of evolution in the brain. Many species communicate using sounds and tones but only humans are able to develop abstract language or use double entendre or humor. The evolution of language is closely linked to the development of handedness. At the beginning human beings spoke using their hands and by making certain sounds. Then they freed their hands up to carry out other tasks, thus improving their ability to use their mouths for language.

Your brain was prepared and predisposed for language from the very day you were born. However, it seems this predisposition does not materialize without social experience. Therefore, language development is also the result of evolution and programming in our brain. It starts with pregnancy and develops during childhood. Talking to infants a lot is one of the stimuli that helps develop their language skills. Later on in life we can always improve these skills and learn new sounds and languages but probably with greatly reduced capacity.

Some children don't acquire language skills by the usual milestones and this can be a cause of major concern for their parents. But, does this mean they will have developmental difficulties or problems learning to read in the future? What are the telltale signs?

Join me now as we explore this incredibly complex human skill

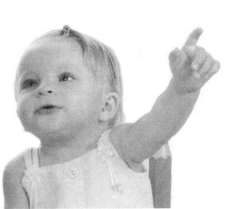

«Language is a symbolic process of communication, thought and formulation».

De Quiros y Schrager

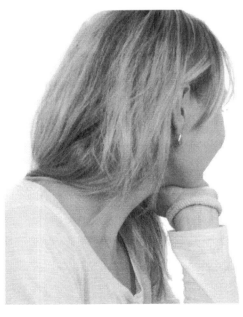

Lucy is trying to communicate with her mother. Language is a uniquely human skill involving verbal and non-verbal aspects.

The history of language

When do human beings start to show signs of language? Communication is present from the moment life is created in the maternal womb. Initially it is biochemical through the substances that pass between the mother and fetus. At birth another type of communication appears which is non-verbal at the outset.

Vision, touch and smell become the mediators of this communication between mother and infant, which will open up to the other senses. When the primitive reflexes integrate at 4 months the maturation of intention begins in the brain. Until then an infant can only grab something if the object touches his hand; he has no intention of grabbing it, but rather it is an automatic reaction. In terms of his mouth, feeding is automatic too; if something touches the infant's face, he turns his head and lips in that direction in order to suck when he subsequently feels the nipple. If you put a finger into an infant's mouth, he will suck that too thanks to the primitive reflexes that guarantee his survival, regardless of his will. At the 4 month stage, the infant begins to «want» and to develop voluntary movement of his hand and mouth towards whatever takes his interest, showing that he wants to suck this or that.

The first more or less articulated sounds appear quite quickly; little babblings that will turn into raspberries at the 6-month stage.

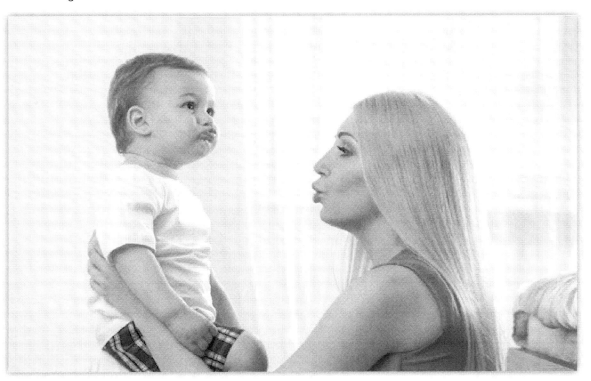

Michael talks non-stop but without using words. Raspberries are a wonderful way to train for using words in the future.

According to Gesell, one of the pioneers of research into child development, an infant acquires his social condition at 6 months. This is the beginning of the long process of integrating into society. According to some lines of psychological thought, it is at this point that the infant conceptualizes the father figure. At 6 months the quality of his verbal and non-verbal expression increases. He will begin to point at things and the wide range of sounds he makes will start to turn into his first words at 9 months. In fact, the first thing an infant does is babble and the inception of verbal language will activate with his ability to understand and pronounce simple words which are almost always nouns that refer to things or people; water, ball, dad, mom, etc.

Infants then progress to two-word sentences with basic grammar. Their speech is telegraphic at this stage. After the age of three a child has a wider grammar that allows him to build sentences which include verbs and words he can combine to express what he wants.

Although the entire human brain evolves from the very first moment, during the first year of life most of this development takes place in the subcortical part in what is known as the «lower» brain. The subcortical or more basic part of the brain deals with automatic functions, while the cortical part, the higher more advanced and eminently human part will develop further from the second year on. But everything in the human being is built on past precedent. The nervous system as a whole develops from the simplest and, indeed, oldest structures and functions both ontogenetically (in a person's development from gestation) and phylogenetically (in the development of the human being through the evolution of the species).

> Although the entire human brain evolves from the very first moment, during the first year of life most of this development takes place in the subcortical part, in what is known as the «lower» brain.

Imagine the following everyday scenario; you are walking down the street with your phone, sending and receiving text messages. The most advanced part of your brain, the cortex, is at work transforming your thoughts and emotions into words that represent the mand that can be recognized by the linguistic "map" of the person receiving our messages. We are able to use certain ways of speaking with those closest to us that could be misinterpreted by others. This is linguistic coding. At the same time the cortex is dealing with language, a huge amount of work is going on in the most archaic part of your brain represented by the spinal cord or the brainstem (the «lower» brain).

A number of structures of this other part of the brain control your gait, the way you put one foot in front of the other and the cadence and span of each step you take. They are in charge of maintaining your balance, even monitoring the peripheral visual information about what there is to the sides of the telephone and behind it, things you are not even aware of. They collect the vestibular perceptions responsible for informing your brain about your head movements so that the image of the words on the phone remains clear. This wouldn't happen if the cervico-ocular adjustment reflexes didn't function properly. Equally, you think about the words, but not about the finger tapping out the spaces. Working out the exact amount of pressure to place on the letters of the keyboard is a voluntary action, but one that is highly modulated by the «lower» brain.

In short, to some extent speech, as an advanced feature, depends on the automatic processes functioning properly. Another example of this can be seen in what happens to your speech when you are learning to drive. When you learn to drive and have to focus on the pedals, changing gears, the steering wheel, traffic and traffic lights, you find you can't even speak. In fact, how often have you said to a fellow passenger; «Don't talk to me now, I'm trying to...» when attempting to park in a difficult spot or during your first solo drives after passing your test? After a while, as these functions become automatized by the «lower» brain, you can talk on the phone and even gesticulate whilst driving (using the hands-free mode, of course).

Language is the cortex's domain whilst verbal expression, a more basic oral communication function in which simpler structures of the nervous system can be used, is not. Talking is not the same as possessing language. Saying or listening to a phrase is not the same as comprehending its ultimate meaning, being able to imagine or understand deep inside what it means or feeling touched by the emotion those words convey. From another perspective it is grammar that sets our language apart from other forms of animal communication. Many other species communicate via calls, shouts, grunts and multiple sounds at different vibration frequencies. But grammar makes language infinitely creative and the sky is the limit in terms of combing words to express new ideas.

> Talking is not the same as possessing language. Saying or listening to a phrase is not the same as comprehending its ultimate meaning, being able to imagine or understand deep inside what it means or feeling touched by the emotion those words convey.

How does language work?

Language operates as a specific mental organ in the brain and is physically located in specialized areas of the cortex. In addition, the fact that the brain is separated into two hemispheres is very important, since language is lateralized in the brain. The left hemisphere is the most verbal side and this is where language can be found in practically everyone, even in left-handed people. The right brain is also responsible for hearing and language, but deals more with prosody. Prosody includes speech elements that are not phonetic units such as vowels or consonants, but that provide an emotional content to the language. Accent, intonation and musicality are controlled by the right hemisphere.

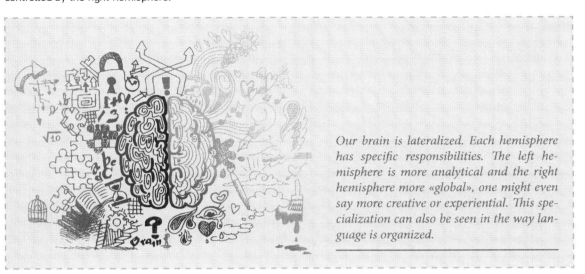

Our brain is lateralized. Each hemisphere has specific responsibilities. The left hemisphere is more analytical and the right hemisphere more «global», one might even say more creative or experiential. This specialization can also be seen in the way language is organized.

Language is located around a central area in the left hemisphere, between the frontal, temporal and parietal areas. There are several specific areas in this zone: Wernicke's area which is next to the auditory cortex at the side of the brain and is responsible for comprehending speech; and Broca's area, located a little further forward very close to the motor cortex, which is in charge of language syntax. It is close to the motor cortex because it is responsible for activating the muscles of the mouth and tongue that can generate the sounds that express what we want to say.

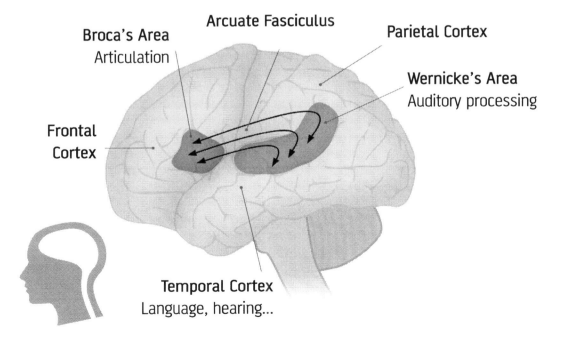

The diagram shows the areas in the left hemisphere of the brain associated with language..

The articulation of sounds is a precise, voluntary action. Even if your speech is so automatic that you are able to talk nineteen to the dozen while doing something else, you still know what you are saying (well, maybe not everyone does). In other words, it's not possible to say something that we don't want to say (except on certain occasions when we say something we shouldn't... but that is more a matter for Freud and could fill the pages of another book!)

The voluntary function of activating the muscles of the mouth requires support from unconscious, automated muscle functions. Try saying this sentence aloud for example: «This book is very exciting and educational». No, don't just think it, say it out loud. Now, afterwards think whether you were breathing in or out as you said it. You were aware of each phoneme but as you will see, not so aware of breathing. Well, it's impossible to make any sound if no air comes out. Okay, now trying saying it as you breathe in, (as if you were sucking air in). What was your voice like? No doubt like something from beyond the grave. Not to mention the difficulty modulating your voice. In the background you brainstem is ensuring that the automatized processes don't interfere with the voluntary ones. Whilst you are busy saying the sentence using your cortex, the most primitive area of your brain deals with the details. Only these details are very important. Some neurologically immature children are incapable of making sounds because their breathing doesn't adjust automatically and they have to learn to exhale first and then pronounce.

The level of coordination between comprehension and speech must be extremely high.

As you can well imagine, comprehension and speech must be highly coordinated. Similarly, there is a communication highway known as the arcuate fasciculus between Wernicke's area and Broca's area, hence, when we want to speak, Wernicke's area sends the structure of what we want to say to Broca's area. Neurology has a pretty good understanding of this channel but it is possible that it may not be fully developed in children under the age of 4 and that they may use other substitutes. For example the thalamus which may act as a distributor of sensory input as well as other input reaching the brain.

The frequencies in the voice spectrum increase when infants handle large objects compared to when they handle small ones.

Interestingly, the frequencies of the voice spectrum increase when infants handle large objects compared to when they handle small ones. This suggests that manipulation has something to do with language. In fact, Broca's area seems to be involved in representing both the arm and the mouth. This is one of many lines of research that support the hypothesis that human speech evolved from hand gestures to a mirror system which included mouthing as hominids evolved. Speech probably became the dominant mode of expression with the emergence of Homo sapiens around 170, 000 years ago. Until then it may have been based on hand and arm gestures. Despite the pervasiveness of speech, hand gestures continue to accompany speech in a number of situations. For example, deaf people use them; we use them to write and they are prevalent in certain cultures and societies. There is growing evidence that speech originated from gestures and not vocalization. Subsequently it seems to have developed as a mirror neuron system for perception, imagination and carrying out manual tasks. In humans it also involves the Broca's area. Ultimately, Broca's area became central to the organization of speech articulation.

There is growing evidence that speech originated from gestures and not vocalization.

Auditory processing and speech

Right from the word go a child listens to the sound environment in which he lives for spatial awareness, to integrate with his social setting, detect hazards and learn to speak. Each deviation in his verbal perception will result in the sound being reproduced incorrectly, likely in the way he perceived it. Sound reception and auditory processing can have a significant bearing on learning disabilities and reading and behavioral disorders.

When we screen for auditory processing, auditory discrimination is assessed in both ears, not just with one specific sound. It's what we call binaural integration (assimilation of input from both ears). If we perceive the sound input from both ears differently, our hearing lacks «sharpness» and this causes confusion. Have you ever had one ear blocked and the other not? It's an unpleasant feeling, right? Just imagine what it feels like to be in a place with lots of background noise and to have this feeling permanently.

Another aspect to consider is the intensity with which we perceive low (background sound) and high-pitched sounds. If there is a significant variation, we will present auditory figure-background problems, or, in other words, difficulty in differentiating a specific sound from other similar ones. Auditory maturity curves improve up to the age of 10 where we find curves similar to those of adults. At younger ages we perceive acute sounds more intensely and this triggers the search reflex. As a child matures, the auditory curve levels off and he can start to sustain his attention for longer periods. But, if our curves are impaired, we will experience difficulties when there is a lot of background noise. This happens to a lot of children with attention deficit and associated auditory impairment.

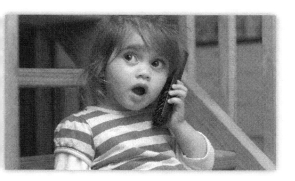

Lily is an expert in communication. The quality of our hearing and how we process the information we hear plays an important role in language.

Sound reception and auditory processing can have a significant bearing on learning disabilities and reading and behavioral difficulties.

When a child reaches school age, difficulties in auditory perception become a tremendous burden for him. Whereas his parents don't mind repeating a word he misunderstands, his teacher speaks at a normal pace, constantly using new words that the child will have to repeat and record in his memory. Poor auditory lateralization may cause him to perceive certain letters or groups of letters the wrong way round. He must place the phonemes he perceives in the right sequence if he is to grasp each word as a whole. Then he must put each word in the right place in the sentence and he will have difficulty grasping the meaning and the message within that sentence. He can do it but only by making a colossal effort which quickly exhausts him and causes him to lose concentration. Moreover, he will need much more time to do his homework leading to further exhaustion.

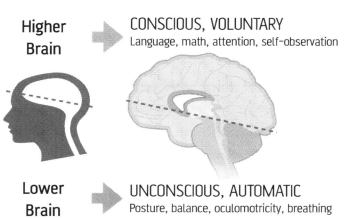

Higher Brain → CONSCIOUS, VOLUNTARY
Language, math, attention, self-observation

Lower Brain → UNCONSCIOUS, AUTOMATIC
Posture, balance, oculomotricity, breathing

«There is an almost constant parallelism between the precise quality of our perception of the external sound world on the one hand and, on the other, our way of being, behaving and reacting».

Guy Berard

The diagram shows our two brains: the higher one for voluntary, uniquely human skills and the lower one for the automatic operation of our most basic functions.

Problems with language development

Just as occurs with many other brain functions like vision, language develops in a very specific, crucial period; an early stage in which the child must experience language, otherwise brain maturation will not be activated in the neurological structures that control it. And the reality is that not all children develop language functions properly.

Simply put, problems with language development may relate to sound reception, sound and language processing and, last but not least, producing speech sounds. In a nutshell, these are problems of input, processing and output. But as it is a comprehensive, interrelated process, it is likely that if there are problems in one of these three areas, the other two will suffer the consequences. So, if I don't hear well, it is likely I won't process properly or will only do so with great effort. If I don't process language properly, I will reproduce sounds that are incorrect or respond out of context and therefore my response will be inappropriate. In the same way, development aphasia is a language processing disorder, but obviously the symptoms only become apparent through speech. From a clinical point of view it is very hard to differentiate. It is also possible that some problems are related to an impairment in processes that are closely linked, such as visual processing in developmental dyslexia (specific reading disorder).

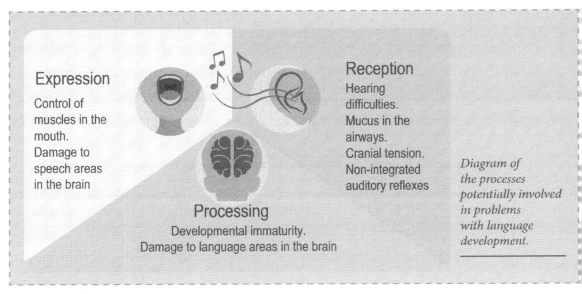

Expression

Control of muscles in the mouth.
Damage to speech areas in the brain

Reception

Hearing difficulties.
Mucus in the airways.
Cranial tension.
Non-integrated auditory reflexes

Processing

Developmental immaturity.
Damage to language areas in the brain

Diagram of the processes potentially involved in problems with language development.

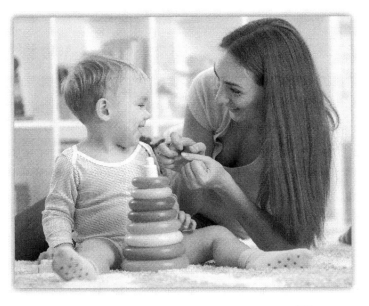

Liam is playing with his mother and loving it! He is communicating with her verbally and non verbally. Her hand actions mirror her words and this helps him to understand. However, it is important she verbalizes using the richest vocabulary and most vibrant tone possible for her baby.

Problems with sound reception: input

It appears that the human being has an innate capacity for language, but infants need external stimuli too in order to develop language. The way parents vocalize creates imprints (brain maps) that help the child to vocalize correctly as he grows up. His parents' voices and the voices of others around him trigger brain connections for the development of verbal expression and language. If he doesn't receive the right stimuli or if problems in his vestibular system prevent him from perceiving them correctly, both his processing and subsequently, his speech, will be affected.

We have a habit of modifying and simplifying our language and sometimes exaggerating our intonation when we talk to children. We refrain from using certain words in an attempt to make our interactions more infant-friendly although this way of communicating with children may prevent them from reaching their full potential. Yet it also seems that vocalizing slowly and using mime and gesturing helps create better vocalization later on. Speech therapists use it as part of their treatment because there are also elements of vision and movement in language.

If a child doesn't receive the right stimuli or if problems in his vestibular system prevent him from perceiving them correctly, both his processing and subsequently, his speech, will be affected.

Likewise, there are certain problems that can affect how well infants and children perceive and process sounds. The Pre-school to Elementary School stage is characterized by mucus. In fact, small children seem to have mucus almost 24/7. Sometimes it can make them breathe through their mouths and form big bubbles in their nostrils when they exhale. During this phase you are constantly chasing after your child with a handkerchief. Otitis usually strikes between the ages of 2 and 4 and there are several key reasons for this. Firstly, it could be immunological. Mucus is a protection system that triggers the immune system to deal with possible threats. During this period a child's immune system undergoes a major training process which is why coming into contact with other children and substances not encountered previously at home, activates the mucous membranes to deal with a possible infection.

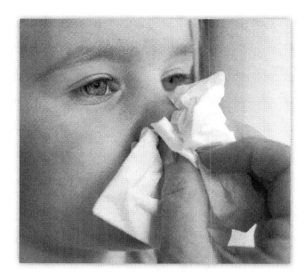

The continued presence of mucus alters our hearing and can accelerate the onset of otitis. Respiratory physiotherapy is highly effective in draining mucus and teaching parents the correct way to perform nasal washes.

The second factor which is also immunological could be the hypersensitivity some children have to dairy products. The excessive consumption of milk has long been associated with the production of mucus in the respiratory tract, although this cannot be explained by the allergy paradigm and there is very little medical evidence to prove this causality. The incidence of true allergy to the protein in cow's milk is 2-3%. Although cow's milk is a very nutrient-rich food, it is also a very controversial food and, contrary to what people usually think, it's not something humanity always had access to. Human beings have been as we know them today for the best part of a million years but it was only with the development of livestock production around 10,000 years ago that milk became part of our staple diet. In western countries milk still forms part of the basic recommendations for children, but this isn't the case in all cultures. In eastern countries, the Amazon and Polynesia, milk is not part of the population's staple diet and there is no record of children having more health problems because of it (leaving aside other aspects such as hygiene or social development). In fact, in the entire history of mankind there has never been one universal diet eaten by all human beings, including the more than 20 species of hominids that have been present over the last 5-7 million years.

The third factor in the high incidence of otitis in childhood is the bony architecture of the face. The Eustachian tubes which are the drainage tubes leading from the ear to the larynx, have less of a slope than in adults, and obviously, are smaller in size. This makes drainage difficult. These tubes let air from outside into the inside of the eardrum thus equalizing the pressure of the inner and outer ear. Moreover, if our airways and sinuses are full of mucus, it is much easier to develop inflammation and infections. From the age of 4, the face undergoes a morphological change that also affects the way these drainage routes slope and the frequency of otitis tends to decrease. Meanwhile it is essential parents know how to perform regular nasal irrigations in the correct manner. The most popular way of squirting syringes full of physiological saline up the nose is neither ideal nor comfortable or effective. Nasal irrigation requires a continuous stream of fluid, not sudden squirts. With effective respiratory physiotherapy techniques, a pediatric physiotherapist should be able to get rid of mucus not just in the upper tracts, but also in the bronchial tubes. Many parents begin to see the light at the end of the tunnel the moment a physiotherapist starts to help free their child of mucus.

Meanwhile it is essential parents know how to perform regular nasal irrigation in the correct manner.

Finally, the amount of mucus and the influence it has on the episodes of otitis has a lot to do with the way in which the sinuses and the palate have developed. If the face has not been able to broaden out sufficiently and the palate is high or narrow, the space behind the nose will be much smaller and this can easily lead to an accumulation of mucus and swelling of the adenoids. Enlarged adenoids are also associated with breathing through the mouth, snoring and otitis but they can also be the result of excess mucus and limited space with swelling and repeated infections. This is why it is essential that an infant's face grows and broadens properly as he develops, so that there is sufficient air space behind it. Pediatric physiotherapists specializing in PIMT can evaluate and treat the infant's skull and face and support their development.

Returning to the subject of otitis, as we saw earlier the first 4 years of life are vital for programming many systems. One system that is particularly sensitive to this need for early programming in life is the auditory system. We hear different types of sounds and our brain is programmed to process them properly and to repeat them correctly later. If our airways are full of mucus and our ear is under pressure from poorly drained mucus, the two sides of the eardrum don't have equal atmospheric pressure and it can't vibrate properly. As a result, the sound we perceive is distorted and the sounds we register are different. Subsequently, a child starts to mispronounce

some sounds; it appears he can't hear certain conversations or tones of voice properly and, something which will become more relevant later on, it seems he doesn't understand what he hears in certain situations.

Problems processing

Even if sounds are perceived correctly, other factors are necessary in order to process and learn language properly. Firstly, we need to understand that although there are specific areas for the development and execution of language, the whole nervous system is responsible for language in a global context, not just certain areas of the brain. Although the spinal cord may not appear to have anything to do with communication or language, it too plays a very important role by informing the nervous system about posture, arm and hand movements and breathing, all of which are heavily involved in both verbal and non-verbal communication. Remember that it is very difficult to talk if you are unable to speak and exhale at the same time.

There is a very interesting study on five year olds with severe and moderate language and speech disorders which is helpful for understanding the relationship between language and the overall development of the nervous system. The research showed that the children had obvious difficulty with gross motor development tasks such as leg strength, jumping ability or hand-grip strength.

Language processing may be affected by damage to the areas of the brain responsible for language. However, if this damage is caused perinatally and compensated, it is very difficult to find the lesions in MRI scans or other imaging tests.

The most common form is developmental aphasia probably caused by damage to Wernicke's area in the left hemisphere of the brain. A diagnosis is reached by thoroughly examining the child's medical records from birth and sometimes by carrying out neuropsychological procedures and special tests. The main symptom is speech delay and difficulty understanding speech. Developmental aphasia isn't always directly related to academic performance but it does have a bearing on social development.

Dyslexia may be the result of damage or dysfunction in a different area of the left hemisphere between the parietal and temporal lobes. The main characteristic is a visual perceptual impairment and the effect this has on hearing and speech on the one hand and visual perception in cognitive processes on the other. In dyslexia, the main symptom is difficulty with reading and writing combined with left-right confusion.

The two hemispheres of the brain are connected by numerous pathways that form the corpus callosum and it is essential they work together. It is worth remembering that the left hemisphere is responsible for language and is more analytical, and the right hemisphere is in charge of the body map and spatial relations. Difficulties with reading and writing can be linked to problems with the body map and spatial relations as well as poor communication between the right hemisphere which locates letters in space or a left-right relationship, and the left hemisphere which gives them sound and meaning.

Speech impairment

Even if we perceive and process sounds properly, in order to be able to produce sounds the shape of our mouth and the position of our teeth and tongue must be right and our mouth and tongue muscles must work closely together. Some infants experience difficulty latching on correctly the first time they breastfeed, and midwives play an important role in helping mothers during this crucial period. If an infant suffers a traumatic birth involving their head being under tremendous pressure for a long time, they may experience damage to the nerves which emerge from the back of the skull and are responsible for the mouth and tongue muscles and swallowing. They are the hypoglossal nerve (cranial nerve XII) and the glossopharyngeal nerve (cranial nerve IX). Damage to these nerves can result in difficulty sucking or fatigue and the infant appears to tire of sucking straight away and falls asleep.

There are different ways of spotting potential cranial disorders in these nerves. For example, you may notice the infant's lips are asymmetrical when he cries or that his tongue is lateralized; up to 12 weeks an infant can only move his tongue up and down which is the exact movement he needs to push the nipple and extract the milk. Lateralization of the tongue before this stage is a sign of cranial nerve dysfunction. Again, early intervention with PIMT will allow the infant to breastfeed successfully, integrate the primitive reflexes associated with the mouth correctly and speak properly later on.

Some children have difficulties with verbal expression. However, the telltale sign they have a problem with speaking and not processing is when it also affects their eating. For example, children who find chewing difficult or painful and mealtimes become arduous affairs for their parents; children who have difficulty swallowing or who refuse to eat certain food textures, etc. As you can imagine, if the problem affects the coordination of the muscles in the mouth, this has an impact on everything the mouth does, not just on language.

As you can imagine, if the problem affects the coordination of the muscles in the mouth, this has an impact on everything the mouth does, not just on language.

The specialists who help children with these kinds of disorders are speech therapists. However, they can be of even greater help if specialist physiotherapists administer treatment to the child's cranium either beforehand or simultaneously.

Specific reading disability.... rather than calling it dyslexia

Developmental dyslexia is a medical diagnosis that refers to a major, specific difficulty with reading skills that cannot be explained by a lack of general intelligence, opportunities to learn, general motivation or sensory acuity. As we will see later on in the chapter on learning disabilities, a diagnosis of developmental dyslexia runs the risk of labelling the child. Therefore, in our opinion, it would be better to apply the broader term used in education and refer to it as a «specific reading disability». Statistics say that between 10 and 17% of people in developed countries could be affected. The data varies greatly because the diagnostic criteria for defining dyslexia versus an overall language disorder or an attention disorder also vary.

Developmental dyslexia is a medical diagnosis but it would be better to apply the term «specific reading disability».

The first fundamental difference that needs to be established is whether there is difficulty decoding written letters to sound (accuracy or fluency when reading aloud) or with comprehension (the ability to understand what we read). These are two very different types of reading disability, although both depend on the development of oral language. Decoding difficulties can be referred to as developmental dyslexia relating to problems with oral language development, with the development of skills relating to speech and sound (phonological awareness) or visual skills. On the other hand, comprehension difficulties are also linked to difficulties with oral language though more associated with understanding the meaning of words or assimilating grammar.

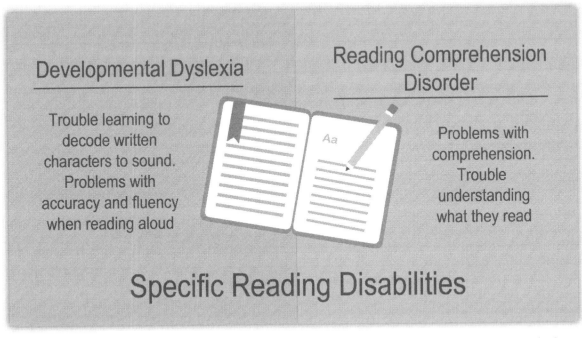

It is important to differentiate between decoding and comprehension difficulties, though they may both play a role in language development.

Many children with specific reading disabilities also have attention and hyperactivity issues or motor coordination problems. This makes it really difficult to diagnose and requires a new paradigm for learning disabilities as discussed earlier; one with a more comprehensive vision of the child that takes their neurodevelopment into account and embraces a more biopsychosocial approach.

Contrary to what many people think, the process of learning to read doesn't begin when the child starts school, it starts much earlier, in the preschool years. You could say that it begins in the first months of life, with the development of hearing, language (the first sounds we make), and vision. Learning to read is one of the keys to education as we know it in the developed world and children who have difficulty reading get caught in a spiral of academic failure. Attempts have been made to discover the factors that may cause a child to develop reading disabilities. Familiarity with letters and sounds, the vocabulary the child uses, his ability to mimic sentences and tell stories are all important signs in predicting if a preschooler will experience reading disabilities.

Developmental dyslexia is often associated with changes in phonological awareness, the ability to recognize and work with the sounds of spoken language. Phonological Theory is the classical and most widely accepted theory amongst educational experts and it is still the prevalent theory today. One hypothesis is that a lack of phonological awareness hinders the ability to convert the map of sounds from their equivalent visual letters, causing a blockage in reading fluency. However, the difficulty in science when two phenomena coincide is establishing if one is the cause of the other, or if they are both the result of the same, unknown problem. Methodological concerns about the research and the absence of positive results in reading skills despite an improvement in phonological awareness, have led some researchers to uphold other hypotheses which co-exist alongside the main one. These include; auditory processing, attention deficit and several theories that blame the visual system such as the magnocellular-dorsal deficit theory and visual crowding.

The magnocellular theory is based on the fact that children with dyslexia have problems in the visual pathways that process movement and depth, while the visual crowding theory sustains that children with dyslexia also have difficulties recognizing written characters when they are surrounded by other similar ones (and we are not talking just about letters). Both the movement that is undoubtedly sensed when the eyes move over a text and the ability to recognize a letter amongst other similar ones, are obviously important aspects of reading. It shouldn't be difficult to accept that several decodings are necessary; the first one being visual.

Faced with this situation, specialists can adopt one of two opposing stances: selective fanaticism or open cooperation. Many experts become obsessed with their own theory, sometimes to justify the priority of their work over that of others. However, successful specialists always work as a team and have an open outlook. It doesn't take an Einstein to figure out that no human being, specialist, or theory has a 360º vision of reality. It is clear that the human being is a set of interrelated biological systems (and much more besides) and in the same way, the brain's role in successfully communicating different areas that correspond to different systems is undeniable. From this perspective it should be relatively easy to understand that the areas of vision which gather written input, do not connect well with the areas of language that try to interpret them and give them an associated sound and meaning. It is a communication problem between the visual, on the one hand, and the phonological (or the auditory or responsible for associating what we see with what we know and give it meaning), on the other. But in which children is this problem linked slightly more to one side than the other? How can we tell?

Faced with this situation, specialists can adopt one of two opposing stance: selective fanaticism or open cooperation.

Would it not be better if optometrists and hearing and language specialists worked side by side doing everything in their power to clear the way for the other? Surely this would be the most comprehensive and honest help we could offer a child with difficulties? Or can just one specialist single-handedly cure a health problem? There is no drug in the world that can fix a health problem on a lasting basis unless the individual in question makes lifestyle changes too.

Would it not be better if optometrists and hearing and language specialists worked side by side doing everything in their power to clear the way for the other?

Finally, all that remains for me is to remind you that purely human cognitive skills like reading and writing rely on the neurological development of the «lower», automatic brain, the one in charge of sensorimotor programming. And this development requires the infant to complete the necessary stages of its development and receive the appropriate stimuli. In the case of specific reading disabilities that concur with attention or coordination issues, it is essential we build a solid base, the foundations of the building. The developmental physiotherapist can provide the terrain so that vision and language specialists can build their part. Nobody would start work on the roof without first checking that the foundations and pillars of the building were sound. Those of us who work successfully in neurodevelopment always rely on a good team made up of different experts.

What can you do?
HELPFUL PRACTICAL ADVICE

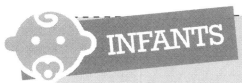 INFANTS

- Stimulate your baby's rooting and sucking reflexes. Don't simply «latch» him onto the bottle or your nipple, allow him to do some searching on his own. This will help considerably in developing his mouth and the sensorimotor programs linked to it. You can do this by gently touching around his lips with the nipple or bottle nipple so that he actively moves his head, lips and tongue in search of food. This is a simple but essential form of stimulation.

- Gently stroke the palms of his hands as he breastfeeds. This will activate the Babkin reflex which aids suction. The Babkin reflex forms part of the neural substrate which maintains the motor skills of the mouth and relates them to the hands.

- If your baby has trouble breastfeeding and also suffers from colic or irritability, find a pediatric physio-therapist specializing in PIMT to check his neck and head. The nerves that control the mouth muscles emerge from the back of the skull and in slow or difficult births they may have been under pressure during birth. In infants, most cases of colic are related to neck pain, particularly when they are accompanied by irritability and show up at unspecified times during the evening. This can be treated very easily with specialized physiotherapy.

- Speak to him affectionately with vibrant tone of voice, but at the same time ensuring you vocalize clearly. Your facial gestures should mirror your words. Many infants are confused when their parents say «No honey, you mustn't hit» with a big smile on their face. Human beings rely more on non verbal language and mimicry (both hand and mouth) than on words. You don't have to be angry to pull a face that matches your words, especially when you want to correct behavior. This works with older children too. The same goes for positive language.

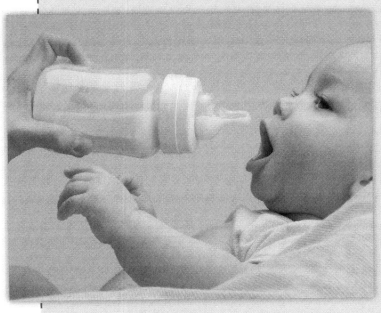

Make the most of each feed to stimulate your baby's rooting reflexes. They have a major influence on his neurological development.

- Keep his upper airways free of mucus. Learn how to perform a nasal irrigation using a steady flow rather than a syringe. Ask a pediatric physiotherapist to show you how. Keeping his airways clear prevents the development of otitis, improves breathing and sleep, prevents auditory perceptual disorders and allows the bones in the face to develop properly.

- If your baby suffers from bronchiolitis or lower respiratory tract conditions, ask a pediatric physiotherapist to perform respiratory physiotherapy on him as soon as possible. There is no question that this is immensely beneficial for your baby as he is developing. The same goes for older children with respiratory problems. People don't realize just how helpful it can be.

- It seems a pacifier can be helpful during the first year. Some studies suggest it can prevent sudden infant death syndrome. However, after the first year it can have drawbacks including an increased risk of developing ear infections. Slowly but surely you should gently wean him off it. You can give him other «substitutes» like a comfort blanket or soft toy that he can suck on to soothe himself while smelling the reassuring scent of his own saliva or the maternal odor of his mom. Under no circumstances should he be allowed to replace it with his thumb as this will deform his palate and teeth. If this happens, remove his thumb immediately before it becomes impossible to break the habit. Some children may use their thumb as a way of stimulating their palate to release pressure in the head. Again, we recommend you consult a pediatric physiotherapist specializing in the orofacial region. He will be able to check that all is well.

OLDER CHILDREN

- Keep older children's upper respiratory tracts clear of mucus too. Learn how to perform a nasal irrigation using a steady flow rather than a syringe. Ask a pediatric physiotherapist to show you how. Keeping their airways clear prevents ear infections from developing, improves breathing and sleep, prevents auditory perceptual disorders and allows the facial bones to develop properly.

- Talk to your child using the widest possible range of vocabulary. Don't limit your language to make it easier for him. On the contrary, the greater the stimulation, the faster we learn. The wealth of sounds and words he hears from you during his pre-school period will have a bearing on his language development later on, unless of course has other disorders. Seize the opportunity to introduce a second language while he is still small. There's no time to lose. From the age of 6 or 7 it will be more difficult for him to recognize and reproduce new sounds.

- Encourage your child to tell you stories about things that have happened to him. Let him tell you things, ask him questions and let him explain things to you, what is this or that for? This is particularly important in trauma cases or when children have experienced extremely stressful situations. Let him share it with you and allow him to tell you the same thing over and over as often as he needs to, reassuring him at the end that you understand and that he is safe now. Telling stories also helps him to learn how to sequence events and structure time as well as encouraging him to visualize. Ask him questions about his stories using the different sensory channels as this helps him to become aware of what he sees, hears and feels, as well as of all his senses.

- If your child barely speaks, get help as soon as possible to check he is developing properly and make sure he doesn't have difficulties in other areas such as social relationships, independence, fine motor skills and motor skills in general. The sooner he receives stimulation, the better the outcome will be. Get a developmental physiotherapist to carry out the assessment and recommend the best specialists to help your child. Once his overall development has been assessed, a speech therapist's skills will be essential.

- If your child mispronounces some sounds or if it seems he can't hear properly sometimes or that certain sounds bother him; if he has gone through periods where he had a lot of mucus and nasal or ear congestion, his auditory processing may be incorrectly programed. This usually happens between the ages of 2 and 4. Around the age of 5 (under the age of 5 the test is not very reliable), a specialist audiologist should carry out a qualitative review of his hearing. If there are signs of hearing loss or deafness it is important you contact an otolaryngologistal though certain aspects of pronunciation or hypersensitivity will require different types of audiometry. A hearing and language expert and other auditory training specialists will be able to help him. This may also be useful in the case of certain language problems.

- If you were unable to accompany your child in his early stages of development because you weren't aware it was necessary or because of other difficulties he may have had (illnesses, hospitalizations, etc.), don't panic it can all be programmed later. The brain is an amazing thing and sometimes has the ability to find alternative ways to build or repair itself. If you consider that your child's difficulties are related to language development, there are several specialists who can be of tremendous help. Speech therapists, speech, language and hearing experts and psychologists will all be able to stimulate and enhance his communication and language development. There are some amazing specialists in these areas. Never give up hope – there is always a way to help your child progress!

BIBLIOGRAPHY

Regarding the neurobiological basis of learning disabilities:

> Krishnan S, Watkins KE, Bishop DVM. Neurobiological Basis of Language Learning Difficulties. Trends in Cognitive Sciences; 2016.

Regarding how the development of handedness could contribute to the development of language:

> Michel GF, Babik I, Nelson EL, Campbell JM, Marcinowski EC. How the development of handedness could contribute to the development of language. Developmental Psychobiology. 2013;55(6):608-20.

Regarding how grammar makes language infinitely creative:

> Eliot L. What's going on in there? How the brain and mind develop in the first five years of life. Bantam Books; 1999.

Regarding the evolution of the Western diet and its health implications:

> Bartley J, McGlashan SR. Does milk increase mucus production? Med Hypotheses. 2010 Apr;74(4):732-4.

> Cordain L, Eaton SB, Sebastian A, Mann N, Lindeberg S, Watkins BA, et al. Origins and evolution of the Western diet: health implications for the 21st century. The American Journal of Clinical Nutrition. 2005;81(2):341-54.

Host A, Halken S. Cow's milk allergy: where have we come from and where are we going? Endocr Metab Immune Disord Drug Targets. 2014 Mar;14(1):2-8.

Regarding auditory training:

Bérard G. Reeducación auditiva para el éxito escolar y el bienestar emocional. Biblioteca   Nueva; 2010.

Regarding how infants change their speech according to what they touch:

Bernardis P, Bello A, Pettenati P, Stefanini S, Gentilucci M. Manual actions affect vocalizations of infants. Exp Brain Res. 2008 Feb;184(4):599-603.

Regarding the relationship between language and gestures:

Corballis MC. Language as gesture. Hum Mov Sci. 2009 Oct;28(5):556-65.

Rizzolatti G, Arbib MA. Language within our grasp. Trends Neurosci. 1998 May;21(5):188-94.

Regarding the relationship between developmental disorders and language disorders:

Müürsepp I, Ereline J, Gapeyeva H, Pääsuke M. Motor performance in 5-year-old preschool children with developmental speech and language disorders. Acta Paediatr. 2009 Aug;98(8):1334-8.

Regarding the definition of developmental dyslexia:

Habib M. The neurological basis of developmental dyslexia: an overview and working hypothesis. Brain. 2000 Dec;123 Pt 12:2373-99.

Regarding dyslexia and specific reading disabilities:

Hulme C, Snowling MJ. Developmental disorders of language, learning andcognition. Chichester, UK: Wiley-Blackwell; 2009.

Hulme C, Snowling MJ. Reading disorders and dyslexia. Curr Opin Pediatr. 2016 Dec;28(6):731-5.

McCardle P, Scarborough HS, Catts HW. Predicting, explaining and preventing children's reading difficulties. Learning Disabilities Research & Practice. 2001;16:230-9.

Peterson RL, Pennington BF. Developmental dyslexia. Lancet. 2012;379(9830):1997-2007.

Regarding the phonological deficit hypothesis in dyslexia:

Galuschka K, Ise E, Krick K, Schulte-Körne G. *Effectiveness of treatment approaches for children and adolescents with reading disabilities: A meta-analysis of randomized controlled trials. PLoS One. 2014;9(2):e89900.*

Hornickel J, Kraus N. *Unstable representation of sound: A biological marker of dyslexia. Journal of Neuroscience, 2013;33:3500-4.*

Vellutino FR, Fletcher JM, Snowling MJ, Scanlon DM. *Specific reading disability (dyslexia): What have we learned in the past four decades? Journal of Child Psychology and Psychiatry. 2004;45:2-40.*

Regarding the visual deficit hypothesis in dyslexia:

Gori S, Facoetti A. *How the visual aspects can be crucial in reading acquisition? The intriguing case of crowding and developmental dyslexia. Journal of Vision. 2015 Jan 14;15(1):8.*

Stein J. *Visual contributions to reading difficulties: The magnocellular theory. En: Stein J, Kapoula Z, eds. Visual aspect of dyslexia. Oxford, UK: Oxford University Press; 2012.*

Stein J, Walsh V. *To see but not to read: The magnocellular theory of dyslexia. Trends in Neuroscience. 1997;20:147-52.*

Whitney D, Levi DM. *Visual crowding: A fundamental limit on conscious perception and object recognition. Trends in Cognitive Science. 2011;15(4):160-8.*

Reading the development of language in the classroom:

Álvarez C. *Las leyes naturales del niño. La revolución de la educación en la escuela y en casa. Aguilar; 2017.*

Chapter 8

Children and pain
Pain is programmed too

Iñaki Pastor Pons

Infants, children and young people often complain of pain, generally caused by headaches, stomach aches, muscle aches, growing pains, etc. However, just as with adults, how often and how intensely children feel pain and how they adapt to it can vary greatly. For some children, pain can be chronic or severe and take a huge toll on the day-to-day life of the whole family. This is why pain is fast becoming a top priority for scientists, as on the one hand they seek to identify the factors that may influence the experience of pain and, on the other, establish if these factors can be acted upon to make it more manageable.

Neuroscience is advancing rapidly in its understanding of the mechanisms that produce or perpetuate pain in chronic pain sufferers. There are more and more studies on the subject and little by little we are beginning to understand some aspects that until recently were completely unknown.

Nowadays there is general consensus that, although pain usually appears as a result of injury or tissue damage (though it isn't always clear that there is a physical cause for it), quite often the frequency or intensity cannot be explained by physical causes alone. This means that the amount of tissue damage is not proportional to the pain the person experiences.

One of the fundamental aspects in the quest to understand pain is the existence of "modulators". These cause people with the same injury to suffer significantly more, or less. What are these modulators? Modulators can be their own past experiences or those of people close to them; their fears; beliefs about pain; a fear of the unknown; sociocultural aspects or a fear of the consequences this pain may cause in the person's life. When one or more of these modulators is active, the individual may feel much more or much less pain than another with a comparable amount of damage. It is as if an alarm bell goes off inside their brain telling them just how dangerous this pain could be for them.

The most powerful modulators are probably our own experiences in early life, even before we are able to speak, in addition to those of our parents or those close to us when we were children. In a household where one of the parents suffered headaches, years later you will very likely find that some of their children do too. The same applies to back pain and other types of pain. This is an environmental problem, not a genetic one because our early experiences in life shape the way we face a particular situation for the rest of our lives.

It is important to understand how our attitude towards our own pain and that of our children, patients and students will shape the way they experience pain in the future. This may seem strange, but read on because it could turn out to be a watershed moment for you and your loved ones.

When do we start to feel pain?

Neonates have the so-called heel prick test done when they are just a few hours old. Even at this stage an infant's grimace tells us that she is able to feel pain. In line with other sensory responses, pain is one of the most developed senses an infant experiences. The ability to feel pain probably develops around the third trimester of life in the womb.

The medical profession has only become fully aware of neonates' sensitivity to pain in the last few years. Before this, whilst it was obvious that infants clearly reacted to painful experiences, it was thought that they were incapable of really feeling them because the cerebral cortex was very underdeveloped. This is why all kinds of invasive procedures were carried out on them without using anesthesia or analgesia, including operations.

Now that we know that the cortex starts to work before birth, it is clear that many aspects of pain sensitivity are already perceived even by premature infants. This has led to a rethink when it comes to treating infants.

So, what do infants feel when confronted by a painful stimulus? Well, they cry, of course, and there is evidence that they cry harder than they do when they are hungry or in discomfort. Typical reactions include grimacing and adopting certain postures, as well as other responses such as an increase in the stress hormones in the blood, accelerated breathing or heart rate. What seems clear is that the ability to locate pain in the body is something that develops rapidly in the first years of life as your brain maps become more accurate.

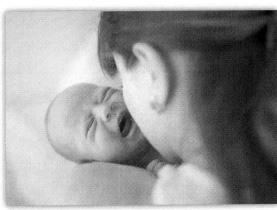

The way Mason cries when he is in pain is clearly different to the way he cries when he is hungry. The challenge is to figure out what is causing him distress in order to help him.

It is important to treat pain in infants. Although there is no precise way of diagnosing pain in neonates, we must find the source and alleviate their suffering so it doesn't become chronic. This is important because pain interferes with growth, leads to a distorted perception of pain in the future and impairs cognitive and behavioral development.

It is important to treat pain in infants

Even though there is no conscious memory of the first years of life, infants possess other types of memory that affect learning models. Painful events can have an impact on certain patterns of emotional or physical responses and, in the long term, on their minds.

What is not so obvious to many people is the need to treat infants who cry uncontrollably because of back or neck pain.

Clearly infants must be protected from painful experiences both during diagnostic procedures and operations. What is not so obvious to many people is the need to treat infants who cry uncontrollably due to back or neck pain. The difficulty diagnosing these cases means they are often confused with purely digestive problems like colic (bear in mind that the digestive function depends on the vagus nerve which stems from the back of the head). In our experience, Pediatric Integrative Manual Therapy (PIMT) is hugely beneficial in treating the colic and resulting pain these infants suffer. We have found that it not only improves areas such as posture control and movement on the official scales of development but also levels of calmness and quality of sleep.

Pain… is it a good thing?

So, what is pain? Well, probably something that everyone is familiar with but that each of us would describe in a totally different way. Pain is one of the great mysteries of life and one of the most powerful motivators of human behavior. Some say that it is an alarm bell from the area that has been injured, but what about those major accidents where people feel no pain? Did you know that in an accidental amputation the person feels no pain until they see the wound or are out of danger? Others will say that it is your body's way of telling you there is something wrong. Still others will say that it is unimaginable agony. Some will say it is punishment for your sins or something that tests your faith.

A scientist would say that it is a particular pattern of brain activity. Scientists agree that pain is an unpleasant physical and emotional sensation in the body that causes us to change our behavior to protect ourselves. No one in the world of science believes any longer that the intensity of pain is equal to the amount of damage done to the tissue.

An unpleasant physical and emotional sensation in our body that makes us want to change our behavior to protect ourselves.

You may have heard someone exclaim «this pain is killing me», «it feels like I'm being stabbed» or «I could rip this leg off». Who in their right mind could think that pain is a good thing? But the fact of the matter is that it's a very good thing: a quantum leap of nature. Now you are thinking: «This guy has gone completely crazy...». Allow me to explain...

For many years now I have seen people with pain on a daily basis as part of my job as a physiotherapist; in fact this is the main reason they came to see me. But once I had a visit from a girl who had been practically paralyzed from the waist down following an accident. After several operations they had been able to recover some of the nerves so she could just about walk with the help of crutches. What she had lost was the sensitivity in her legs, and as a result, any sensitivity to pain. She once told me how she had stood next to a hot stove without realizing that she was getting burnt. She was only aware of the danger because of the smell of burning flesh; her own flesh. Can you imagine that? How must she have felt when she looked down and saw her flesh burning and the bone almost visible? And so I ask you again: is pain a good thing?

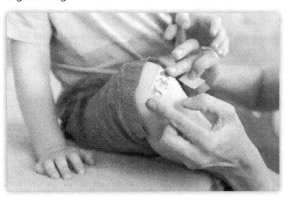

James has fallen. The comments his mom makes and the way she applies the band-aid will have an effect on how much pain he suffers.

Yes, pain is one of our most advanced and key defense mechanisms. It is one of the greatest evolutions of natu-re, because not only does it activate the muscles to flee aggression, but it also triggers neuro-hormonal activity for an enhanced adaptation and survival response. It also includes systems of prognosis and learning so that we don't get close to the source of danger. Pain is one of nature's wonders but for it to do its job of protecting you, it must be a truly unpleasant experience of the worst possible kind. Only an unpleasant experience and feeling will allow it to fulfil its protective function of keeping you away from the source of pain. Should the sound of a fire alarm be soft and melodic to make people exit from a building as quickly as possible? Of course not, for it to be of any use it must be as unpleasant as possible.

Pain is one of your most advanced, key defense mechanisms.

You don't have anything as specific as a pain receptor. However, you do have nerves that specialize in detecting potentially dangerous changes in temperature, chemical balance and pressure. These danger detectors or nociceptors send alerts to the brain, but do not send pain as pain is produced in the brain itself.

Pain depends on how the brain assesses a large amount of information from the environment through the sensory pathways and from our mind (such as expectations, previous experiences, culture, social norms or beliefs). Of course, all the danger receptors distributed around the body are the brain's sensors. When there is a sudden change in the state of the tissues, these sensors are our first line of defense: they alert the brain, mobilize inflammation mechanisms, launch their own immune system cells into the blood and begin the process of tissue repair.

In order to understand how we become aware of pain and how it works in real life in people with real pain, we can apply the simple principle that any credible evidence that the body is in danger and that protective behavior would be beneficial, will increase the probability and intensity of pain. On the other hand, any indication that the body is safe will decrease its likelihood and intensity. It is as simple and as complicated as that.

There are several studies that provide a practical illustration of this relationship between the perception of danger and the intensity of pain, but one, I feel, is particularly enlightening. Several groups of people in different environments were touched on the hand with a very cold piece of metal (-20 degrees). The stimulus was clearly very painful as it had the potential to burn them. One group was shown a red light whilst the other group a pale blue light. Subsequently they were asked about their experience and their responses measured according to the unpleasantness and intensity of the pain. The group shown the red light experienced significantly more pain in a more unpleasant way. Interesting, isn't it? Notice that both groups received the same painful stimulus at the same time, on the same hand, but their perceptions were completely different.

People today are afraid of pain

We live in a society and at a time in history with some very interesting characteristics compared to other eras. Technologically we are very advanced and in some countries people enjoy a high quality of life and security allowing them to develop their personal and professional projects. Some writers say that we are becoming a hedonistic society in search of pleasure and entertainment. Of course, the indications are that this type of lifestyle is hard to reconcile with pain.

In the world ranking of the 100 best-selling medicines carried out by IMS Health, anti-inflammatories and analgesics occupy pole position. We are very fortunate that medicine can make our lives freer from suffering. But there is something we need to understand. Inevitably, every person in the world will suffer pain at some point in their life and probably more than once. As a parent you will not be able to protect your children from feeling either the physical or emotional pain they will experience for all kinds of different reasons and at different points in their lives. All you can do is help them to live these experiences in the best possible way, through love and understanding.

As a parent you will not be able to protect your children from feeling either the physical or emotional pain they will experience for all kinds of different reasons and at different points in their lives. All you can do is help them to live these experiences in the best possible way, through love and understanding.

When a child falls and hurts herself, most parents are inclined to rush over in alarm whilst nervously repeating: «It's nothing honey, it's nothing!». They pat all around the affected area hoping desperately that their child isn't in any pain. Often at the first sign of even the slightest fever, children are given Paracetamol or Ibuprofen in an attempt to alleviate even the slightest symptoms or discomfort.

At our clinic, where we treat many infants and children every single day with extremely gentle and surprisingly effective techniques, we see them cry during treatment. Not because it hurts but because they have to lie down, or because they can't move around as much as they would like, or they don't understand what is happening to them, or simply because they are hungry. It is surprising just how many mothers and fathers we see suffering because of this, despite the fact that the child is simply complaining and that they are present in the room and can see for themselves that it is a safe, caring environment. The interesting thing is that many other infants and children fall asleep during exactly the same treatment.

It is a sobering thought that many parents cannot stand to see their child in any pain or discomfort, even when it is for their own good. I have witnessed a mother crying because her child was complaining during (completely pain-free) treatment: at the end, she jumped off the treatment table and came happily over to give me a drawing and a kiss. Is this a good way to teach children about pain? Is this the best way to help them to cope with future experiences which will no doubt be much more unpleasant than 20 minutes of gentle handling on a treatment table? How on earth will they cope with having vaccines or other much more invasive medical procedures?

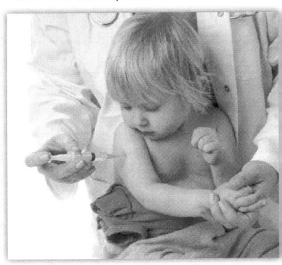

Charlotte keeps a close eye on the needle but she doesn't seem too scared. We experience pain many times in our lives. How can you prepare your children for this?

What we see at our clinic and what all the pediatric physiotherapists that I train tell me is that children of calm, trusting parents cry much less and are much more relaxed during treatment.

Could it be that we are bringing our children up to be «incapable» of experiencing any discomfort in life? Could we be programming them to be chronic patients in the future?

Sometimes only the parents of children who have experienced severe illness and pain can really show us the courage and determination required to face what life throws at us. On reading the draft of this book, the mother of a wonderful child who comes to our center with brain damage (she has another son with very serious developmental problems who had to spend long periods in intensive care), said to me: "Iñaki, you have to talk about the importance of infusing children's lives with joy and wonder». What a beautiful life lesson! Thank you!

On reading the draft of this book, the mother of a wonderful child who comes to our center with brain damage (she has another son with very serious developmental problems who had to spend long periods in intensive care), said to me: «Iñaki, you have to talk about the importance of infusing children's lives with joy and wonder». What a beautiful life lesson! Thank you!

It is a fact that the tendency to perceive unfamiliar situations in a negative or threatening way plays an important role in adults with chronic pain. So, in an unfamiliar situation like a visit to a pediatric physiotherapist's office where they are unsure if their child is going to experience pain in spite of the kindness shown towards her, this negative perception is a sign of the parents' predisposition to chronic pain. The interesting thing is that a study of adolescents, who catastrophize about pain or who have suffered many episodes of pain in a given period of time, shows they will not only interpret pain in a negative way but social situations too. What made the initial impact on these children and adolescents to cause them to have negative perceptions and catastrophic thinking? It would be reasonable to assume that it was probably their parents' attitude, wouldn't it?

The things children hear

Parents aren't always aware of the impact their words have on their children's intellectual and emotional development. This is true when they are speaking to their children but even more so when they leave comments hanging in the air in their presence, even when they are not talking directly to them. You know perfectly well that children's minds are like sponges and they mirror everything they see and hear. You know that the important thing is not what you tell them to do, but the example you set. They will unconsciously mimic your behavior in the future so it would be a good idea to stop and consider which aspects of yourself you would like them to develop and pay more attention to what you say and do.

They will unconsciously mimic your behavior in the future so it would be a good idea to stop and consider which aspects of yourself you would like them to develop and pay more attention to what you say and do.

We all experience aches and pains, they are an inevitable part of being human. Unfortunately, some people suffer terrible pains for different medical reasons and others experience sporadic pain for entirely different, and usually less serious, reasons. It is not uncommon for an adult to have a sore back or neck at some point in their life. Previous trauma, stress, poor posture or an additional workload can cause the body to protest whether it has cause to or not.

Science knows that, in spite of what everyone may think, the pain a person experiences is never proportional to the tissue damage caused. In his theory of the mechanism of pain in the sixteenth century, Descartes left us with the misconception (according to modern neuroscience) that pain is directly proportional to the tissue damage. But this couldn't be further from the truth. Pain is never proportional to actual tissue damage. A minor illness can cause enormous pain and yet people rarely describe the pain of serious injuries, such as amputations, as being awful. Quite the opposite, many amputees refer to feeling a blow and only later do they realize they are missing a finger or a limb.

Pain is never directly proportional to the actual tissue damage caused.

Several studies have shown how pain depends on context and previous experience. The place, the moment and the people around you can substantially change your experience of pain. However, it's not only your current situation that has an impact on the way you experience the pain of a certain injury but previous ones too, which you may not even recall. These historical, family or social determinants are called pain modulators. Regardless of the true state of the tissues, pain modulators are determinants that can make the brain believe the pain is very dangerous. Furthermore, we know that pain can be activated or increased in intensity by anything that provides the brain with credible evidence that the body is in danger and needs protection.

There are different pain modulators but the family is one of the main ones. When a small child is continually hearing her mother complaining about having headaches and describing the symptoms in lurid details, she is changing the type of relationship she has with the child as a result of the pain, without them knowing or understanding that they are not responsible for it. This creates a strong modulator in the child's subconscious. Consequently, from the child's perspective, a headache is very dangerous, and this emotional experience can become rooted in her experience of pain.

The family is a great pain modulator. It can mean the difference between the child's experience of pain being bearable or totally unbearable in the future.

The odds are that the child will suffer from headaches as an adult, and that, if she does, her pain will be much more intense and disabling than if she had shoulder or knee ache. We should not talk about our pain in front of our children in a dramatic or catastrophic way. It would be better to tell the adults we live with when the children are not around. It is very different for a child to hear «Mommy's going to have a little lie down» than «Leave me alone, my head is about to explode» or even worse: «Shut up, you're giving me a headache!».

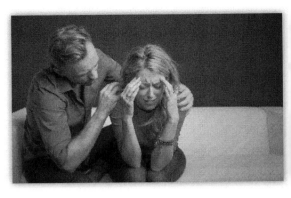

Pain is linked to our existence, it is part of life. But it can also be hard-wired based on our early experiences in life.

There may well be families that undergo great suffering because of illness, but wherever possible, it is preferable to protect our children from catastrophic messages and feeling guilty about their parents' pain. When we are in pain and have had enough, such as in cases of chronic pain, our way of relating to others generally changes. People are usually in a worse mood, their patience wears extremely thin and they become irritable. However it is unlikely that a child will be capable of interpreting this in the right way if they receive messages that are difficult to integrate and if the parents' relationship towards them changes. Clearly, it is very important to understand how parents' chronic pain affects their children.

At the Center for Pediatric Pain Research (IWK Health Center, Halifax, NS, Canada) they conducted a review and synthesis of different studies on pain, physical and psychological health, and family functioning in children of parents with chronic pain compared with children of parents who did not have chronic pain. The results were quite clear. The children of parents with chronic pain scored worse in various areas and we can see how these children are more prone to experience pain themselves. It is surprising to note that newborns of mothers with chronic pain have poorer weight gain, spend more time in intensive care due to health problems and have a higher mortality rate.

From a more psychological perspective, children of parents with chronic pain were more prone to internalized disorders such as anxiety or depression, or externalized, for example, hyperactivity, and poorer social skills compared to children of parents who don't suffer from chronic pain. Family life and functioning was also poorer. Oddly enough there was one positive aspect that these children developed better: compassion and understanding towards other people experiencing difficult circumstances. Interesting isn't it?

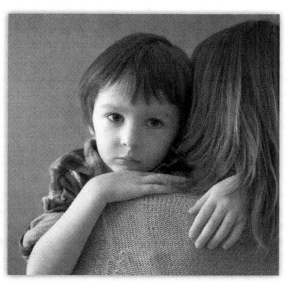

Oddly enough there was one positive aspect that these children developed better: compassion and understanding towards other people experiencing difficult circumstances.

Noah isn't feeling well and is being held by his mom. The stories he's heard about other peoples' sicknesses have scared him.

There are many other determinants or modulators. The stories we hear at home about other people's pain and how it affects them are some of the most important ones.

«Do you remember my colleague, Jason? He's had back pain for weeks and they've just operated on him. He might never work again or even walk for that matter. It's awful».

«Did you hear about my cousin? Remember she had a pain in her leg? Well, it turns out it was cancer. What's going to become of her?».

If a child is listening to any of these stories and is unable to understand the specific context of the person they are talking about (which even adults do not fully understand), a subconscious threat detection modulator may be created in her mind. If she hears this story repeated several times at home the modulator will become firmly embedded. At some point when the child is older, she will suffer back or leg pain. Who hasn't experienced back pain from a strain or a knock or due to poor posture? When this occurs in the future, the child, who is now an adult, will experience pain far beyond what she would suffer if this modulator were not active in her brain. Somewhere in her subconscious a warning signal will go off about the gravity and danger this pain poses. Of course, she won't make the connection with the stories she heard so often at home, she will just feel a great deal more pain. Curious isn't it?

Once again, we are talking about programming. Everything in humans is programmed. When we are children, everything we feel and everything that happens to us or that we hear or do conditions our development, our life-experiences and our possibilities in the future. It is vital we avoid trivializing other people's suffering based on pure speculation about situations we do not know enough about. And, even if we do, what possible good can it do for a child to hear the unfortunate fate of someone in pain?

The healing power of stories about pain

From ancient times, stories and tales have been used to heal the sick. Some stories came from mythology. Other stories tried to offer a divine reason for the illness or teach the patient how to fight their own demons. This is because human beings are strongly influenced by stories. Stories are messages that go directly to a person's subconscious mind. Just like a Trojan horse that invades their subconscious without the conscious protector setting off the alarms, blocking its entry, arguing or even asking questions. Today, anyone wishing to develop their public speaking skills to influence or motivate others must be an expert in story-telling.

Stories are one of the tools that modern neuroscience proposes for treating and managing pain. Stories enable people to conceptualize pain in a new way by reaching them at an emotional level, sparking a change in beliefs and allowing the story to be embedded in their memory. This doesn't mean that the child shouldn't know what is going on and what's wrong with her. The truth is a necessity for every human when understanding their illness, but stories can help reduce suffering. The aim of the stories is not to mask the pain or trick the child, but to remove the fear.

The book by Australian physiotherapists Lorimer Moseley and David Butler, Explaining pain, marked a paradigm shift at a global level in the way we help people with pain. Their work which is based on hundreds of cases, has led them to develop a new approach to the knowledge, understanding and belief that a person has about their pain. One of the simplest ways to reduce the intensity of pain and achieve modulationis to explain what it is. It is also one of the easiest ways to prevent chronic pain from developing.

The aim of physiotherapists around the world is to teach people about pain as this type of intervention really helps to change their beliefs about it whilst at the same time making it less dangerous. It has the immediate effect of decreasing the intensity of the pain. This means interacting with the patient in a calm, friendly way whilst at the same time being empathetic. Metaphors are very useful for this. Metaphors can be defined as understanding and experiencing one kind of thing by talking about another which shares similarities or has an association with the situation described. It is believed that they provoke thoughtfulness and increase the potential to reorganize previous beliefs or prejudices.

In a paradoxically simple way, reading short stories and tales as metaphors for key areas of the biology of pain, can produce measurable changes in suffering and reduce the catastrophic thinking associated with feeling unwell, as well as improving a person's ability to function.

In short, using therapeutic strategies to explain pain leads to rapid changes in the beliefs and attitudes associated with it, as well as reducing the actual pain experienced during movement. When this is coupled with other therapeutic strategies and actions, explaining pain can lead to a reduction in (perceived) pain and improved functioning, along with greatly improved coping mechanisms for resolving problems which may occur later.

Using therapeutic strategies to explain pain leads to rapid changes in beliefs and attitudes linked to pain and reduces pain during movement.

Stories enable people to conceptualize pain in a new way by reaching them at an emotional level, sparking a change in beliefs and allowing the story to be embedded in their memory.

All of this is even more important when we are talking about children. Not just as a means of helping them with their painful experience, but also to avoid them programing pain in the wrong way, something that would affect their experience of pain for the rest of their lives. Not to mention the implications this has for preventing the kind of catastrophic thinking that leads to pain in adult life.

It is essential parents know how the child's nervous and emotional systems work in relation to pain so they can prevent their children from becoming chronic patients in the future. There is no doubt about it, experiencing pain is «unpleasant» but there are some fundamental aspects that could significantly contribute to the process in a constructive way, with the net result of less suffering for the child.

So, what should we say to children when they are in pain? How should we behave when they, or we, are in pain? These questions are vitally important for their future... and yours.

SUMMARY

Infants, children and young people often complain about pain which is generally caused by headaches, stomach aches, muscular pains, growing pains, etc. But there are also many children who suffer from terrible diseases or undergo surgery which causes them pain and discomfort even though it is designed to help.

There is currently wide consensus that, although pain usually appears due to an injury or tissue damage (although sometimes it is far from clear there is a physical basis), the frequency or intensity is often not easily explained by physical causes. This means that the amount of tissue damage caused and the amount of pain the person suffers are not proportional.

Arguably, the most powerful pain modulators are our own experiences in early life (even before we can speak), together with those of our parents or the people close to us when we were children.

Pain is one of nature's wonders but for it to do its job of protecting you, it must be a truly unpleasant experience of the worst possible kind. Only an unpleasant experience and feeling will force you away from the source of the pain.

The use of therapeutic strategies to explain pain and telling stories about it, leads to rapid changes in the beliefs and attitudes associated with it, reducing the pain experienced during movement. When this is coupled with other therapeutic strategies and actions, explaining pain can lead to a reduction in (perceived) pain and improved functioning, along with greatly improved coping mechanisms for resolving problems which may occur later.

As a parent you will not be able to protect your children from feeling either the physical or emotional pain they will experience for all kinds of different reasons at different points in their lives. All you can do is help them to live these experiences in the best possible way so that they affect their lives as little as possible.

What can you do?
HELPFUL PRACTICAL ADVICE

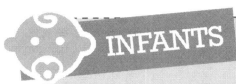

INFANTS

- If your baby is irritable, doesn't sleep and cries incessantly, if it is impossible to calm her down and she twists and turns restlessly yet the pediatrician cannot find any specific problem or illness, then take her to a pediatric physiotherapist (at the end of the book you will see how to find one). Don't wait. The pediatrician may well assure you there is nothing to worry about, that your baby does not have a specific illness. But she is suffering for some reason. Quite often it is due to neck, back or tummy problems that can be treated very effectively in expert hands. A physiotherapist will be able to help her and alleviate her pain very quickly. It is not a good idea for infants to suffer pain on a constant basis without relief as this could influence their behavior and the way they program pain in the future.

- Use skin-to-skin contact, a reassuring hug or even a song to calm her down when she has aches and pains, bangs and bruises. Even if you think she can't understand every word you say, explain to her that you know how she feels and that you are there for her. Try to be calm and comforting.

OLDER CHILDREN

- When your children accidentally harm themselves, don't be unnecessarily alarmed; don't shout or get upset, keep calm, especially if it is clear there is no real threat to the child's health or safety. A small bump or fall should be treated naturally, as just another life-experience. Most likely this fall won't be their first or their last. Give the child a warm hug, offer them support and protection but steer clear of anxious pain-avoidance behaviors. You can explain to her that it is normal for it to hurt because her body has been hurt and is healing inside. You can explain that it hurts to make sure she is careful with that part of her body and looks after it so it doesn't get injured again and can heal properly. Of course you should follow the doctor's instructions should it be necessary to call one, and avoid self-medicating prematurely for no good reason other than to alleviate the discomfort. Remaining calm and collected as you deal with her pain will help your child much more than getting upset and flustered trying to make her pain go away as quickly as possible. Have you noticed what young children do when they fall or hurt themselves? Quite often they don't cry as soon as they fall over but they look for you and as soon as they reach you they begin to cry inconsolably. Do you think that the expression on your face and the words you use have no impact on their experience of pain?

- Teach children at home, or at school if you are a teacher, that pain is basically good. It is extremely unpleasant but its function is to protect us and help us to heal. Thanks to this pain we can avoid hurting ourselves even more and wait before using that part of the body again allowing it to heal. Thanks to the pain and connected with it, there is tissue inflammation after a blow or damage to the skin. It is good thing for children to know that this is the body's way of healing so that they are not afraid of the experience. I am sure you can find educational resources to help you. One good example is the TV series called "Once upon a time... the human body" but there are probably more state-of-the-art materials or ideas you can develop yourself with drawings or stories. Learning that there are unpleasant experiences in life that are beneficial to us is something that helps people evolve and stops them from developing an overly superficial outlook on life.

- When the child is in slightly more intense pain due to some illness or injury, it may helpful for her to understand that pain is never directly proportional to the damage done. This is one of the fundamental concepts of «pain education» but it is extremely difficult to explain to a child, particularly when perhaps you, the parent or teacher, don't believe it yourself. That is why it is a good idea to use stories to reduce pain. Lorimer Moseley always tells the story of a man who picked him up when he was hitchhiking on a road somewhere in the middle of nowhere in Australia. After chatting and getting to know each other for a while, the driver pulled out a huge knife and swiftly stabbed himself in the leg in front of Lorimer who was totally distraught by what he had just seen. He couldn't believe it and didn't know how to react. He was also terrified he'd met a madman or a psychopath. Then the driver burst out laughing and showed him the leg was made of wood due to an amputation he had suffered in the past. He told him he loved to play that trick on everyone he met. This simple story has an effect on a person's subconscious. Somehow, you open your mind to the belief that the pain you feel does not mean that you have something serious, nor is it proportional to the problems you may have. Maybe you can find your own story adapted to the children around you and most importantly, written in a fun and if possible, surprising way, in language they can understand. A book about stories and pain written by physiotherapist Carlos López Cubas (Cuentos analgésicos, Ed. Zérapi), includes tools for children and can give you some very good ideas.

- Don't catastrophize about pain or talk about it thoughtlessly in front of the children at home. Try not to moan about it when they are around. The truth is that it is better not to moan or complain about anything as the chances of living a better life increase considerably for people who do not complain because they feel they are in charge of their own lives, not victims of fate. Don't talk in a dramatic way about your own aches and pains in front of children and avoid making bold or dramatic statements. If you have to talk to your partner or other adults at home about an illness or pain, find some privacy away from the children. They will not interpret things like you, nor understand what is serious and what isn't, unless you can explain it calmly using metaphors, which is very difficult when you are in severe pain. And above all, do not let your pain change the way you interact with them unless they fully understand that they are not responsible.

- Be aware that you cannot prevent your children, students, nieces and nephews or any other child that is dear to you, from suffering pain in their life: it could be as a result of an accident such as a fall; maybe due to an illness; most likely emotional pain due to a problem in a relationship. Whatever the cause, we can only hope that they are minor setbacks though some people do experience a lot of physical suffering for different reasons during their lifetime. You will not always be able to prevent their pain, but there is one thing you can do which is invaluable: you can make a big difference to how these children experience pain not only as children but also as adults. According to your children's first experiences of pain with you, how you explain things to them, how you reassure them, how you help them to trust their body and its mechanisms of protection and healing, you can rest assured that when they experience pain later in life, it will be much less intense and they will cope with it in a much calmer way. Of course, it's quite probable that you will be able to prevent them from becoming adults with chronic pain, with all the limitations this brings. You have more influence over their future than you think.

BIBLIOGRAPHY

Regarding what pain is and how to understand it better:

Blakelsee S, Blakeslee M. El mandala del cuerpo. El cuerpo tiene su propia mente. La Liebre de Marzo; 2009.

Craig AD. A new view of pain as a homeostatic emotion. Trends Neurosci. 2003 Jun;26(6):303-7.

Moseley L, Butler D. Explicando el dolor. Noigroup Publications; 2010.

Moseley L, Butler D, Beames TB, Giles TJ. The graded Motor Imagery Handbook. Noigroup Publications; 2012.

Regarding neonates' sensitivity to pain:

Eliot L. What's going on in there? How the brain and mind develop in the first five years of life. Bantam Books; 1999.

Regarding the relationship between pain and development:

Bouza H. The impact of pain in the immature brain. J Matern Fetal Neonatal Med. 2009 Sep;22(9):722-32.

Van Ganzewinkel CJ, Anand KJ, Kramer BW, Andriessen P. Chronic pain in the newborn: toward a definition. Clin J Pain. 2014 Nov;30(11):970-7.

Walker SM. Biological and neurodevelopmental implications of neonatal pain. Clin Perinatol. 2013 Sep;40(3):471-91.

Regarding the need to treat infants for neck or back pains:

Biedermann H. Manual Therapy in Children. Churchill Livingstone; 2004.

Fabry G. Clinical practice: the spine from birth to adolescence. Eur J Pediatr. 2009 Dec;168(12):1415-20.

Regarding the relationship between pain and danger perception:

Arntz A, Claassens L. The meaning of pain influences its experienced intensity. Pain. 2004;109:20-5.

Bayer TL, Baer PE, Early C. Situational and psychophysiological factors in psychologically induced pain. Pain. 1991;44(1):45-50.

Heathcote LC, Koopmans M, Eccleston C, Fox E, Jacobs K, Wilkinson N, et al. Negative interpretation bias and the experience of pain in adolescents. J Pain. 2016 Sep;17(9):972-81.

Moseley GL, Butler DS. 15 Years of Explaining Pain – The Past, Present and Future. J Pain. 2015 Jun 4;16(9):807-13.

Moseley L, Arntz A. The context of a noxious stimulus affects the pain it evokes.Pain. 2007;133:1-3, 64-71.

Regarding the differences between children whose parents suffer chronic pain and those who do not:

Higgins KS, Birnie KA, Chambers CT, Wilson AC, Caes L, Clark AJ, et al. Offspring of parents with chronic pain: a systematic review and meta-analysis of pain, health, psychological, and family outcomes. Pain. 2015;156:2256-66.

Regarding how to explain pain to really help those suffering from it:

Traeger AC, Moseley GL, Hübscher M, Lee H, Skinner IW, Nicholas MK, et al. Pain education to prevent chronic low back pain: a study protocol for a randomized controlled trial. BMJ Open. 2014 Jun 2;4(6):e005505.

Traeger AC, Hübscher M, Henschke N, Moseley GL, Lee H, McAuley JH. Effect of Primary Care-Based Education on Reassurance in Patients with Acute Low Back Pain: Systematic review and meta-analysis. JAMA Intern Med. 2015 May;175(5):733-43.

Regarding children of parents with chronic pain:

Christy EM. Why Does Mommy Hurt? Helping children cope with the challenges of having a caregiver with chronic pain, fibromyalgia, or autoimmune disease. Denver, CO: Outskirts Press; 2014.

Erdreich S. Parenting with chronic pain.Slate. 2015 Jan. Disponible en: http://www.slate.com/articles/life/family/2015/01/parenting_with_chronic_pain.html

Sturgeon J, Zautra A. Resilience: A new paradigm for adaptation to chronic pain. Current Pain and Headache Report. 2010;14:105-12.

Regarding the power of stories and metaphors in pain relief:

Gallagher L, McAuley J, Moseley GL. A randomised controlled trial of using a book of metaphors to reconceptualise pain and decrease catastrophising in people with chronic pain. Clin J Pain. 2013 Jan;29(1):20-5.

López Cubas C. Cuentos analgésicos. Herramientas para una saludable percepción del dolor. Editorial Zérapi; 2011.

Moseley GL. Painful Yarns. Metaphors and Stories to Help Understand the Biology of Pain. Australia: Dancing Giraffe Press; 2007.

Regarding how to explain pain as a therapeutic tool:

Meeus M, Nijs J, Van Oosterwijck J, Van Alsenoy V, Truijen S. Pain physiology education improves pain beliefs in patients with chronic fatigue syndrome compared with pacing and self-management education: a double-blind randomized controlled trial. Arch Phys MedRehabil. 2010;91(8):1153-9.

Moseley GL. Combined physiotherapy and education is effective for chronic low back pain. A randomised controlled trial. Aust J Physiother. 2002;48:297-302.

Moseley GL. Evidence for a direct relationship between cognitive and physical change during an education intervention in people with chronic low back pain. Eur J Pain. 2004;8(1):39-45.

Moseley GL, Nicholas MK, Hodges PW. A randomized controlled trial of intensive neurophysiology education in chronic low back pain. Clin J Pain. 2004;20(5):324-30.

Van Oosterwijck J, Nijs J, Meeus M, Truijen S, Craps J, Van den Keybus N,et al. Pain neurophysiology education improves cognitions, pain thresholds, and movement performance in people with chronic whiplash: a pilot study. J Rehabil Res Dev. 2011;48(1):43-57

Chapter 9

Attention, learning and behavioral disorders
A modern day epidemic

Iñaki Pastor Pons

The current situation of children with attention and learning disorders could arguably be defined as dramatic or, at the very least, widespread. The story behind the figures (approaching 20% according to some authors), tells us that about one in every 5-6 children has difficulties focusing on activities or acquiring literacy skills. Aside from these figures which are alarming in themselves, we know that in Spain the education system is failing over 30% of students, twice the average of other European countries. This is an indication that the problem very probably lies not so much with the children, as with the society they live in. Many children with attention deficit are medicated using really aggressive active ingredients with potentially worrying side effects that are still unknown in the long term. It is true that some children need and benefit from this kind of medication. But is there nothing else we can do? And as if this were not bad enough, different studies have linked learning disabilities to the risk of mental health problems in the future, such as anxiety or depression, among others.

So what is causing this situation? And why is this happening? Is it a global health problem? Is it an education policy issue, such as the age at which children should start learning to read and write or the way learning takes place in schools? Does the problem lie with the teaching methods or educational approach? Does it have to do with how these children have developed from birth? Could these problems be prevented?

As you can see, there are more questions than answers. It is imperative not only that medical and psychoeducational sciences gain more in-depth knowledge of the real causes and factors involved, but also that there is a paradigm shift on the part of professionals and institutions. We need to move away from labelling towards an understanding of learning disabilities as an expression of neurodevelopmental immaturity. This paradigm shift will pave the way for a much more comprehensive perspective of the problem; offering new pointers for the assessment and treatment of these disorders within an interdisciplinary framework that takes into account biological, psychological and social aspects.

If you are the parent of a child with learning disabilities, I want you to think of this chapter as a message of hope. It is true that as a society we still have a plenty of work to do but there are more and more experts who are doing a fantastic job with these types of children and getting terrific results. Join me now as we discover how to help them find their wings!

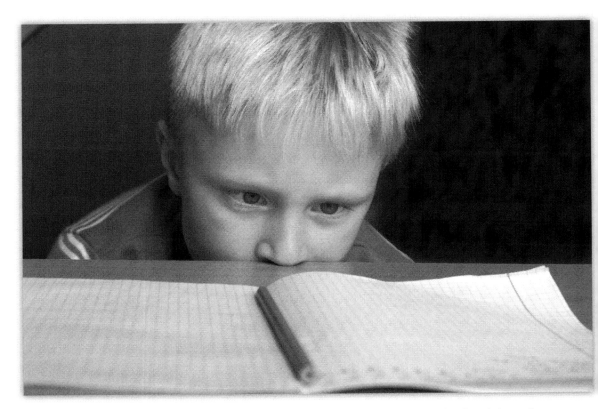

John finds his homework overwhelming. It's an enormous strain for him because he doesn't have the necessary neurological resources for optimal visual and auditory processing. His nervous system is immature. Attention deficit and learning disabilities are a serious problem in our society and should give us all pause for thought.

Intelligence and development

Not that long ago it was commonly believed that the key to a child's academic future was related to his intelligence. Intelligence is a complex issue that hasn't really been fully understood until now and possible interpretations were defined from a psychological perspective (cognitive, learning and relational capacity), a biological perspective (the ability to adapt to new situations) and an operational perspective (measured by intelligence tests).

However, there are actually different types of intelligence: logical-mathematical, spatial, relational, emotional, etc. With the help of different tests we can calculate a child's general intelligence quotient (IQ). At the outset, IQ tests were used to predict school performance and a measurement called «general intelligence factor» was derived from them. This measurement has been used to justify genetic theories whereby intelligence is fixed when a human being is born and cannot be changed. These tests were fashionable a few years ago and myriad psychoeducational exams were carried out in many schools.

IQ tests are carried out less and less these days, probably for three main reasons:

a. The danger of labelling children.

b. They don't really measure intelligence in the truest sense.

c. Gifted children don't always «perform» well at school.

a) The danger of labelling children

By determining their general intelligence factor, we run the risk of labelling children and limiting their supposed future academic potential which is anything but predictable. For some psychologists this seemingly scientific view of intelligence has legitimized social prejudices. One factor that may have helped in this practice being phased out was the discovery of the «Pygmalion effect» in education. The Pygmalion effect helped to explain how one person's belief can influence the performance of another. This is a fundamental truth and should be required reading for both teachers and parents alike. In fact, it probably holds true for anyone wanting to get the most out of the people around them.

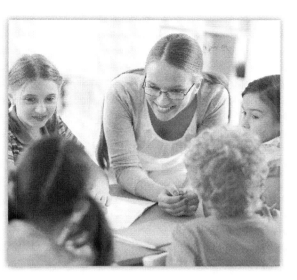

This teacher's belief in her students' potential and her positive view of them can spur them on to incredible heights. Everyone who works with and for children should always keep this in mind.

Two researchers, Rosenthal and Jacobson carried out a study involving teachers and students. The teachers were given a list of the IQ of the students they were going to have during that year, making it clear which students had above average intelligence and which below, but with no mention of treating them differently or asking them to perform different tasks. After a few months it was clear that the brightest students were the ones who improved the most in the tests. So far, so good. To a certain extent it is logical to think that the brightest students would make the most progress. What is interesting is that the list given to the teachers was false. The IQ scores had been allocated randomly to the students in the two groups. Had they given the students they considered to be the brightest, the most stimuli? Perhaps they had given them more time to answer. More to the point, these students probably responded differently because they were treated differently, thus confirming the teachers' expectations. In conclusion, the beliefs you have about your children or your students, even those you have about your co-workers or your employees will have a direct impact on their performance and development in the future.

This is great news for us parents! What an easy way to help our children! All we have to do is believe in them! So much cheaper than a support teacher, right?

The beliefs you have about your children or your students, even those you have about your co-workers or

employees, will have a direct impact on their performance and development in the future.

b) They don't really measure intelligence in the truest sense

Some experts criticize the fact that people have a different concept of intelligence than that measured by the tests and that other circumstances influence the outcome too such as; mood, tiredness, certain physical abilities or prior exposure to similar tests. Perhaps it would be better to consider intelligence as the potential each person possesses to a greater or lesser degree, instead of as a measurement to be monitored and built upon. This is the basis for the theory of multiple intelligences developed by Howard Gardner and his view that intelligence is the ability to solve problems or develop products that are highly regarded in a particular culture. It seems far simpler and better suited to real life.

Perhaps it would be better to consider intelligence as the potential each person possesses to a greater or lesser degree, instead of as a measurement to be monitored and developed.

By taking the different types of intelligence into account you get a more comprehensive view that is much better suited to real life than a mere psychometric test score. It provides a perspective of intelligence as a living thing which can be developed and, whilst it may be conditioned by a particular genetic inheritance, it is fundamentally influenced by the environment. Think back to the chapter on «Bonding through touch» where we saw that infants who are not caressed enough can develop intellectual disability. This gives you an idea of the extent to which the environment can have a positive or negative influence. As a child grows up, teaching methods should enhance learning by taking into account his unique potential as an individual – because a child's potential is highly dependent on how the learning process is implemented and what his neurological development is like.

c) Gifted children don't always «perform» well at school

Another problem with considering IQ as something that is predictive or preventive of how a child will perform at school or a young person in their studies, is that it does not always follow that the smartest do the best, in fact quite the opposite. Many gifted children fail badly at school. So why is this? On the one hand, it is possible that gifted children require different stimuli from the rest of the class to keep them interested and motivated, and there is debate as to whether these children should follow adapted school programs. But, on the other hand, and this is essential for something we will look at in more detail later on, gifted children must relate to their environment, to people, texts, the language they hear or to the pencils and school equipment they use, through their body. What, I hear you ask, does the body have to do with academic performance when we're referring to their intelligence? Well, as Sally Goddard, one of the world's leading experts on learning disabilities linked to neurodevelopment says: «Although all learning ultimately takes place in the brain, it is often forgotten that it is through the body that the brain receives sensory information from the environment and reveals its experience of the environment». Antonio Damasio explains it very clearly: «This is Descartes' error: the abyssal separation between body and mind [...] the separation of the most refined operations of the mind from the structure and operation of a biological organism».

Therefore, in learning disabilities it is not just the child's intelligence that counts; what really counts is the child's neurodevelopment. The degree of maturation of his nervous system will determine the way the child interacts with the environment and other children and how he interprets all the information he receives from the world outside. It will also define the way he is able to perform in this environment after he processes the information. This is part of a conceptual framework called the neurodevelopmental framework, which is based on the medical diagnosis and an assessment of the maturation and development of the nervous system.

In learning disabilities it is not just the child's intelligence that counts; what really counts is the child's neurodevelopment.

For example, how good is the child's vision and how smooth and precise are his eye movements? This has a direct impact on how the child integrates written information and the time, effort and precision he requires to take this information in. Vision has a bearing on the quality and performance of the way the brain processes this input too, including memory and the ability to relate this information to information the child already has. It is unlikely that a child with poor visual and oculomotor skills (not just in terms of vision but also in terms of controlling eye position and movement) can perform well academically even if he is gifted. Just to be clear, we are not talking about a child who is blind or visually impaired. There are plenty of children with learning disabilities who have good visual acuity or «vision correction» (thanks to glasses, for example) who have not developed proper control of their eye movements, the ability to focus, visual perception of shape or depth or visual memory. In other words, they have not developed the visual skills essential for learning. Do you remember the chapter on the visual system?

«Although all learning ultimately takes place in the brain, it is often forgotten that it is through the body that the brain receives sensory information from the environment and reveals its experience of the environment».

(Sally Goddard).

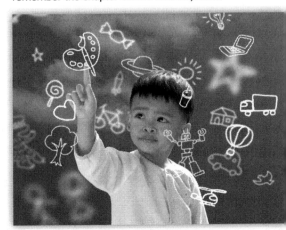

Mark is good at problem solving and coming up with worthwhile solutions for the society he lives in. That is true intelligence!

Intelligence is the ability to solve problems or develop products that are
highly regarded in a particular culture.

This example involving the visual system can be applied to all the other sensory systems. It is unlikely that a child with poor hearing capacity (we are not just talking about deafness here, but also an inability to process the information he hears) will perform well academically. And on it goes, the list is endless... It is unlikely that a child with poor balance control, sense of his own body, vestibular function, cerebellar function, postural control, etc. will perform well academically. If he does, it will be the result of his own tremendous effort.

Consequently we are looking at a new, additional dichotomy: intelligence on the one hand and development on the other. If we look a little closer, we see that intelligence has a more intellectual connotation and development a more physical one. As we saw in the opening chapters, neurodevelopment is built on the physical stimuli the body must receive, such as movement or touch, (although the nervous system must also be healthy and intact). Isn't this a new and interesting way of interconnecting the «body» and «mind»? Both are closely connected, since there are types of intelligence that can only develop if the body gathers and processes environmental input properly. Together, they are vital for academic performance and learning and schools should assess both when faced with a child with learning disabilities (and perhaps it should even be done before they start school).

The difference in development between children with problems of intelligence and children with developmental problems is considerable (if this kind of radical differentiation is even possible). It is very difficult to change even the slightest intellectual disability with intervention (the more serious the delay the more difficult it is), although special educational measures can be put in place to develop the child's full, albeit limited potential. However, with the appropriate interdisciplinary help, a neurodevelopmental problem can improve significantly (especially if the child has normal intelligence and a safe, loving home environment). At our clinic we help children with major learning and attention issues on a daily basis, and in just a few months see surprising changes in them; as long as their parents adopt a constant approach to the program of exercises and treatments the child needs (which often involves several professionals).

In conclusion, chronological age and intelligence are not the only criteria for success in learning and developmental and physical exams are usually only carried out if the-

re is some sort of medical problem. This is resulting in mismanagement of what is in fact a significant problem, since most cases of children with learning disabilities are not severe enough to require early intervention services (i.e. for brain damage, genetic syndromes, etc.), yet are not good enough to «perform» to the best of their ability in school. How many children are left in no-man's-land with no neurodevelopmental assessment? How many of the clinical signs that no doubt appeared were ignored? How many times have we heard it said about a child who doesn't reach his developmental milestones «Don't worry, he'll get there!»?

Chronological age and intelligence are not the only criteria for success in learning.

If neurodevelopmental assessments or at least screening tests are not carried out by qualified professionals, such as developmental physiotherapists, early in a child's life, we run the risk of not taking action at the most effective time. The fact is that a 5 or 6-year old child with difficulties probably showed signs of developmental immaturity as an infant. If these signs had been spotted, simple, effective, low-cost prevention and stimulation measures could have been put in place.

Labels? No thanks
Evolving towards a new conceptual model of learning disabilities

The term «learning disability», was first coined in the 1960s. On the whole it was used to refer to children who could not be classified as blind, deaf or mentally retarded..., but who had learning disorders linked to visual or auditory impairments or difficulties with motor coordination or adjusting to the environment.

The term itself has as many meanings as experts who use it. For their part the experts have been trying to provide greater diagnostic resources, but in a scenario where there has been a lack of clearly unified criteria that would allow everyone to understand each other. Notably, there has been, and continues to be, a disconnect between the medical diagnosis and functional assessments carried out by experts from non-medical professions such as physiotherapy, occupational therapy, psychology, psychopedagogy, optometry and speech therapy. This is one of the consequences of the health sector not working as a team, a decision which can no doubt be traced to a country's institutional policies. The countries with the best health care are those where health programs are planned by multidisciplinary teams made up of representatives from different health professions.

The countries with the best healthcare are those where health programs are planned by multidisciplinary teams made up of representatives from different health professions.

This divide between the medical diagnosis and functional assessment (which is usually not as scientific) doesn't just occur with learning disabilities, but with other health problems too. And unless both assessments are taken into account, people are left to face their discomfort and distress feeling confused and misunderstood. Take a common example such as back pain. Someone with back pain goes to the doctor and, after a brief examination and some imaging tests the doctor determines that it is not caused by a physical problem like a herniated disk or an inflammatory disease. The doctor attributes the pain to a muscle contracture and the patient leaves the surgery with a prescription for anti-inflammatories.

So far, so good, this is an essential step. However, an important part of this individual's health care is missing; they require a functional examination and an analysis of how the different joints and muscles operate. This should involve a postural assessment of the quality and quantity of both general movement and individual joints, as well as a postural assessment of the individual's professional and recreational activities, etc. One approach is to carry out a medical examination using validated international scales to quantify the function based on recognized criteria of normality. The physiotherapist responsible for carrying out this assessment will no doubt discover certain impairments or «dysfunctions» in the way the individual moves, works, treads..., and, using their professional know-how and tools of the trade, will be able to help them and have a direct impact not only on the consequences but on the causes too. It is essential to have both assessments (medical and physiotherapy), if someone really wants to solve their health problem on a lasting basis. It is quite possible that the opinion of other experts will also be required. This is the joy of an integrated vision and it clearly provides better overall healthcare for the user.

The same is true of learning and attention issues, sometimes diagnosed as developmental dyslexia or attention deficit disorder (ADD). In these cases, the diagnosis or medical perspective alone, whilst fundamental, is not enough to understand and help the child. The same goes for the brilliant psycho-pedagogical assessments carried out by psychologists, educational psychologists and counselors in schools. These assessments are essential and help to give a true picture of the child's situation, allowing educational resources to be put in place to help and guide him and reassure his parents. However, it is not enough.

A new paradigm is required for understanding and addressing learning disabilities. This new paradigm is based on three models or conceptual frameworks:

1. Neurodevelopmental spectrum model
2. Biopsychosocial model.
3. ICF functioning model (WHO)..

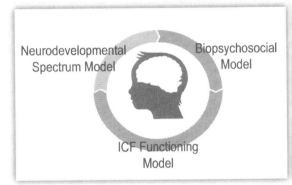

A diagram of the models that comprise the new paradigm of learning disabilities which should redirect our understanding and approach to this major problem. This new vision is necessary both for institutions and policies and medical and educational experts.

A new paradigm is required for understanding and addressing learning disabilities.

Neurodevelopmental spectrum model

In simple terms, the neurodevelopmental spectrum model helps us to comprehend that the child's evolution and acquisition of cognitive skills (and not just the cognitive ones) depends on the degree of development and maturation of the nervous system.

It is clear from the way an infant develops that the acquisition and development of cognitive abilities is closely linked to physical abilities. As an infant's posture develops, he is able to make better use of his hands. As his hands, mouth and eyes encounter real world objects through movement, his intelligence is able to develop and he can begin to adapt to his environment. Motor skills are always linked to learning processes and no one should be in any doubt that knowledge originates through deliberate, coordinated motor activities.

As Piaget said, «all cognitive mechanisms are based on motor activity» (on movement), but not just any kind of movement; they are based on coordinated systems of movement that seek a result or an intention. You could say that movement is tantamount not only to life, but to maturation, development and intelligence too. Infants who were not stimulated, touched or carried around enough can experience serious cognitive development problems together with learning disabilities, impaired emotional processes and poor social skills in the future.

> *Movement is tantamount not only to life but to maturation, development and intelligence too.*

Cognitive processes follow a certain order, even in language acquisition: motor skills develop first, followed by perceptual skills and last but not least, symbolic processes.

As the more basic motor activities become automatic, the higher cortical levels can be used for other learning processes. The highest level of cognitive functioning can only occur when the most basic bodily functions are covered and no longer require the intervention of the higher resources. To understand this a little better, imagine a child with reading problems. He reads very slowly, skips words and lacks comprehension. The task of reading is carried out by the highest cortical processing centers. If we carry out a basic balance test on this child and find that he has serious difficulties maintaining his balance, it is easy to understand that balance is a much more vital basic function than reading. You can't do anything if you are unsteady as anyone who has suffered vertigo or a severe bout of dizziness will tell you.

The first thing the nervous system does is secure our balance. If it is unable to do this with the neurological structures in charge such as the spinal cord, brainstem or

cerebellum, it will have no choice but to resort to higher resources to ensure this basic process is covered. As a result, the cortex that is occupied with balance control will be unable to develop higher-level cognitive functions at full capacity, whether reading or math. Evidently, sustained attention is also impossible.

To put it another way, how well would you be able to read on a bus that is constantly stopping and starting and making you lose your balance? How well will a person be able to concentrate if his car has just been rear-ended and he feels dizzy and unsteady?

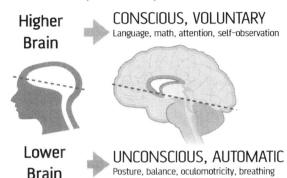

Higher Brain → CONSCIOUS, VOLUNTARY
Language, math, attention, self-observation

Lower Brain → UNCONSCIOUS, AUTOMATIC
Posture, balance, oculomotricity, breathing

A diagram showing the didactic division of the brain into higher and lower processing centers. For the «higher» brain to function properly, the «lower» brain must keep the automatic functions going and these in turn must be programmed correctly.

Cognitive processes follow a certain order, even in terms of language acquisition: motor skills develop first, followed by perceptual skills and, last but not least, symbolic processes.

If our automatic motor control does not work properly, our cognitive processes won't either, no matter how many hours we dedicate to the subject or how much pressure we are put under. In fact, this will only increase our level of frustration and exhaustion and, consequently produce rejection. Exactly the same thing happens if the motor control of our eye movements has not been integrated properly through sufficient maturation of the vestibular system and correct information from the neck muscles. It takes so much cognitive effort just to move and position the eyes, that it is extremely difficult to assimilate what we are reading.

It is not just the automatic regulation of motor control (movement) that is important either, it is essential that we properly regulate and process what we feel too. As a child reads, his nervous system is bombarded by a plethora of information entering his sensory pathways: the sound of other children moving or talking; his classmates' movements that are picked up by his peripheral visual field; his clothes chafing against his skin; the pressure of the seat or backrest on his skin; sensations from the book or the table through his hands; memories and emotions he has; feelings of hunger or thirst, etc. Countless amounts of information reach the nervous system and must be processed without this diverting the child's attention from what he is doing. After a quick risk assessment, a mature nervous system will inhibit much of this information and process it behind the scenes.

> *It's not just the automatic regulation of motor control (movement) that is important, it is also vital that we properly regulate and process what we feel too.*

For example, a child with hyperacusis (excessive hypersensitivity to certain sounds) cannot block out specific sounds he hears at a very painful frequency. This triggers an alarm in the brain that diverts his attention and causes him to abandon reading as soon as the first sound reaches him whether it comes from the classroom, the street outside or the floor above, hindering the learning process. His skin may also be hypersensitive, either in general or in certain areas such as the lower back, where many children react automatically to any form of touch with a reaction similar to a primitive reflex (found in infants) known as the Galant reflex. Had there been correct maturation of the nervous system and muscles and lumbar vertebrae free from tensions and blockages (an occurrence that is more common than people think), this would have been inhibited. Any kind of touch will cause the child to «freak out», move, or change his position as if he had ants in his pants.

Some children experience generalized hypersensitivity due to a trauma that may have occurred during the prenatal stage (e.g. a stressful experience the mother had), the perinatal stage (e.g. a very traumatic birth) or childhood (e.g. a stressful experience both physically and emotionally). This hypersensitivity, amongst other symptoms, could be an expression of Post-traumatic Stress Disorder (PTSD). If this is the case work protocols and therapies are available to help. These may be physical, to desensitize and harmonize the form and intensity with which the child feels and perceives; psychological, via EMDR (Eye Movement Desensitization and Reprocessing); or sensorimotor psychotherapy. Pioneering approaches to trauma intervention usually involve the body to treat emotions.

In all these cases, but particularly those in which the trauma occurred during the preverbal period (including prenatal or perinatal stages), it is very important to involve the physical side in the treatment as the somatic memory stores an imprint of traumatic experiences. In the same vein, the body is an infinite provider of resources for integrating everything we experience because it has self-regulatory tools which can be stimulated with the right treatment. This way we are addressing every aspect: the emotional side (sadness, helplessness, lack of faith that things will turn out ok); the cognitive side (negative or debilitating thoughts); and the physical side (images, sounds, movements, muscular pains, hypersensitivity to certain stimuli, etc.), and fully integrating the experience.

Some children suffer generalized hypersensitivity with other emotional, cognitive or physical symptoms due to a trauma that may have occurred during the prenatal, perinatal or postnatal stage.

In short, the nervous system's sound automatic management of sensorimotor processes provides the foundations for cognitive development. Mª Jesús López Juez clearly describes it as the «need to organize an effective bottom-up system» that is fast, automatic and capable of guiding and organizing actions based on the way the lower brain works. This will enable an effective top-down system to develop, capable of controlling emotional impulses and providing self-awareness, reflection and planning; key tasks for paying attention and learning in school.

Hence the surprise experienced by staff at many schools when they see an improvement in the reading and comprehension of the children we treat with manual therapy, exercises at home and reprogramming of sensorimotor systems, and the general feeling that they are more mature and focused. Their surprise is plain to see. Sometimes a child who does more «physical exercise» improves their reading more than a child who is given an additional two hours reading support. Of course we are not suggesting they should just run around after a ball, but it is certainly significant that children with learning disabilities are taken out of physical exercise to spend more time sitting in front of a book. Only those who have experienced this can judge how effective it really is.

Sometimes in the case of children with severe motor impairments such as cerebral palsy or paraplegia you may find the following paradox; the cognitive function for learning has a better footing than in other children with milder motor disorders. There are several hypotheses for this. The first is that the brain can always develop parallel ways of learning. Additionally, if the child's innate cognitive function is good, to a certain extent it will be able to make up for physical limitations. The older a person is, the clearer this is.As we age our mental processes become freer of our body and are able to develop independently from it. Take Stephen Hawking for example, the renowned astrophysicist, scientist and public figure who had a serious degenerative disease called amyotrophic lateral sclerosis (ALS). He was practically paralyzed, but this did not stop his mind from being creative. Of course he was a healthy child. The disease developed much later.

The second hypothesis is that for cognitive performance to be reduced, the cortical part of the brain must attempt to compensate deficit in the «lower» brain such as when we try to fix our gaze or maintain our balance. If the physical problem is so serious that there is nothing the «higher» brain can do to keep things functioning properly, then, paradoxically there are fewer «symptoms» or cognitive limitations. As strange as it may seem, a child with poor balance has much greater difficulty reading than a child in a wheelchair who is paralyzed in both legs. This paradox can also be found in the symptoms of certain physical problems such as small-angle strabismus which can cause headaches and balance disorders, while more severe strabismus does not trigger any similar symptoms.

The biopsychosocial model

When talking about the health and well-being of a child it is important to include the biological, psychological and social perspectives. This approach takes into account the child's physical, behavioral and developmental status while using medical services (such as glasses, orthotics, medication for asthma, psychotropic drugs, etc.), rehabilitation services (physiotherapy, occupational therapy, speech therapy or optometry), educational support (special needs support, psychopedagogy) and behavioral support (psychology).

This model also allows us to determine the child's strengths and challenges in his everyday life and to see the child holistically, bearing in mind that certain interventions may disrupt his normal environment or routines and require additional measures to be put in place. For example, if a health problem requires the child to rest at home for a long period of time, certain measures will have to be put in place (from an academic, social and health perspective) to avoid the possible drawbacks of being at home: social isolation, skipping school, lack of exercise, etc.

According to this model, it would make no sense to carry out an isolated intervention that might destabilize the whole child. Needless to say, once again we favor a comprehensive, interdisciplinary approach.

This model allows us to determine the child's strengths and challenges in his everyday life and to see the child holistically.

In 2004, the National Research Council and the Institute of Medicine proposed an approach to the health and well-being of children called Kaleidoscope. This model covered biological considerations, behavior, the physical and social environment, as well as the policies and services available to the child. Again this is a holistic approach which, unfortunately, is not always reflected in our health policies and the work of certain specialists. Many experts in the fields of health and education now base their work on this model.

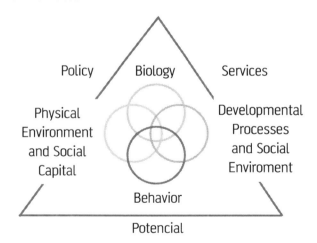

Kaleidoscope model (2004) that takes into account not just physical and behavioral aspects but social environment and health policies too.

The ICF model designed by the WHO

The third model was developed by the World Health Organization (WHO) in 2011 and is called the International Classification of Functioning, Disability and Health (ICF).

On the back of this ICF framework the WHO developed an ICF for Childhood and Youth (ICF-CY). The ICF is designed to record the characteristics of child development (that word again) and the impact of their environment. The ICF-CY can be used by all those interested in the health, education and well-being of children and young people, and provides a common and universal language for use in clinical practice, public health and research. This same language facilitates the documentation and measurement of health and disability in children and young people.

The ICF model establishes that conditions of health and well-being are determined firstly by body functions and structures, by activity and also participation. Allow me to further develop each of the three points that the World Health Organization proposes in its ICF-CY framework for health in childhood and youth.

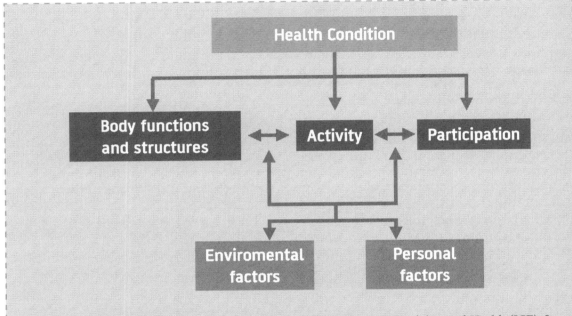

The WHO's Model for the International Classification of Functioning Disability and Health (ICF). Its aim is to ensure that health policies and specialists take into account the functional status associated with health conditions as well, not just the impairment, disorder or illness itself.

Body function and structures

Clearly, in order to understand a child's problem we need to assess his body structure and how it works. The first step perhaps is to find out if he has a specific health problem; something that might show up in an imaging test, a blood test or other kind of medical test. Secondly, as discussed earlier, we need to find out if his body works properly; whether his vision, hearing, perception of his own skin or body (proprioception), balance, coordination, swallowing or speaking, among others, allow the child to develop to his full potential.

Activity

Just because a child can swallow doesn't mean he can eat; just because his joints and leg muscles are «healthy» doesn't mean he can run; just because he has «healthy» eyes doesn't mean he can read, etc. Activity is not just about having healthy body structures and physiological function, it also requires a correct perception of the environment and the ability to relate and adapt to it. We regularly see lots of children who, despite having made a full recovery, still daren't put weight on their leg or walk on it. The health specialist can't simply focus his attention on the muscle, joint or organ in question, but instead must help the child to use his body for a relevant or necessary activity. This is not as straightforward as it may sound and it's not just that the child is afraid; all too often there is also an altered perception of the environment and of oneself after an illness or trauma.

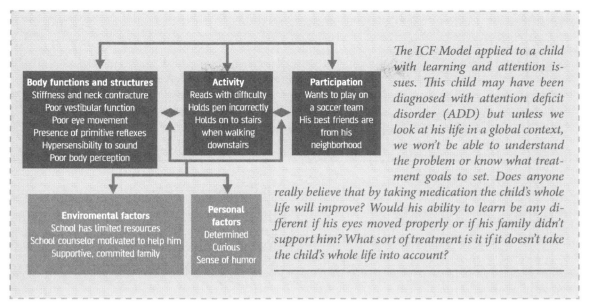

Body functions and structures
Stiffness and neck contracture
Poor vestibular function
Poor eye movement
Presence of primitive reflexes
Hypersensibility to sound
Poor body perception

Activity
Reads with difficulty
Holds pen incorrectly
Holds on to stairs
when walking
downstairs

Participation
Wants to play on
a soccer team
His best friends are
from his
neighborhood

Enviromental factors
School has limited resources
School counselor motivated to help him
Supportive, commited family

Personal
factors
Determined
Curious
Sense of humor

The ICF Model applied to a child with learning and attention issues. This child may have been diagnosed with attention deficit disorder (ADD) but unless we look at his life in a global context, we won't be able to understand the problem or know what treatment goals to set. Does anyone really believe that by taking medication the child's whole life will improve? Would his ability to learn be any different if his eyes moved properly or if his family didn't support him? What sort of treatment is it if it doesn't take the child's whole life into account?

Participation

Participation is the great novelty in terms of health in the World Health Organization's vision and it is something that all health professionals are slowly starting to embrace. You see, not only must the structure and function be healthy and the child be able to carry out an activity, but the WHO considers that the highest attainable standard of health is to be able to carry out said activity whilst interacting with others. This concept is as revolutionary as it is beautiful. It is not just a case of having healthy throat muscles and being able to chew and swallow, but being able to chew and swallow whilst eating with others. We see many such cases at our clinic. I remember one particular boy with learning and developmental disorders whose greatest ambition was to run faster. We always make a point of asking children what they would like to improve as we feel it is important. The boy's parents felt he was clumsy and always tripping up. He wasn't good at physical activity, almost as though he had been born in the wrong body. Needless to say he found reading, writing and paying attention challenging and this was why they brought him to see us. His self-esteem was in tatters and the problem was becoming increasingly complex both socially and emotionally. When he started to make progress, the first thing his parents noticed was that his balance and coordination improved. His movements were much more fluid. We asked him, «In what ways do you feel better?». Do you know what he was most pleased about? He said: «My friends choose me to play football now». How amazing; now participation was possible because he was able to develop as an individual in an activity with others.

The WHO considers that the highest attainable standard of health is being able to carry out an activity whilst interacting with others.

Personal and environmental factors

As well as structure and function, activity and participation, there are many factors that can affect a child's development and how he adapts to academic or social demands. These are classified as personal or environmental factors. A child has a series of innate personal abilities such as curiosity, capacity for hard work and intelligence. At the same time he is part of a family, school and social reality that can greatly facilitate or block his development.

By taking the personal and environmental factors into account we are able to understand the global nature of the child's situation much better and consequently to act in a more effective and be spoke way. Environment is key to the development of human beings. Educating the family, training the professionals who come into contact with the child or improving educational and social policies would have a dramatic effect on the well-being and development of children

What will his health look like in 5 years' time thanks to this treatment?

To conclude, when we assess a child and his learning, attention and behavioral issues, it is not just the medical diagnosis that counts, even though the problem needs to be identified and given a name. We must also accurately assess the extent to which his nervous system was able to mature at the right time, in other words, the degree of neurodevelopment he has. This needs to be done in a biopsychosocial framework, taking into account his behavior, ability to undertake an activity and participate with others in that activity. Moreover, firstly we need to look at the social and family environment and the health services and policies around that child so that we can develop his potential in the reality he lives in. The broader the vision we have of the child or the young person, the higher the chance of effective action and lasting results.

I'm sure the following will make it even clearer; if your back hurts and the only treatment is to take anti-inflammatories, what do you think your health will be like in 5 years' time? Not just your back either – because you didn't actually do anything to improve the way it functions or discover what was causing the pain – but the health of your digestive system too after taking medication for so long.

Don't you need something instead of painkillers? How about physiotherapy, more exercise, improved posture, improving your diet, managing your family or professional responsibilities better, sleeping more or taking more holidays? Or at least some combination of these factors.

If eating makes you feel heavy and you struggle to digest food properly, once illness has been totally ruled out, do you think that taking a gastric protector is your only option? What do you think your health and digestive system will be like in 5 years' time? Shouldn't you find out if something you are eating is making you ill, if you could improve your diet, or at least have more regular mealtimes, etc.? Perhaps eating more slowly and chewing more would help? Surely some of the above would help you to lead a healthier life in the future?

It seems pretty obvious doesn't it? Well, by the same token, if the only treatment given to a child with an attention disorder whether hyperactive or not, is psychiatric drugs, what do you think his outcome will be over time? Surely there is something else we can do to help him?

Of course there is. First and foremost a neurodevelopmental assessment should be carried out; we need to evaluate the quality of his visual and auditory input and how it is processed; the psycho-emotional aspects he may be experiencing; the quality of his sensorimotor organization starting with a study of his vestibular system which, as we saw earlier, is the basis for eye function and muscle tone and is essential in neurodevelopmental terms; the type of academic intervention he receives; the age he started to read and write which may have been too soon for him; the amount of time he spends outdoors or watching TV and playing video games, etc., etc.

If the only treatment given to a child with attention disorder, whether hyperactive or not, is psychiatric drugs, what do you think his outcome will be over time? Surely there is something else we can do to help him?

At the same time, wouldn't it be helpful to teach parents how to manage frustration, boost self-esteem and encourage their child's development? Of course it would.

We can only help children maximize their full biopsychosocial development if we adopt a broad, holistic approach. Would you settle for less for your child?

We can only help children maximize their full biopsychosocial development if we adopt a broad, holistic approach. Would you settle for less for your child?

SUMMARY

Intelligence is not the best parameter for predicting the learning disabilities a child may have. In fact, by calculating their IQ we run the risk of labelling children. This score doesn't really measure intelligence in the truest sense and the reality is that gifted children do not always «perform» well at school.

The beliefs you have about your children or your students will have a direct impact on their performance and development in the future.

A paradigm shift is needed to enable us to detect, prevent, understand and better support children with learning disabilities.

This new paradigm should be based on the neurodevelopmental spectrum model, a biopsychosocial model and the map created by the WHO to better understand and guide clinical processes, the International Classification of Functioning, Disability and Health (ICF).

What we really need is a map of the child showing the whole picture, not just a label.

When a child has learning disorders, a medical diagnosis is not enough. A neurodevelopmental assessment should be carried out; we need to evaluate the quality of his visual and auditory input and how it is processed; the psycho-emotional aspects he may be experiencing; the quality of his sensorimotor organization starting with a study of his vestibular system which, as we saw earlier, is the key to correct eye function and muscle tone and is essential in neurodevelopmental terms; the type of academic intervention he receives; the age he started to read and write which may have been too soon for him; the amount of time he spends outdoors or watching TV and playing video games, etc., etc

What can you do?
HELPFUL PRACTICAL ADVICE

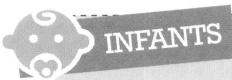

INFANTS

- If your child is still a baby keep an eye on his development, learn about the milestones he should reach each month. Check with your pediatrician and if you see signs of a lack of head or postural control, or irritability, ask a neurodevelopmental physiotherapist to carry out at least one developmental screening test and advise you on the type of stimulation he requires. In some cases these tests should be ongoing throughout the child's development to ensure that everything is going to plan as sometimes certain small changes can develop at specific ages. Throughout this book you will find plenty of advice about how to offer your child the ideal stimuli so he can reach his maximum potential and how to forestall minor developmental problems and mild learning disabilities.

OLDER CHILDREN

- At the age of 5 all children should undergo comprehensive screening by a developmental optometrist. Behavioral optometrists are a good option. They are vision experts and very familiar with the visual skills required for learning. They are also aware of the need for a multidisciplinary approach and the majority work alongside physiotherapists trained in PIMT. If you detect a specific problem such as strabismus or some kind of eye disease it is vital you also get a medical diagnosis from an ophthalmologist.

- Keep an eye on your child to see if he is sensitive to unexpected sounds. Telltale signs he may have an auditory processing problems include; covering his ears or over-reacting to certain sounds; trouble focusing when there is background noise, or difficulty pronouncing certain sounds correctly. This can have a major impact on his language and literacy development. You may want to consult a hearing expert who specializes in screening for learning disabilities. There are various methods available offering systems for assessing and treating auditory processing disorders. The most well-known ones include; Tomatis, Berard, Sena and Johnson. There are some differences between them and a hearing and language specialist will be able to recommend which one suits your child best. Neurodevelopmental physiotherapists and optometrists can also help you to find a center that specializes in this type of screening and treatment. Just as with vision, a medical diagnosis is vital if there is the slightest suspicion of hearing loss, deafness or respiratory illnesses.

- Play with your children as much as possible: on the floor and outside. Playing on the floor allows them to complete the stages of development they didn't integrate as infants. Being in contact with nature makes us happier and more human.

- Put firm limits on screen time. This must be done as early as possible so they grow up knowing that it is normal. Let them make up their own games, be active, inventive and even get bored. They need to know how to use technology but too much screen time can be harmful for their neurological development on different levels. If you spend time with them and play with them they will feel better supported and this will obviously make it much easier. In his book *Homo videns*, Giovanni Sartori warns of the dangers of children growing up addicted to the TV and videogames, something that seriously hampers their personal and cultural growth. Scientific studies show that increased TV time in children is associated with poorer relationships with their parents and other children and the negative effects become more apparent during adolescence.

- Encourage your child to be independent and responsible. At the beginning it may just be a case of him always putting his shoes together when he takes them off. Be clear and uncompromising that he must do it himself if he is able to whether it be tidying up his toys, looking after his own clothes, or taking his plate or glass into the kitchen. This needs to start as soon as possible so that he grows up knowing it is normal.

- Allow your children to contribute to the family's well-being by helping out at home. Doing chores helps them to develop as people, encourages them to be responsible and boosts self-esteem. Again, it is important to establish these routines as soon as possible so that they grow up knowing this is normal.

- Make sure your children sleep well. Studies show that good development is linked to getting the right amount and quality of sleep. It isn't the only factor but it is a major one. Get him into good habits from the start by sticking to a set bedtime. If an infant has trouble sleeping, it is often due to physical discomfort that can be treated by a specialist physiotherapist. Don't just accept it – seek help.

- If your child has been diagnosed with developmental dyslexia, attention deficit disorder or any other type of disorder, don't give up or just accept the label. Don't settle for just one kind of treatment as it won't guarantee to help him develop to his full potential in the future. Sometimes medication is essential. However, it isn't merely about disguising the symptoms or ensuring he passes all his exams at school; it's about allowing him to develop to his full biopsychosocial potential and, of course, be happy. As we saw earlier, children who experience difficulty with reading often having trouble concentrating; many are also clumsy, have poor balance, hypersensitivity to sounds; a certain impulsiveness; trouble managing frustration, etc. We are not just referring to issues with reading or paying attention either. Developmental immaturity comes in many forms which are not always taken into account during the «diagnosis». Try looking at the problem from a new perspective by standing back and remaining calm as you track down the help you need. One sign of a good developmental specialist is if he works side by side with other experts; they don't need to work in the same center but they should be in constant communication and take decisions by consensus. There are increasingly more, better trained professionals out there who can help you!

- Notice to what extent your child's disorders are behavioral, if, for example, he has anxiety, unexpected aggressive reactions or trouble empathizing. It may be necessary for a child psychologist to assess his emotional development in order to advise you on the best way to support him. If this psychological help is coordinated with help from other professionals like developmental physiotherapists, all the better because what people always need is help that is both top-down (mind to body) and bottom-up (body to mind).

- If your child had problems with his neurological development and you were unable to accompany him in the early stages of his life because you weren't aware that it was necessary or perhaps because of other difficulties he may have had (illnesses, hospitalizations, etc.), don't panic. It can all be programmed later. The brain is an amazing thing and sometimes has the ability to find alternative ways to build or repair itself. There are some amazing specialists who can help your child with his developmental, learning and attention issues. Never give up hope – there is always a way to help your child progress!

BIBLIOGRAPHY

Regarding how and when the term learning disabilities was first coined:

Tannhause MT, Rincón ML, Feldman J. Problemas de aprendizaje perceptivomotor. Editorial Médica Panamericana; 1996.

Regarding the statistics on learning and attention issues in Spain:

El aprendizaje en la infancia y la adolescencia: Claves para evitar el fracaso escolar. Cuadernos Faros. Sant Joan de Déu. Observatorio de salud de la infancia y la adolescencia; 2010.

Regarding intelligence:

https://es.wikipedia.org/wiki/Inteligencia

Gardner H. Inteligencias múltiples. Paidós; 2003.

Schlinger HD. The myth of intelligence. The Psychological Record, vol. 53, 2003.

Regarding the need for physical development for optimal learning:

Damasio A. El error de Descartes. La emoción, la razón y el cerebro humano. Editorial Crítica; 2010.

De Quiros JB, Schrager OL. Fundamentos neuropsicológicos en las discapacidades de aprendizaje. Editorial Médica Panamericana; 1996.

Goddard Blythe S. Attention, Balance and Coordination. The ABC of Learning Success. Wiley-Blackwell; 2009.

Thinking goes to school. Piaget's theory in practice. Oxford University Press; 1975.

Piaget J. Perception, motricité et intelligence. Enfance. 1956;2:9-14.

Piaget J. Les praxis chez l'enfant. Revue Neurologique. 1960;102:551-65.

Regarding the Pygmalion effect:

Sánchez Hernández M, López Fernández M. Pigmalión en la escuela. Editorial Universidad Autonómica de la Ciudad de México; 2005.

Regarding vision and academic performance:

Vergara P. Tanta inteligencia, tan poco rendimiento. ¿Podría ser la visión la clave para desbloquear su aprendizaje? Ed. Pilar Vergara; 2008.

Regarding the range of developmental problems and their causes:

Accardo PJ. Capture & Accardo's Neurodevelopment Disabilities in Infancy and Childhood. Volume I: Neurodevelopment Diagnosis and Treatment. 3rd ed. Paul H Brookes Publishing; 2009.

Regarding the need for a biopsychosocial model:

Stein RE, Silver EJ. Operationalizing a conceptually based noncategorical definition: a first look at US children with chronic conditions.Arch Pediatr Adolesc Med. 1999 Jan;153(1):68-74.

Regarding the neurodevelopmental spectrum model:

De Quiros JB, Schrager OL. Fundamentos neuropsicológicos en las discapacidades de aprendizaje. Editorial Médica Panamericana; 1996.

Regarding the ascending and descending systems in the organization of the central nervous system:

López MJ. Principios básicos de Neurodesarrollo infantil. Mª Jesús López Juez; 2017.

Regarding the ICF model by the World Health Organization (WHO):

Cieza A, Bickenbach J, Chatterji S. The International Classification of Functioning Disability and Health as a conceptual platform to specify and discuss health-related concepts. Gesundheitswesen. 2008;70:47-56.

Clasificación Internacional del Funcionamiento, de la Discapacidad y de la Salud: versión para la infancia y la adolescencia: CIF-IA. Organización Mundial de la Salud; 2011.

Regarding the importance of getting enough quality sleep:

Gruber R, Wise MS. Sleep Spindle Characteristics in Children with Neurodevelopmental Disorders and Their Relation to Cognition. Neural Plasticity. 2016;3:1-27.

Regarding the risks and dangers of excessive screen time

Richards R, McGee R, Williams SM, Welch D, Hancox RJ. Adolescent screen time and attachment to parents and peers. Arch Pediatr Adolesc Med. 2010 Mar;164(3):258-62.

Sartori G. Homo videns: la sociedad teledirigida. Ed. Taurus; 1998.

Chapter 10

Classifying learning disabilities without labeling

Iñaki Pastor Pons

We saw earlier how learning disabilities can be a clear sign of immaturity in the way a child's nervous system has developed and that a comprehensive approach is required to provide her with as many strategies as possible to help rebuild it. However, it is equally true that we need to know something about how the main disorders are classified.

To begin with, the problem is by no means easy because, for example, a teacher's classification will differ to that of a doctor. A neurodevelopmental specialist's classification will differ again. The question is whether the classification is more useful to science than it is to the individual involved. It is essential there is a correct diagnosis so that protocols for medical treatment can be established. However, these protocols will only be effective if the diagnosis is based on causes and not just on symptoms or signs. A diagnosis also helps target welfare aid to selected groups of children who need more help or assistance.

On the other hand, medical protocols should be open and supported by an assessment of the disorders that could benefit from physiotherapy, psychology, occupational therapy, optometry or speech therapy programs. These evaluation and treatment programs are delivering superb outcomes in children's functioning (function, activity and participation) and the family care provided.

We will attempt to shed some light on the subject to offer you a clearer, more comprehensive overview. Our aim is to do this without resorting to over simplifications which might categorize children according to limiting or even crippling diagnoses and run the risk of labeling them for life.

If you are the parent of a child with learning disabilities, you would be wise to read on.

Is classification always based on the cause?

All medical diseases are defined using different points of view. For example, a disease can be defined based on a change observed in the structure (e.g. a certain kind of cyst), how the symptoms occur (e.g. migraine), on a deviation from the norm (e.g. hypertension) and on a cause (e.g. infection by one bacteria or another).

Symptom-based diagnoses don't provide guarantees about the potential causes and, therefore, the possibility of any alternative treatments. Even more importantly, these diagnoses don't provide scope for prevention. How can you prevent something if you don't know what caused it or even have a working hypothesis?

Symptom-based diagnoses don't provide guarantees about the potential causes and therefore, the possibility of any alternative treatments.

There are many reasons a child can develop attention and learning disorders, some of which are well known because they are linked to other health and psychological problems or social issues. Others are a lot less familiar because they affect apparently healthy children who have adequate family and social support. Top Argentine researchers, De Quiros and Schrager, propose two groups of learning disabilities. On the one hand, primary learning disabilities, which very specifically affect particular human achievements (language, literacy and numeracy, among others) and, on the other, secondary learning disabilities where there are specific biopsychosocial problems that indirectly affect specific human achievements too.

Let's look at a few examples to get a better idea. A child with brain damage, blindness, psychotic behavior, or who is malnourished or abused, will probably have some degree of learning disabilities. However, these disabilities are secondary to the specific problems affecting the child's physical, mental and social health. In these cases, not only is the child's reading or writing affected but he may also have other problems that require help, whether it be medical treatment or welfare assistance. These are classed as secondary learning disabilities

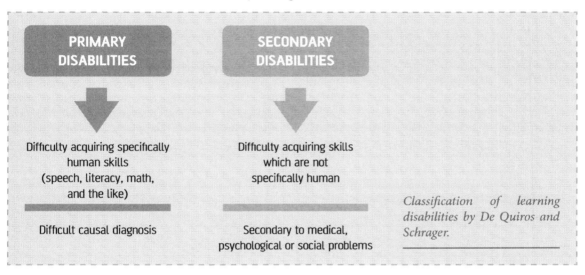

Classification of learning disabilities by De Quiros and Schrager.

A child may also have significant, specific difficulty with language, literacy and numeracy skills which cannot be explained by a deficit in her overall intelligence or because she has missed opportunities to learn, lacks general motivation or sensory acuity. In other words, the child does not have a specific health problem, yet she fails to acquire specifically human skills. As you can imagine, it is a lot harder to talk about causes in this second group. And if the causes are missing, what we will find in this group is a myriad of very different sub-classifications and theories.

A child may have significant, specific difficulty with reading, writing, language or numeracy which cannot be explained by a deficit in her overall intelligence or because she has missed opportunities to learn, lacks general motivation or sensory acuity.

I don't know if you know children with learning disabilities but you probably do. Do you think their problem is well defined? They may have a medical diagnosis or a label, but does anyone really understand what is wrong with them? Once again, we are faced with the dilemma of using a «heading» in order to define problems instead of a model such as the ICF or neurodevelopmental specimen models we saw in the previous chapter.

According to Bessel Van der Kolk, one of the world's leading psychiatrists in childhood disorders and trauma:

> The first serious attempt to create a systematic manual of psychiatric diagnoses occurred in 1980 with the release of the third edition of the Diagnostic and Statistical Manual of Mental Disorders, the official list of all mental diseases recognized by the American Psychiatric Association (APA). The preamble to the DSM-III warned explicitly that its categories were insufficiently precise to be used in forensic settings or for insurance purposes. Nonetheless, it gradually became an instrument of enormous power. [...]

This manual is the most definitive resource for the internationally agreed classification of «mental problems». Psychiatrists, psychologists and lawyers around the world have a copy on their bookshelves. Doctors in particular, rely on this classification to establish treatment protocols with medication in children with learning disabilities and many other disorders.

He goes on to say...

> DSM labels quickly found their way into the larger culture [...] A psychiatric diagnosis has serious consequences: Diagnosis informs treatment and getting the wrong treatment can have disastrous effects. Also a diagnostic label is likely to attach to people for the rest of their lives and have a profound influence on how they define themselves [...] None of these diagnoses take into account the unusual talents that many of our patients develop or the creative energies they have mustered to stay alive. All too often diagnoses are mere tallies of symptoms, [...]

> With DSM-V psychiatry firmly regressed to nineteenth century medical practice. Despite the fact that we know the origin of many of the problems it identifies, its «diagnoses» describe surface phenomena that completely ignore the underlying causes.

> [...] Even before the DSM-V was released, the American Journal of Psychiatry published the results of validity tests of various new diagnoses, which indicated that the DSM largely lacks what in the world of science is known as «reliability» - the ability to produce consistent, replicable results. In other words, it lacks scientific validity...

In 2011, the British Psychological Society complained to the APA that the DSM identified situations «located within individuals» and neglected the «undeniable social causes of many of these problems».

Is there such a clear difference between a child with dyslexia, ADD (Attention Deficit Disorder), developmental immaturity or attachment trauma? This poses a differential diagnosis and assessment problem for all health and education professionals and it affects a lot of children. Normally it is the teachers and counselors in schools who are most aware of this problem. They are the ones who, in the absence of clear criteria from our educational and health system, do an admirable job identifying and helping these children. However, we work side by side with them on a daily basis and they often talk about their confusion and the lack of training and support they experience.

In the absence of clear criteria from the education and health system, teachers, educators and counselors are the ones who do an admirable job identifying and helping these children.

Whereas serious neurodevelopmental problems (such as a syndrome of genetic or metabolic etiology, or cerebral palsy) are relatively easy to diagnose with appropriate intervention and support from early infancy, milder impairments to the central nervous system (especially those involving the «lower» brain) are often misinterpreted by both professionals and parents and attributed to poor parenting or the child's personality.

The DSM-IV manual states that:

> The specific diagnostic criteria ... are meant to serve as guidelines to be informed by clinical judgement and are not meant to be used in a cookbook fashion.

It also says:

> The clinician using the DSM-IV should therefore consider that individuals sharing diagnosis are likely to be heterogeneous [...]. This outlook allows greater flexibility in the use of the system, encourages more specific attention to boundary cases and emphasizes the need to capture additional clinical information that goes beyond diagnosis.

It is important to note the DSM-IV's warning about the choice of treatment:

> Making a DSM-IV diagnosis is only the first step in a comprehensive evaluation. To formulate an adequate treatment plan, the clinician will invariably require considerable additional information about the person being evaluated beyond that required to make a DSM-IV diagnosis.

Therefore it is essential we study the «functioning» of a child with learning disabilities as this opens up promising treatment options and avoids simply using medication, even if the medication seems advisable.

Educational classification

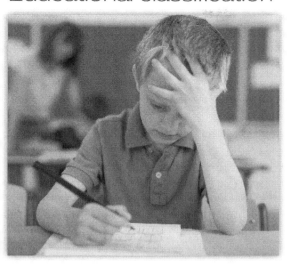

Robert struggles with math. His teacher is aware and does everything she can to help him make progress. However, he needs to undergo an exhaustive neuro-developmental assessment to find out if his nervous system lacks maturity and if so, why?

Learning disabilities are classified in different ways, some of them more official than others. One of the most helpful ways is the one used by teachers and counselors. On the basis of this educational classification they can be grouped into the following types:

- School problems (SP).
- Low school achievement(LSE).
- Borderline intellectual functioning (BIF).
- Specific learning disability (SLD).
- Attention deficit hyperactivity disorder (ADHD).

The first three types (SP, LSE and BIF) may correspond to secondary difficulties, as discussed earlier i.e. they may be linked to the child's physical and psychological health, or environmental problems (family, society or educational system).

Within the category of specific learning disabilities (SLD), the following are identified in relation to the specific difficulty involved:

- Reading-based learning disability.
- Writing-based learning disability.
- Math-based learning disability

One of the advantages of this classification versus the more «scientific» classifications is that it avoids the overuse and abuse of labels. As far as a biomedical researcher is concerned, a reading-based learning disability is dyslexia; a writing-based learning disability is dysgraphia and a math-based learning disability, dyscalculia, etc. It must be the tendency medicine has to classify and label things. On the one hand it provides clarity so that we all understand each other and, on the other, it makes writing action protocols easier. The downside is the sort of classification that pigeonholes a child; the type where one simple word can lead to prejudice and limit recovery if the child considers the diagnosis part of her identity.

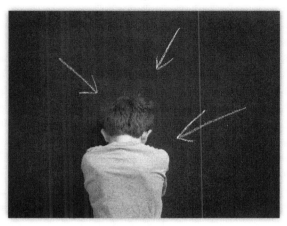

Attention and learning disabilities inevitably result in children comparing themselves with others and undergoing considerable social pressure. We need to develop ways of pre-empting these issues and of optimizing the child's abilities.

All these disabilities can be classed as neurodevelopmental disorders and children who suffer from them usually also have balance problems, a lack of coordination, poor proprioception, sensory impairments and low muscle tone, all of which indicates that development of the nervous system was non-optimal. Treatment aimed at reprogramming and improving the child's sensory and motor bases has an immediate effect on their performance at school. Moreover, educational adaptations can be developed to further enhance their performance.

Attention deficit hyperactivity disorder (ADHD) is another story altogether. Two characteristics are present in ADHD, attention deficit and impulsivity or motor hyperactivity. These two main symptoms have led to several subtypes: children for whom inattention is most prevalent, children for whom hyperactivity / impulsivity is the dominant factor and children with a combination of the two symptoms. The disorder is much more common in boys than in girls. The neurobiological basis of ADHD is complicated to understand because some of the behavioral aspects, such as deficits in working memory, cognitive flexibility and attention, are common to and present in other disorders. There are also some aspects shared with autistic spectrum disorders (ASD) and other behavioral problems, such as attachment issues, which has led some lines of psychological research to call for clearer criteria for differential diagnosis.

On the other hand, as the symptoms are very subjective (they are assessed based on the perception of the observer, parents or teachers, and not by observation through analysis or objective testing), there is a real risk that many cases diagnosed as ADHD are in fact not. This is something that many teachers, counselors and professionals dedicated to treating neurodevelopmental disorders complain about on a daily basis. This overdiagnosis is yet another consequence of the failure to carry out comprehensive neurodevelopmental assessments. Further still, although ADHD may have a strong hereditary component, some studies have linked this disorder to environmental factors such as prenatal lead and nicotine exposure.

> *There is a high risk that many cases diagnosed as ADHD are in fact not.*

Methylphenidate is the medication most commonly used to treat children and adolescents with ADHD. However, despite its widespread use, it's only now that the first systematic review studies about its benefits and risks are starting to emerge. It seems that, according to teachers and parents, methylphenidate can improve the symptoms and the general behavior of the child and adolescent with ADHD, however, the amount of improvement is still unclear. There is also some evidence of certain side effects, such as sleep problems and reduced appetite, although long-term studies are lacking. Again, this raises the question, besides medication, is there anything else we can do to help a child with this neurodevelopmental disorder?

Methylphenidate is the medication most commonly used to treat children and adolescents with ADHD. However, despite its widespread use, it's only now that the first systematic review studies about its benefits and risks are starting to emerge.

Autism spectrum disorder (ASD) is another kind of disorder, although it is not usually linked to the rest of the learning disabilities in the classifications. Let's take a quick look.

Autism is a neurodevelopmental disorder characterized by a lack of social reciprocity, communication and the presence of repetitive interests and / or behaviors. In order to receive the diagnosis a child must exhibit at least three of the following traits

- Abnormalities in social interaction
- Abnormalities in language used for social communication
- and abnormalities in symbolic/imaginative play before the age of 3

If a child does not fulfill all these criteria, she requires a different diagnosis such as Asperger's Syndrome, among others.

Distinctive social behavior includes: avoiding eye contact; difficulty regulating and controlling their emotions and understanding the emotions of others; and having a very limited range of activities or interests. ASD is not a simple problem and it is thought there are different genetic and non-genetic risk factors. It generally manifests in the first 3 years of life in the form of social behavior disorders with children often displaying unique perceptual skills, a certain degree of clumsiness and insomnia.

There is growing interest in the area of sensorimotor processing disorders in the evaluation and treatment of autistic spectrum disorders. As we explained earlier, the way we feel and process what we feel, and the way we move, are the best expressions of the maturity of our nervous system. Exciting possibilities are opening up in the treatment of ASD thanks to the sensory integration based approach used in occupational therapy and the work of pediatric neurodevelopmental physiotherapy.

Neurodevelopmental evaluation. What is required?

So, as we are seeing, learning disabilities that are not secondary to a medical cause or social problem are a sign of a delay, immaturity or poor neuro development. Regardless of whether the child is diagnosed as having a specific learning disability (SLD), or attention deficit disorder with or without hyperactivity (ADD or ADHD), we need to know how her nervous system has developed and how it was programmed

Regardless of whether the child is diagnosed as having a specific learning disability (SLD) or attention deficit disorder with or without hyperactivity (ADD or ADHD), we need to know how her nervous system has developed and how it was programmed.

Different learning disabilities, such as dyslexia, dyspraxia, ADD or autism spectrum, share common impairments of perception, organization and execution of controlled movement. This points to common ground in terms of neurological development and requires in-depth assessment. It is vital that children undergo neurodevelopmental assessments as infants, but this rarely happens. Sadly, all too often the risk factors pointing to potential learning disabilities and developmental immaturity are ignored.

The neurodevelopmental assessment should involve a comprehensive review of the child's prenatal history (pregnancy, medical problems during pregnancy, etc.), the circumstances surrounding her birth (premature birth, low birth weight, instrumental delivery, health complications, etc.) and the child's health during the first years of her life (medical history, repeated infections, sleep quality, nutrition, etc.). Some of the risk factors for developing learning disabilities can be linked to a child's prenatal, perinatal and postnatal history. For example, children born prematurely or with a very low birth weight are much more likely to underperform at school and experience difficulty regulating their emotions and paying attention. It is also important to check if they achieved the key stages of development and hit milestones at the right time (whether they walked before or after 18 months, when they said their first words, etc.).

Premature babies and those with a very low birth weight are much more likely to underachieve at school and experience difficulty regulating their emotions and paying attention.

The number of cases of children whose developmental immaturity only becomes apparent when they start school raises some troubling questions: is it only possible to detect that a child has attention and learning disabilities when she starts to learn to read and write? Is there really no way of identifying and preventing her problems at an earlier stage?

The truth is that there are early signs that a child's neurodevelopmental maturity is not optimal, and we are not just referring here to autism spectrum disorder where it is clear early on that the child is not interacting. In a large study on childhood conducted in the UK that took into account health, educational and sociological factors, they concluded that children with poor motor skills at 9 months would also be behind in their cognitive development and display worse behavior at the age of five. If we were paying attention we would see the signs and risk factors early on in life. Just imagine the advantages.

Children with poor motor skills at 9 months will also be behind in their cognitive development and display worse behavior at the age of 5.

There are in fact numerous screening tests and assessment scales to determine whether an infant or child is achieving all the neurodevelopmental stages correctly. Some of these tests are even designed for infants barely a few weeks old. Most of these tests look at aspects such as fine motor skills, gross motor skills, autonomy, social behavior and language. The problem is that these tests are only administered to children with very severe delays or if there are neurological diseases such as cerebral palsy or specific syndromes. However, all infants and children should undergo neurodevelopmental assessments by pediatricians, pediatric neurologists or pediatric neurodevelopmental physiotherapists, to detect possible signs of delay and implement prevention and stimulation programs where necessary with physiotherapy and occupational therapy. At the very least this could be carried out at home by parents who are informed, trained and motivated to do it.

All infants and children should undergo neurodevelopmental assessments by pediatricians, pediatric neurologists or pediatric neurodevelopmental physiotherapists, to detect possible signs of delay and implement prevention and stimulation programs.

Furthermore, different tests should be carried out to establish the child's sensorimotor status. A thorough neurodevelopmental assessment takes time and cannot be reduced to a couple of tests and assumptions based simply on a child's behavior.

Additionally, a physical examination of the child's neck and skull should be performed to detect contractures and spinal rigidity that could result in a lack of balance control or affect eye movements. The neck is central to the development of infants and children as this is where the first movements that guide postural maturation and vision develop. Many infants experience torticollis or have preferential head positions that are a sign of a neck problem. On the one hand these children develop flat head syndrome (plagiocephaly), and on the other, they have difficulty with postural control, the development of arm and hand functions, and the maturity of their balance and oculomotor control is affected. These last two factors, balance (as we saw earlier in the chapter on the vestibular system), and the control of eye movement and position, are absolutely essential for staying focused and developing effective learning.

The main areas that need to be assessed include:

- Anthropometric measurements (such as the head circumference in babies).
- Balance.
- Gross motor coordination.
- Fine motor coordination.
- Cerebellar function; for example, in the ability to make precise rhythmic movements or to keep muscles tense without making uncontrolled movements.
- The presence of primitive reflexes that have not been properly integrated.
- The presence of absent postural reactions.
- Right-left discrimination in relation to themselves or the examiner.
- Organization of laterality.
- Oculomotor control: the presence of smooth pursuit eye movements to track an object and in relation to their head or hand
- Temporal-sequential organization or how the child understands the concept of time, sequences and rhythm.
- A comprehensive eye exam (not just visual acuity).
- A full hearing test (not simply to establish the existence of hearing loss or deafness).
- Visual perceptual motor function or the ability to reproduce or copy geometric figures.
- Cognitive function using a test like the Goodenough-Harris test which reliably determines the cognitive state of a child on the basis of the details they include when drawing a person.
- A psychological interview in the light of behavioral disorders or family or social situations that may affect the child's functioning.

Additionally, a physical examination of the child's neck and skull should be performed.

Finally, we need to check we have gathered as much information as possible about the child's functioning in terms of the three clearly differentiated areas recommended by the ICF-CY (the assessment model proposed by the WHO) we saw in the previous chapter: body function and structures, activity and participation. In addition to this, we must gather information about the child's social and family environment, personal aspects and potential.

This will allow us to set realistic targets for the treatment process. Communication between the different professionals involved in assessing and treating the child's systems (physical, visual, auditory, emotional, etc.) and working under a shared conceptual model, is central to ensuring a successful outcome. The older the child is, the higher the number of experts that will have to intervene in her evaluation and treatment, as neurodevelopmental problems become more complicated as the child grows, thus affecting her physiological systems in a kind of «domino effect».

Let's look at an example. If we take the case of a 3 month old infant who had a long, traumatic birth, difficulty holding her head up, some degree of hypotonia, problems with the correct positioning of her arms or trunk and sleep problems, we can see she is at risk of suffering developmental problems to a greater or lesser degree. After she has been examined by a pediatrician, a neurodevelopmental physiotherapist will be able to completely alter this infant's path in life by providing guidance to her parents, stimulating her development, checking that her sensory and motor programming is correct and treating the dysfunctions in her neck or skull. Poor neurodevelopment can be rechanneled back – toward normality. Even if there are serious hereditary issues and normality is a long way off, early intervention has incalculable benefits that are without doubt much more powerful than any subsequent intervention later on in life.

However, if that same infant grows up and comes to us at the age of 7 with attention, learning and coordination issues, it will be a totally different story. As well as seeking the opinion of a neuropediatrician, a physiotherapist or occupational therapist will need to carry out a full neurodevelopmental assessment and initiate corrective action to rebuild the foundations of the nervous system through a sensorimotor stimulation program. Likewise, an optometrist should examine her vision; a hearing and language expert her hearing; a psychologist the emotional and behavioral issues borne of the frustration and anxiety inherent in learning disabilities (or check if these aspects are among the causes); an educational psychologist should guide the family as to how best to manage the child's frustration and provide learning support, etc. Not all these specialists will be necessary, but it is important to be aware that the later the problem is tackled, the more complex and global the consequences will be.

> *The older the child is the higher the number of professionals that will have to intervene in herevaluation or treatment.*

SUMMARY

Not all diseases and health issues are diagnosed according to what causes them. Diagnoses are often based on a patient's symptoms and behavior and since these are not entirely reliable, it makes prevention even more difficult. This is what often happens when diagnosing attention and learning disorders and why models which are functional maps of the child, like the ICF Model we saw in the previous chapter, are needed alongside the medical diagnosis for effective, individualized treatment.

The DSM (Diagnostic and Statistical Manual) provides both medical and educational classifications of learning disabilities.

The DSM by the American Psychiatric Association (APA) is the main reference for the internationally accepted classification of «mental» disorders, but even it warns of the limitations of using the manual in a "cookbook" fashion and encourages clinicians to collect as much information as possible for a sound therapeutic approach.

The educational classification of learning disabilities is more open and offers more advantages, not least that it avoids labeling children according to their symptoms and offers the most comprehensive functional examination.

While severe neurodevelopmental problems (such as syndromes of genetic or metabolic etiology) are relatively easy to diagnose –with the right intervention and support being provided from early infancy milder impairments to the central nervous system are often misinterpreted by both professionals and parents alike and blamed on poor parenting or the child's personality.

Furthermore, different tests should be carried out to establish the child's sensorimotor status. A thorough neurodevelopmental assessment takes time and cannot be reduced to a couple of tests and assumptions based simply on a child's behavior.

Even if there are serious hereditary issues and normality is a long way off, early intervention has incalculable benefits that are without doubt much more powerful than any subsequent intervention later on in life.

As well as seeking the opinion of a neuropediatrician, a physiotherapist or occupational therapist will need to carry out a full neurodevelopmental assessment and initiate corrective action to rebuild the foundations of the nervous system through a sensorimotor stimulation program.

What can you do?
HELPFUL PRACTICAL ADVICE

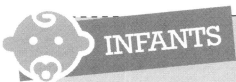 INFANTS

- If your child is still a baby, find out more about the monthly milestones you need to look out for and track how she is developing. Book an appointment with her pediatrician. If you see any signs of a lack of head control when she should be able to hold it up, of poor postural organization, irritability or a lack of communication, ask a neurodevelopmental physiotherapist specializing in PIMT to carry out an assessment to detect any indication of developmental disorders. He will be able to give you detailed advice about the kind of stimulation your child may need. These kinds of validated, reliable assessments are highly recommended throughout your child's entire development because they allow us to check that all is well and monitor the progress of any minor disorders that may develop as she matures.

- Throughout this book you can find multiple recommendations about how to offer your child the ideal stimuli to ensure her maximum development and how to prevent minor developmental issues and learning disabilities. At the end of the book there is a list of references so you can find the physiotherapists and psychologists who can help you.

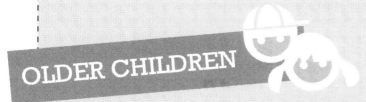

- If your child has been diagnosed with developmental dyslexia (see the article on the terminology used in the DSM-V), an attention deficit disorder or any other disorder and you want to make sure that she develops her full potential, the only option is to look for a team of professionals with a global approach to carry out an optimal functional assessment and draw a clear map of her development. By sticking with the approach of just one professional, we are potentially depriving her of unleashing all her hidden talents in the future. A multidisciplinary team working side-by-side with her family and school can ensure she develops to her full potential in life.

- Tell your child what is wrong with her using clear, positive language. It is important she knows what she has and why, and what she needs to do to make progress. If you focus on «the diagnostic label» she will probably feel «labeled» and «pigeonholed» and it may generate a limiting belief about her abilities and damage herself-concept. Talk to her about her possibilities and approach the issue from the perspective of multiple intelligences. Emphasize what she does well and encourage her resolve and willingness to improve in the things she finds difficult. We are all experts at something.

- Whichever specialist and path you choose, bear in mind that reprogramming the nervous system requires constant, relevant stimulation for a sustained period of time. Relevant, because the nervous system must receive stimuli that can create connections in the brain to allow the child to function in a way that is more closely adapted to the environment. Sensorimotor reprogramming is always necessary. Constant, because no profound changes in the brain will come about from just one session a week. The professionals who work in neurodevelopment will always set work to be done at home. Try to do the exercises at times that have the least impact on family life and be persistent. Sometimes it can take several months. If you encounter any problems ask the professional treating your child to teach you how to perform the exercises better and give you more insight into why they are important. This will help you stay motivated.

- If you were unable to help your child with her development stages and the stimulation of her nervous system during her early years because you weren't aware that it was necessary or perhaps because of other difficulties she may have had (illnesses, hospitalizations, etc.), don't panic. It can all be programmed later. The brain is an amazing thing and sometimes has the ability to find alternative ways to build or repair itself. Never give up hope –there is always a way to help your child progress!

- Help your child to step up and push the boundaries. Evaluate her progress in relation to her own performance and development; never compare her to others. There may be all kinds of disorders that might be affecting the way her brain functions at different levels, but never forget, your child is totally unique. Help her find her wings! Help her to push the boundaries every single day and to stand out from the crowd. No doubt your child will go on to do amazing things in her life and to love in her own special way.

BIBLIOGRAPHY

Regarding the definition of learning disabilities:

Habib M. The neurological basis of developmental dyslexia: an overview and working hypothesis. Brain. 2000 Dec;123 Pt 12:2373-99.

World Health Organization ICD-10. The international classification of diseases, Vol. 10: Classification of mental and behavioural disorders. Geneva: World Health Organization; 1993.

Regarding the limitations of the DSM:

Greenberg G. The Book of Woe: The DSM and the unmaking of psychiatry. Penguin; 2013.

Van der Kolk BA. El cuerpo lleva la cuenta. Cerebro, mente y cuerpo en la superación del trauma. Editorial Eleftheria; 2014.

Regarding the educational classification of learning disabilities:

Romero Pérez JF, Lavigne Cervan R. Dificultades de aprendizaje. Unificación de criterios diagnósticos. I. Definición, características y tipos. Materiales para la Práctica Orientadora. Vol. 1. Consejería de Educación. Junta de Andalucía; 2005.

Regarding the relationship between neurodevelopmental disorders and learning disabilities:

Melillo R, Lensman G. Neurobehavioral Disorders of Childhood. Springer; 2009.

Regarding ADHD:

Castellanos FX, Tannock R. Neuroscience of attention-deficit/hyperactivity disorder: the search for endophenotypes. Nat Rev Neurosci. 2002;3:617-28.

Gallo EF, Posner J. Moving towards causality in attention-deficit hyperactivity disorder: overview of neural and genetic mechanisms. Lancet Psychiatry. 2016 Jun;3(6):555-67.

Milberger S, Biederman J, Faraone SV, Jones J. Further evidence of an association between maternal smoking during pregnancy and attention deficit hyperactivity disorder: findings from a high-risk sample of siblings. J Clin Child Psychol. 1998;27:352-8.

Nigg JT, Nikolas M, Mark Knottnerus G, Cavanagh K, Friderici K. Confirmation and extension of association of blood lead with attention-deficit/hyperactivity disorder (ADHD) and ADHD symptom do-

mains at population-typical exposure levels. *J Child Psychol Psychiatry.* 2010;51:58-65.

Orjales Villar I. *Déficit de atención con hiperactividad. Manual para padres y educadores.* CEPE SL; 2011.

Unal D, Unal MF, Alikasifoglu M, Cetinkaya A. *Genetic Variations in Attention. Deficit Hyperactivity Disorder Subtypes and Treatment Resistant Cases. Psychiatry Investig.* 2016 Jul;13(4):427-33.

Regarding methylphenidate:

Mulder R, Hazell P, Rucklidge JJ, Malhi GS. *Methylphenidate for attention-deficit/hyperactivity disorder: Too much of a good thing? Aust N Z J Psychiatry.* 2016 Feb;50(2):113-4.

Storebø OJ, Ramstad E, Krogh HB, Nilausen TD, Skoog M, Holmskov M, et al. *Methylphenidate for children and adolescents with attention deficit hyperactivity disorder (ADHD). Cochrane Database Syst Rev.* 2015 Nov 25;(11):CD009885.

Storebø OJ, Simonsen E, Gluud C. *Methylphenidate for Attention-Deficit/Hyperactivity Disorder in Children and Adolescents.JAMA.* 2016 May 10;315(18):2009-10.

Regarding autism spectrum disorder and sensorimotor processing:

Bishop SL, Luyster R, Richler J, Lord C. *Diagnostic Assessment. En: Chawarska K, Klin A, Volkmar FR, eds. Autism Spectrum Disorders in Infants and Toddlers. Diagnosis, assessment and treatment. The Guilford Press;* 2008.

Carson TB, Wilkes BJ, Patel K, Pineda JL, Ko JH, Newell KM, et al. *Vestibulo-ocular reflex function in children with high-functioning autism spectrum disorders. Autism Res.* 2017 Feb;10(2):251-66.

Park HR, Lee JM, Moon HE, Lee DS, Kim BN, Kim J, et al. *A Short Review on the Current Understanding of Autism Spectrum Disorders. Exp Neurobiol.* 2016 Feb;25(1):1-13.

Schauder KB, Bennetto L. *Toward an Interdisciplinary Understanding of Sensory Dysfunction in Autism Spectrum Disorder: An Integration of the Neural and Symptom Literatures. Front Neurosci.* 2016 Jun 17;10:268.

Section On Complementary And Integrative Medicine; Council on Children with Disabilities; American Academy of Pediatrics, Zimmer M, Desch L. *Sensory integration therapies for children with developmental and behavioral disorders. Pediatrics.* 2012 Jun;129(6):1186-9.

Regarding learning disabilities due to non-optimal development:

> *Accardo PJ. Capture & Accardo's Neurodevelopment Disabilities in Infancy and Childhood. Volume I: Neurodevelopment Diagnosis and Treatment. 3rd ed. Paul H Brookes Publishing; 2009.*

Regarding learning disabilities and primitive reflexes:

> *Goddard Blythe S. Attention, Balance and Coordination. The ABC of Learning Success. Wiley-Blackwell; 2009.*

Regarding how at 9 months you can predict the problems there will be at the age of 5:

> *Hansen K, Joshi H, Dex S, eds. Children of the 21st Century: The first five years. Policy Press; 2010.*

Regarding learning disabilities in premature or low birth weight children:

> *Squarza C, Picciolini O, Gardon L, Giannì ML, Murru A, Gangi S, et al. Learning Disabilities in Extremely Low Birth Weight Children and Neurodevelopmental Profiles at Preschool Age. Front Psychol. 2016 Jun 28;7:998.*

Regarding screening for developmental immaturity:

> *Davies NJ. Chiropractic Pediatrics. 2nd ed. Churchill Livingston-Elsevier; 2010.*

> *Goddard Blythe S. Assessing neuromotor readiness for learning. The INPP developmental screening test and School intervention programme. Wiley-Blackwell; 2012.*

> *Goddard Blythe S. Neuromotor Immaturity in Children and Adults. The INPP Screening Test for Clinicians and Health Practitioners. Wiley-Blackwell; 2014.*

Regarding how parental behavior can cause hyperactivity or create security:

> *Jacobvitz D, Sroufe LA. The early caregiver-child relationship and attention-deficit disorder with hyperactivity in kindergarten: a prospective study. Child Dev. 1987 Dec;58(6):1496-504.*

> *Werner EE, Smith RS. Overcoming the Odds: high risk children from birth to adulthood. Cornell University Press; 1992.*

Chapter 11

Pediatric physiotherapy
Helping human development

Iñaki Pastor Pons

The aim of physiotherapy is to assess and treat human dysfunctions in virtually all areas of medicine. Among others: rheumatology, traumatology, the musculoskeletal system, pulmonology, urogynecology, cardiovascular medicine, and pediatrics in particular.

Pediatric physiotherapy has been, and continues to be, an extremely valuable tool for treating children with very severe neurological disorders or respiratory pathologies such as bronchiolitis and other diseases of the respiratory tract. Less is known about the role of physiotherapy in the neurological development of healthy children who have «problems», learning disabilities, issues with coordination or behavior and socialization. These children often have mild to moderate neurodevelopmental disorders.

Pediatric physiotherapy is committed to improving continuously to help children and their families with the different health issues that little ones can face. It goes without saying that our profession is evolving all the time to adapt to the needs of an ever changing society and the findings of ground breaking scientific research. We would like to underscore current developments in two particularly interesting areas.

On the one hand, pediatric physiotherapy is progressing thanks to concepts such as PIMT (Pediatric Integrative Manual Therapy) by applying the kind of manual therapy so effective in treating musculoskeletal dysfunctions in adults, in the field of pediatrics. This represents a major step forward in treating children with; pain, torticollis, infants with colic and irritability, sleep or swallowing disorders, head deformities such as plagiocephaly, otitis, craniofacial trauma, growing pains, sports traumas, etc.

On the other hand, the emergence of developmental physiotherapy within the wider field of pediatric physiotherapy is enabling us to screen children with neurodevelopmental disorders who have attention, learning, coordination or behavior disorders, and help them by adopting an integrative biopsychosocial approach. From a professional perspective, developmental physiotherapy implies a commitment to helping a large group of children (we are talking around 20%) who are doomed to school failure, and, to a lesser degree, to developing social or behavioral disorders with all the suffering this entails for the individual and their families. It really is a commitment to them and their families. In this sense, teaching and training activities for other professionals in the fields of health and education, as well as parents, is an unavoidable challenge for developmental physiotherapists in the fight to prevent many disorders that could be treated or, at the very least, their consequences reduced, with suitable, timely intervention.

Pediatric physiotherapists are well prepared to help you and your child. You can count on us. Stay with me now to learn more about how we can help you.

A paradigm for a more integrated pediatric physiotherapy

It is amazing to see how pediatric physiotherapists around the globe are working to give children with health problems a better quality of life. There is outstanding pediatric physiotherapy work going on in the fields of respiratory illnesses and neurology for children with brain damage or genetic or metabolic syndromes.

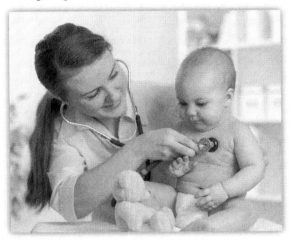

Pediatric physiotherapists working in the field of respiratory illnesses use a stethoscope to locate mucus and apply suitable methods to help the infant or child expel it. The quality of breathing and infection prevention depends on this work.

Over the years many effective methods of neuro-motor rehabilitation have been developed and they coexist with other newer, more integrated approaches backed by growing scientific evidence. Similar advances in the design and implementation of orthopedic aids have proved of invaluable assistance.

The conceptual model most commonly used in neuro-motor physiotherapy is based on a theory of motor control called the dynamic systems theory, which evolved from the work of a Russian scientist named Bernstein. The basis of this theory is that, in order to perform a certain function, the central nervous system must control a number of variables such that even in a repetitive movement like hammering a nail, none of the blows is equal to another. The strength, the joint amplitude in the arm, or the position of the back, changes constantly. In other words, there is no single way of making a movement; the body will adapt to all internal and external conditions to carry out the function in the most efficient and economical way possible. For children with severe motor control disorders such as cerebral palsy where there is spasticity or uncontrolled, involuntary movements, a good strategy is to try to secure the best possible function for that child, bearing in mind the internal conditions associated with his impairment and the external environmental conditions surrounding him. This is an intervention framework based on the dynamic systems theory.

But the dynamic systems theory is not the only theory of motor control. There are others such as the hierarchical theory or the motor program theory which describe how the central nervous system is programmed from the maturation of higher nerve centers that integrate and inhibit previous control models or programs. Even leading experts in the field of motor control such as Shumway-Cook and Woollacott, state in their work on this subject;

> Which is the most comprehensive theory of motor control, the only one that can really predict the nature and cause of movement and that is consistent with current knowledge of the anatomy and physiology of the brain? As you will no doubt appreciate, no theory has it all. We believe that the best theory of motor control is that which combines elements of all the theories presented.

Much of what you have seen in this book is based on programming and hierarchical models of the nervous system. We have clearly seen how, what happens at the beginning of life and the way in which the nervous system begins to function, determines how a child functions and how he will function in the future as an adult, on a physical, emotional or immunological plane, among others. We discussed this topic in the chapter on programming. We have also seen how, to some extent, human beings have several superimposed brains. The newest brain is built on the previous version; it takes control of the higher functions and leaves the previous brain functioning at a lower level, in the «basement» relegated to managing the most primitive and automatic processes. We looked at this in depth in the chapter on the stages of development. Both motor control theories have a large experimental base, and therefore remain as the espoused scientific theories. A really interesting question at this point is, once a nervous system has been programmed, can it be reprogrammed? And, what would it take, how long would it take and what kind of stimuli would it require?

Once a nervous system has been programmed, can it be reprogrammed? What would it take, how long would it take and what kind of stimuli would it require?

In fact, both physiotherapy and psychotherapy, as well as other bio-medical fields that focus on re-educating and rehabilitating different dysfunctions, could not achieve results without somehow changing the way the brain works. The implication being that there is potentially some kind of reprogramming. However, how do we achieve this in the fastest, most efficient, permanent way? This is the real challenge facing science – how to learn more and thus take more effective action.

Physiotherapy and psychology just like other biomedical fields that focus on reeducating and rehabilitating different dysfunctions, could not achieve results without somehow changing the way the brain works. The implication being that there is potentially some kind of reprogramming.

A pediatric physiotherapist must base his decision about which model to use to assess and treat a child on four main variables. On the one hand, the objectives the child and family have. This is perhaps the first point we should consider. We need to fully understand what the family's needs are and what motivates the child. By taking these aspects into account, we can offer more effective help and the family is better able to follow the treatment plan because they feel part of the decision-making process.

Their environmental reality at home or at school is another important factor in the decision making process. The physical environment, which may or may not be adapted, the educational staff who support the child, as well as other aspects relating to the places and people that surround the child, are very important. Sometimes pediatric physiotherapists need to visit the child's home to check that the environment is healthy and stimulating or help the family to organize this environment to ensure the optimal mobility and development of the child.

The child's motivation, the family's objectives, the home and school environment: four very important variables that each individual may experience and develop in a different way depending on their physical, emotional or social reality. Every human being should have a global map that takes into account their own particular and wide-ranging circumstances. This is why the physiotherapist's experience should also be taken into account for decision making purposes. Pediatric physiotherapists are

well prepared to help you and your child. You can count on us.

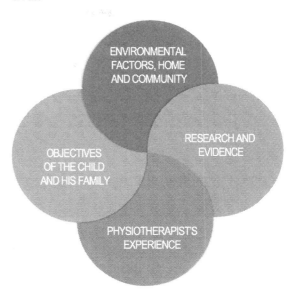

Evidence-informed decision making model. Adaptedfrom Campbell et al., 2006.

The move toward manual therapy in pediatrics

Manual therapy in physiotherapy has made enormous progress over the last thirty years. Many different methods and concepts that are firmly grounded in evidence-based research have been successfully developed around the world for treating musculoskeletal dysfunctions (problems affecting joints, muscles or tissues in general). It is quite possible that at some point in your life you have required the services of a physiotherapist for a back problem and that this specialist used his professional know-how to improve the position of your joints, enhance your mobility or relax the tissues. It is possible that he made effective use of more holistic methods such as global postural re-education (GPR) or perhaps more analytical ones such as orthopedic manual therapy (OMT) derived from the Kaltenborn concept. There are many other treatment systems that also deliver good outcomes.

Despite major strides in terms of the methods of manual physiotherapy available and the contributions they have made to the assessment and treatment of so many problems, none have been developed in pediatrics: as though children and infants never suffered any pain or had spinal joint dysfunction. The number of infants with neck problems following a difficult birth, is no joke. You only need to look at the statistics: the percentage of infants that develop flat head syndrome as a result of neck problems is 19% or even higher. That's almost 1 in 5. Whilst it is inevitable that these methods will require some technical adjustments to take into account the distinctly different anatomy and physiology of the developing child, so far infants and children have been deprived of the benefits of all this excellent work.

Imagine that you have torticollis after twisting your neck or sleeping in the wrong position. It's not hard to imagine the scene because it's something that has happened to all of us at least once in our lifetime. Imagine you go to see a physiotherapist about it. He holds your chest firmly so that you can't move, then turns your head, forcing you to gain range of motion by pushing against your stiffness and pain. He repeats this movement several times. Would you stand for this kind of treatment? The reality is that if you went to see a physiotherapist specializing in manual therapy, he would gently check to see which vertebrae might be blocked or which muscles were causing the dysfunction. He would then carry out a series of non-painful maneuvers that would unlock your neck in a matter of minutes, although it might be necessary to return another day. Well, as strange as it may seem, even to this day in many physiotherapy centers, infants with torticollis still have their heads forcibly turned with no prior joint assessment and without specific, pain-free techniques, even though these would be used in the case of an adult.

The last century saw the fields of osteopathy and chiropractic develop highly effective, ground-breaking pediatric manual treatments. However, they overlooked what we consider to be two key factors; the concept of neurodevelopment and the role families play in treatment. Everything to do with the neurological side requires great perseverance, whether we are talking about brain damage or attention deficit disorder. Craniosacral therapy, particularly the work of John Upledger, has provided us with an amazing set of techniques for harmonizing craniosacral tension in infants and children. However, neurodevelopmental assessment, the stimuli which build the nervous system and the more neuro-orthopedic aspects of pathology, such as an infant's hip or children's feet, have been totally overlooked in spite of their major significance. An infant with torticollis needs his nervous system reprogramming as his limitation prevented him from completing certain important stages of his development; he doesn't control one hand as well as the other; he wasn't able to straighten up or enjoy tummy-time; he doesn't control his eye movements properly; his neck

doesn't function correctly and is locked; he wasn't able to roll over onto his side. In short, he has significant gaps in his neurological development. All this needs taking care of and families need training to create the right environment and necessary stimuli so that their baby can regain all the movements and postures he missed the first time round. It is not enough to simply treat his neck, although clearly, treating it properly is the first step.

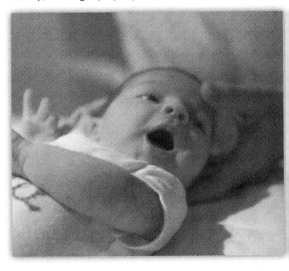

The physiotherapist's expert hands assess Olivia's neck in a gentle, but at the same time highly precise, manner. PIMT is revolutionizing the way we understand pediatric physiotherapy.

Physiotherapy must train families to create the right environment and necessary stimuli so that their baby can regain all the movements and postures he missed the first time round.

Pediatric Integrative Manual Therapy (PIMT) seeks to fill the gap that exists in training and services by providing physiotherapists with the tools they need for the assessment and manual treatment of the musculoskeletal system, the neural system and its membranes, using gentle joint and tissue mobilization techniques. This must always be carried out in line with the child's neurodevelopment and based on scientific and clinical evidence.

The move toward developmental physiotherapy

On the whole, severe neurodevelopmental problems, such as cerebral palsy, are relatively easy to diagnose with the right intervention and support, especially if this begins in early childhood. On the other hand, more moderate impairments of the central nervous system are often misinterpreted by both professionals and parents alike. Some people believe that the child will overcome all the developmental «delays» he has it will just take him a little longer. Not only is this not true but, in some cases, the child gets left even further behind. The problem is also often attributed to personality traits: «It's just the way he is, a bit clumsy». Unfortunately, we know that developmental immaturity in infants carries a high probability of attention, learning and behavioral disorders in slightly older children.

They say that people don't change, but, if we take a close look at human beings, from a biological perspective everything changes all the time. Our body changes, our cells are constantly renewing themselves to the point that in 4 years we have pretty much completely renewed most of the cells in our body. Our physiology changes; the same food won't always suit us at different times in our lives; our muscles are able to cope with widely differing kinds of physical activity depending on our age and the training we have. Our way of thinking and feeling, changes. Once again, age and life experiences give us a very different perspective on life, and a range of different emotions. There is no doubt about it, we do change. But this change is even more dizzying when we are children: our size changes, our maturity, the shape of our bones and our ability to move and to feel. The speed of these changes is frenetic in infancy and childhood. Have you noticed how quickly a flesh wound heals on an infant or a small child? It can be healed overnight leaving no mark, yet in the case of an adult it can take weeks. It is striking how completely different a child's anatomy, the shape of the bones in his body or his head, is to that of an adult.

All of these changes in childhood make it much more complex to assess what is normal or otherwise for an infant or child. The simplest thing, such as an infant holding his head up during tummy-time can be a sign of development in a 3-month old infant, but equally, it can be a sign of a neck problem in a 3-week old infant. Each stage of development takes place at a certain time but even here the normal range changes over time. For example, at six months an infant has a window of around two weeks to learn to roll over, yet when it comes to walking, the normal range is around 3 months, sometimes even longer at 12-13 months.

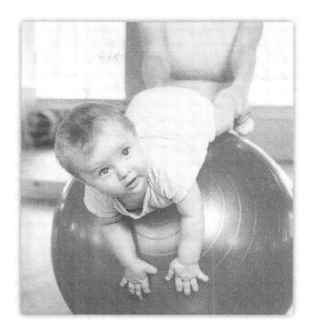

Robert has fun doing stimulation exercises on a ball. Developmental physiotherapy makes use of different stimuli to create more accurate motor patterns and awaken the automatisms that are the building blocks of the nervous system.

In spite of growing evidence, the very fact that there is a normal range during the process of change, has led to the field of Health Sciences and Medicine underestimating the predictive value of neurodevelopmental assessment for future problems, especially with regard to attention and hyperactivity disorders or learning disabilities. For medicine, the normal (note that we are referring to statistical normality here) upper limit for infants to start to walk is 18 months. However, the reality is that infants who start to walk at 17 or 18 months are clearly hypotonic and have developmental problems that are also visible in other aspects of their movements or posture. They are neurologically healthy, but have developmental impairment.

Therefore, health agencies and health professionals need to focus more on setting up a serious developmental assessment for every infant, as well as educating their families about the key stimulation processes required for their children. This stimulation may seek to optimize neurodevelopment or prevent certain problems later on which are bound to have a higher cost for society. But, who should carry out these assessments? There is no doubt in our minds that they should be performed by physiotherapists or pediatric occupational therapists specializing in neurodevelopment. Physiotherapists would also be able to check that there is no stiffness in the infant's neck, head or back that could interfere with his neurodevelopment. There are reliable, validated assessment scales that allow an objective assessment of these tasks. Screening for at-risk cases would mean that professionals would be on the alert and the family prepared to apply the stimuli needed to prevent future problems.

A field known as «developmental physiotherapy» is starting to emerge in several countries thanks to Pediatric Integrative Manual Therapy (PIMT).

Physiotherapy is deeply committed to pediatrics and physiotherapeutic care for children and their families. However, until recently our work was polarized toward children with severe neurological, genetic or orthopedic disorders and some wonderful work is going on in this area. Respiratory physiotherapy in pediatricsis now standard practice in our profession. How many families out there benefit from the help of a physiotherapist in facilitating the release of mucus and allowing children to breathe better and more freely? A field known as «developmental physiotherapy» is starting to emerge in several countries thanks to Pediatric Integrative Manual Therapy (PIMT). Physiotherapists trained in PIMT work with moderate developmental disorders that affect coordination, balance, attention disorders, learning disabilities, immature speech, autism spectrum disorders, children with psychological trauma, and in general neurologically healthy children who don't «function» properly. The suffering these children and their families undergo due to social and family pressures and because they are not meeting expectations, can lead to psychological problems.

Developmental physiotherapy is a branch of the art and science of pediatric physiotherapy and includes various clinical and social factors. It deals with the maturation processes (from fetal stimuli to full growth), in the structure, function, activity and participation of normal children and those with special needs. Its aim is to offer early assessment and effective treatment for conditions involving dysfunctions of the body, mind and personality; and, last but not least, to discover the causes and try to prevent these functionally diverse conditions.

Developmental physiotherapy is a branch of the art and science of pediatric physiotherapy and includes various clinical and social factors.

It deals with the maturation processes (from fetal stimuli to full growth), in the structure, function, activity and participation of normal children and those with special needs. Its aim is to offer early assessment and effective treatment for conditions involving dysfunctions of the body, mind and personality; and, last but not least, to discover the causes and try to prevent these functionally diverse conditions.

Experts in foundations

There are innumerable potential types of neurodevelopmental disorders resulting from: genetic defects, minor organic brain syndromes, the absence of proper programming, damage to the neck and head in the perinatal stage, etc. However, despite the fact that the individualization of treatment is essential, we have a finite number of treatments and reprogramming systems available.

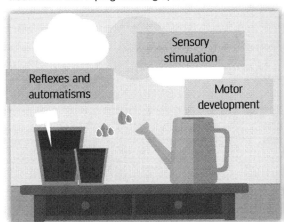

The building blocks of the nervous system are the reflexes and automatic systems that can evolve into more complex programs if the individual receives the appropriate sensory stimulation and experiences movement and posture as nature intended.

Whatever the cause of the disorder or developmental delay, whether it mainly affects the sensorimotor area, cognitive or language areas, the foundations of the nervous system will require reprogramming. In several previous chapters we have seen that for the cognitive part of the «higher» brain to function correctly, the «lower» brain that is in charge of automatic functions (located in the medulla and brainstem), must work properly. The organization and maturation of this part of the nervous system develops mainly in the prenatal phase and during the first few months of life. Certain basic stimuli must activate the brain in this period. Without these experiences, the brain cannot mature optimally. Touch and movement are the main stimuli. Remember that being touched activates many fundamental physiological functions, such as thermoregulation, activation of the immune system or brain mapping of the boundaries of our body and its different parts. It also contributes to emotional and relational regulation and programming. Children who are not touched enough suffer serious developmental problems in cognitive, motor and emotional coordination skills (see the chapter «Bonding through touch»). Head movement activates a basic system for programming the nervous system: the vestibular system. The vestibular system is responsible for organizing balance, spatial orientation, eye movement and regulating stress in the brain. These tasks are essential to establish the foundations for developing the higher, more advanced areas of our brain.

Whatever the cause of the disorder or developmental delay, whether it mainly affects the sensorimotor, cognitive or language areas, the foundations of the nervous system will require reprogramming.

Other floors can be built inside this building, one above the other, using the ground floor as the base. For example, cognitive skills such as attention or literacy are housed on the higher levels of the building.

Pediatric physiotherapists should be experts in assessing how the foundations of the nervous system have been laid and in finding ways to make them solid. Any pediatric physiotherapist specializing in development, such as an expert in PIMT, will prescribe tactile and vestibular stimulation exercises based on the child's age and the extent of the problem. If you were trying to learn a new language or play a musical instrument, would just one lesson a week be enough? Probably not. By the same token, neurological reprogramming can't be effective in just one or two sessions a week either. This is why physiotherapists specializing in PIMT always engage the family's help. In addition to the specialized physiotherapy sessions which deal with the most complex aspects of treatment, the family is given stimulation protocols to follow at home. It is this daily stimulation that will ensure the best results. The reprogramming stimulation must have clearly defined stages and it will require time. Only certain types of exercise will do. Just because an exercise is healthy doesn't mean it is relevant to the nervous system at a particular stage. For example, swimming is a source of excellent physical exercise, but it will probably be ineffective in terms of building foundations in a child who has trouble going down stairs or who can't ride a bike without training wheels. Likewise, if the child's core hasn't been awakened or if his neck is stiff or locked, it is unlikely hand exercises to strengthen fine motor skills will produce results. There is a time for everything and it is the pediatric physiotherapist's responsibility to know when this is.

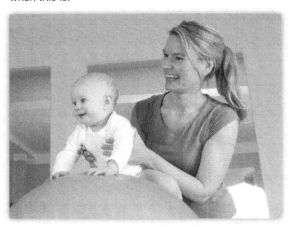

Logan is on cloud nine sitting astride the ball at his physiotherapy session. The physiotherapist's guiding hand helps him discover his body and the precise movement stimulation helps to improve his balance and reactions.

Physiotherapists specializing in PIMT always engage the family's help with stimulation protocols to follow at home.

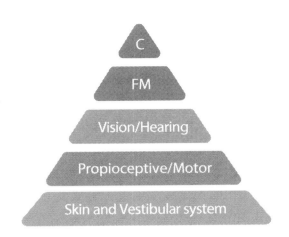

A basic framework showing the stages and goals of stimulation in developmental reprogramming. They are not mutually exclusive as the stroking necessary for skin stimulation also awakens sensations in the deep tissue which in turn stimulates proprioception. Like wise many motor programs provide some tactile and vestibular experiences. Specialists usually start to re-educate vision or hearing when the lower levels are relatively firmly established. However, in some cases it is necessary to intervene earlier to prescribe glasses or reprogram a severe hearing impairment. Fine motor skills (FM) come next and cognitive skills (C), still later.

Primitive and postural reflexes must be integrated

A growing number of studies point to the presence of primitive reflexes –that should have been integrated and inhibited during the first year of life– in children with attention disorders, learning disabilities, immaturity or neurodevelopmental delay.

In recent years several avenues of international research and training in the field of neurodevelopment, have made the role of primitive reflexes in reprogramming the central nervous system (CNS), the focus of their work. Schools like the Institute for Neuro-Physiological Psychology (INPP), run by Peter and Sally Goddard, have been of enormous help to professionals working with children who have developmental delays and learning and attention issues. Correctly applied by competent experts, these methods provide effective pathways for stimulation and reprogramming, although manual physiotherapy is required to unlock the neck, spine and skull.

It is important to stress at this stage that it would be ludicrously simplistic to point the finger of blame at the non-integration of primitive reflexes as the only cause of neurodevelopmental disorders. One of the principles of scientific substantiation is that, the fact two phenomena coexist does not imply that one is the cause of the other. In the same way that just because there are firefighters at fires, it doesn't mean they started them. It would be ridiculous to think that wouldn't it? By the same token, the active presence of primitive reflexes in children with developmental problems does not imply that their presence is the cause of this delay or impairment.

It would be better to see primitive reflexes as an expression of the maturity of the CNS and its level of control. Screening for primitive and postural reflexes is an important part of a thorough neurodevelopmental examination, although it is unclear whether a single assessment of reflexes can offer a comprehensive clinical overview of the child.

Primitive reflexes must form part of the foundations of the nervous system facilitating the myelination of neuronal systems and assisting in neuromotor and sensory functions. They are not the enemy to be defeated.

As Vygotsky says, primitive reflexes must be integrated, not inhibited. They must form part of the foundations of the nervous system, facilitating the myelination of neuronal systems and assisting in neuromotor and sensory functions. They shouldn't be seen as the enemy to be defeated and this kind of thinking makes treatment ineffective. In some cases where there is very severe motor, language and cognitive delay, such an approach can lead to a total lack of results. Not only are they not the enemy, but they are a great ally that must be there in the background to step in and help when something unexpected happens or when there is a significant motor demand. It's simply that they shouldn't be in front-line action as it hinders the effectiveness of the higher motor skills. What would happen if each time I picked up a pen, it triggered a grasp reflex I couldn't control? Firstly, I would struggle to make fine motor movements or a precise pincer grasp as I would have to focus my efforts on keeping hold of whatever I had in my hand without my fist clenching. It would also require a huge amount of energy. However, if I were hanging from a high bar with the risk of falling and hurting myself, I would like this automatic, powerful grasp reflex to give me extra strength to keep me hanging there until help arrived. I wouldn't stand a chance of hanging anywhere for even 5 seconds with my fine pincer grasp.

Primitive reflexes don't always require specific exercises for integration. After years of screening before and after treatment, our clinical expertise tells us that they are often integrated through basic sensory stimulation or when the child recreates certain stages of motor and postural development that he couldn't complete properly when he was an infant. This is understandable because it is possible that reflexes are a sign of a problem and when the problem is solved, the reflex is no longer as visible. Remember that reflexes are an expression of the level of organization of the nervous system, particularly the «lower» brain.

Part of a large team

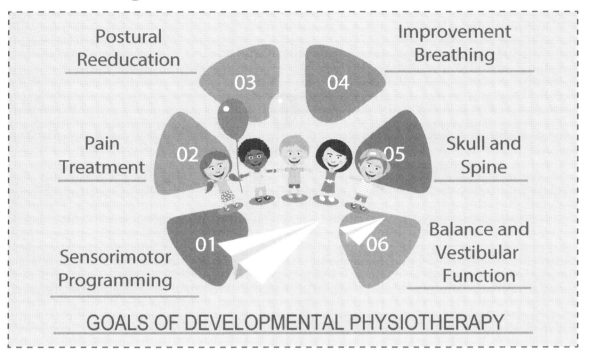

Diagram of the key areas of work in developmental physiotherapy. These areas overlap and complement those of general pediatric physiotherapy and even those of other areas of competence in different professions linked to neurodevelopment.

If we take the definition of developmental physiotherapy described above, adapted from the definition of "developmental medicine" by Sheridan (1980), we see that no professional can single-handedly treat the human body, mind and personality. The body alone requires different professionals to screen its structure and function for a person to achieve their optimal state of health.

Children with moderate or severe neurodevelopmental impairment, whether more on a motor, cognitive or speech level, or a combination of all three, require different professionals to help them heal or adapt. The developmental physiotherapist is responsible for screening and treating motor and sensory impairments (especially vestibular, proprioceptive and tactile impairments); checking there are no mechanical dysfunctions of the spine, skull or joints in the limbs (and if necessary treating them immediately); reeducating posture, improving breathing, treating pain, improving coordination and balance and participating in the design and implementation of orthopedic devices (where necessary, for example in serious motor disorders such as cerebral palsy).

Developmental physiotherapists always work as a team with the child and his family but they are also part of a professional network that includes many other specialists:
- Pediatricians.
- Neuro-pediatricians.

- Behavioral optometrists.
- Speech therapists.
- Psychologists.
- Educational psychologists.
- Podologists.
- Orthopedic technicians.
- Occupational therapists.
- Teachers and school counselors.
- Orthodontists.
- Others.

Not all children will need to see all these specialists if they have a developmental problem, far from it. The specialists they need to see will depend on the type of problem they have. A child with visual impairments that affects his learning or balance would first and foremost need to see a behavioral optometrist. If we are talking about a child with disturbed behavior, low self-esteem or problems of attachment and bonding, the priority will be for him to see a psychologist. In fact, we should screen the neurodevelopmental status of every child and lay the foundations to ensure it is optimal. If a child has severe neurodevelopmental impairment it is hard for specialists to achieve therapeutic goals in their scope of responsibility. It is our job to help the family prioritize and put them in touch with other specialists to ensure that they genuinely receive comprehensive care.

It is our job to help the family prioritize and put them in touch with other specialists.

SUMMARY

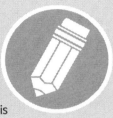

Pediatric physiotherapy has been, and continues to be, a very valuable tool for treating children with severe neurological impairments or respiratory pathologies such as bronchiolitis. The role of physiotherapy in the neurological development of healthy children with mild to moderate neurodevelopmental disorders is less well understood.

A pediatric physiotherapist must base his decision about which model to use to assess and treat a child on four main variables. On the one hand, the objectives the child and the family have. On the other hand, environmental factors such as home or school, scientific evidence and, finally, the physiotherapist's professional experience.

A field known as "developmental physiotherapy" is starting to emerge in several countries thanks to Pediatric Integrative Manual Therapy (PIMT). Physiotherapists trained in PIMT work with moderate developmental disorders that affect coordination, balance, attention disorders, learning difficulties, immature speech, children with psychological trauma, and in general children with joint or muscle pain. Even though they may not be serious, some of these disorders can cause the child and his family to suffer due to social and family pressures and because they are not meeting expectations, all of which can lead to psychological problems.

PIMT provides physiotherapists with gentle, effective manual techniques for use on infants and children. As a result, physiotherapy can provide much more comprehensive treatment for colic, torticollis or head deformities.

A growing number of studies point to the presence of primitive reflexes —which should have been integrated and inhibited during the first year of life— in children with attention disorders and learning disabilities, immaturity or neurodevelopmental delay. These primitive reflexes have to be integrated for the nervous system to function properly.

Developmental physiotherapists always work as a team with the child and the family, but they are also part of a professional network that includes many other specialists.

BIBLIOGRAPHY

Regarding the incidence of infants with flat head syndrome:

Robinson S, Proctor M. Diagnosis and management of deformational plagiocephaly. Journal of Neurosurgery: Pediatrics. 2009;3(4):284-95.

Regarding the dynamic systems theory:

Bernstein N. The coordination and regulation of movement. Londres: Pergamon; 1967.

Regarding the different theories of motor control:

Shumway Cook A, Woollacott MH. Motor Control. Translating Research into Clinical Practice. 4th ed. Wolters Kluwer. Lippincott Williams & Wilkins; 2010.

Regarding evidence-based decision making:

Campbell SK, Palisano R, Orlin MN. Physical Therapy for Children. 4th ed. Elsevier Saunders; 2006.

The move toward manual therapy in pediatrics:

Biedermann H. Manual Therapy in Children. Churchill Livingstone; 2004.

Davies NJ. Chiropractic Pediatrics. 2nd ed. Churchill Livingstone; 2013.

Sergueef N. Osteopathie pédiatrique. Elsevier; 2007.

The move toward developmental physiotherapy:

Accardo PJ. Capture & Accardo's Neurodevelopment Disabilities in Infancy and Childhood. Volume I: Neurodevelopment Diagnosis and Treatment. 3rd ed. Paul H Brookes Publishing; 2009.

Hansen K, Joshi H, Dex S, eds. Children of the 21st Century: The first five years. Policy Press; 2010.

Regarding physiotherapists specializing in foundations:

Barnard KE, Brazelton TB. Touch. The foundation of Experience. International Universities Press; 1990.

Christy JB, Payne J, Azuero A, Formby C. Reliability and Diagnostic Accuracy of Clinical Tests of Vestibular Function for Children. Pediatric Physical Therapy. 2014;26(2):180-9.

Regarding primitive reflexes and learning disabilities:

Konicarova J, Bob P, Raboch J. Persisting primitive reflexes in medication-naïve girls with attention-deficit and hyperactivity disorder. Neuropsychiatr Dis Treat. 2013;9:1457-61.

McPhillips M, Hepper PG, Mulhern G. Effects of replicating primary-reflex movements on specific reading difficulties in children: a randomised, double-blind, controlled trial. Lancet. 2000 Feb 12;355(9203):537-41.

McPhillips M, Sheehy N. Prevalence of persistent primary reflexes and motor problems in children with reading difficulties. Dyslexia. 2004 Nov;10(4):316-38.

McPhillips M, Jordan-Black JA. Primary reflex persistence in children with reading difficulties (dyslexia): a cross-sectional study. Neuropsychologia. 2007 Mar 2;45(4):748-54.

Regarding conceptual models in primitive reflexes and development:

Goddard S. Attention, Balance and Coordination. The ABC of Learning Success. Wiley-Blackwell; 2009.

Masgutova S, Akhmatova N, Shackleford P, Poston V. Reflexes: Portal to Neurodevelopment and Learning. A collective work. Svetlana Masgutova Educational Institute; 2015.

Regarding the role of reflexes in programming the nervous system:

Vygotsky LS. The child psychology. The problems of child development. Pedagogika; 1986.

Regarding play-based physiotherapy:

Håkstad RB, Obstfelder A, Øberg GK. Let's play! An observational study of primary care physical therapy with preterm infants aged 3-14 months. Infant Behav Dev. 2017 Jan 21;46:115-23.

Chapter 12

What we talk about
when we talk about love

How to create a secure,
loving environment for our child

Jara Acín y Rivera

Love stems from a connection between people: from admiration, chemical attraction, respect and acceptance for who the other person is; from a longing to share, to be there for them, to stay in touch; from intimacy, a desire to help them to grow and even to protect them from the dangers of the world. It is something that develops day by day. When we feel loved, we feel noticed, understood, respected, accepted, safe. We are no longer alone in the world: there is someone who loves us. When we love someone, we create a bond we hope will last forever.

So, to paraphrase the title of Raymond Carver's book: what do we talk about when we talk about bonding and attachment?

The relationship you establish with your baby begins with your own bonding history.

I guess you are reading this book because you want to know more about your baby or child: because you want to support her, help her grow and understand her.

What if I tell you that to do so, first you need to know more about yourself? Take a moment now to think about yourself. Are you ready to look within yourself?

- In a critical situation, do you focus on the «hard facts» and approach the solution rationally, or do you trust your gut feeling and act accordingly? Do you think it's safer to trust logic or gut instinct?

- When someone close to you expresses very intense emotions, do you feel intense rejection, emotional overload, and the need to get away? Do you try to play the matter down and try to bring your emotions under control? Or do you feel a strong urge to care for that person, do everything possible to comfort her and help her return to a more positive emotional state?

- Do you feel extremely uneasy and overcome by a sense of helplessness and loneliness when you must leave the people you are closest to?

These and other questions reveal a lot about your attachment style. Read on and you will no doubt find the answers to why your attachment and relationship history is the way it is and how it has a direct impact on the way your baby will relate to herself and others in the future.

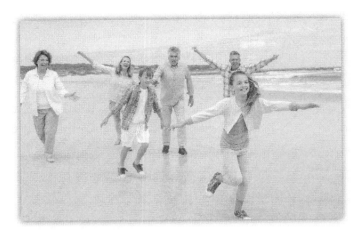

We often hear the terms «bonding» and «attachment» used indistinctly but there are differences between the two. Bonding can start to develop in the early stages of pregnancy and refers to the emotional connection you have with your baby. This is a one-way relationship, from parent to infant and can be extrapolated to other role models in the child's life. Attachment on the other hand, refers to the relationship that the infant builds with her primary caregivers and commences after she is born.

What is attachment?

Attachment is the relationship that is established between an infant and the key figures in her life. She doesn't create just one attachment but rather as many as there are attachment figures. Attachment plays a vital role in human development. Its aim is to regulate the behavior of attachment figures (main caregivers) to keep them close to us. Why is this so important? Because keeping this figure close, helps us to survive.

Through this relationship we learn when and where we can feel safe or, on the flipside, when and where we can expect danger and how to protect ourselves from it throughout our life. It will program our brain, shaping the way we process the information we receive, predisposing us to pay attention to certain stimuli (in the environment and in personal relationships) and triggering alarm bells in some cases.

Are all infants equally prepared for developing attachment behavior? The answer is no. The way it develops in individual infants is influenced by the care their parents can provide, the maturation of their brain, the experiences and circumstances of their lives and what they learn from them. Each human being possesses a unique genetic make-up and the way in which it manifests itself varies widely.

Each human being has a unique genetic make-up and the way in which it manifests itself varies widely.

By the time they are about one year old, infants have established a consistent pattern of strategic behavior to ensure their parent's protective availability. By the end of their second year, rapid neurological changes are taking place (they learn how to talk; walk more confidently; they become aware of others and they are even able to convey different emotions to the one they are feeling!), hence the strategies aimed at proximity maintenance of their attachment figures, become more complex.

It was initially believed that the type of attachment established in early childhood remained stable throughout life. The fact that it programs our way of handling and processing information, as well as responding to dangerous or threatening situations in the most appropriate way –even within a relationship– means that it creates neural pathways which are used time and again and become the preferential route. In other words, attachment directly affects the way our brain develops. There are references in the bibliography in case you are interested in delving deeper into the neurobiology of attachment.

Attachment directly influences how our brain develops.

Nevertheless, this is not set in stone. Current research suggests that even if an individual experiences difficult situations in their childhood, they can still progress towards secure attachment. These findings provide a promising, exciting vision of personal development. Strategies evolve throughout life, influenced by our experiences, the gradual maturation of our brain, the supportive relationships we establish, etc., because the human brain is plastic and has the capacity to reassess the way it views life. We can chart a course that makes us feel safe and at peace with our experiences.

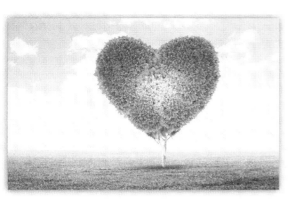

So, what does «parenting for secure attachment» mean?

Raising a secure child involves supporting your children in their personal development by being present in a mindful, predictable way; by offering affection, security and appreciation; by being aware of their needs and attending to them appropriately so they feel seen. They need to know you are there for them; it makes them feel secure and confident. They learn that someone is taking care of them and therefore, the world is a safe place.

It's not just a case of spending time with them either. During this time, you must be in tune with each other too. By playing with them you are helping their growth and bonding which is invaluable. But, to build a secure attachment relationship, you need to go a step further: you must respond appropriately when they need your help.

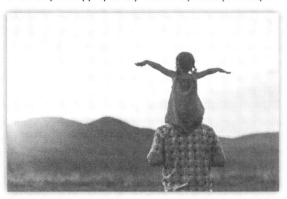

When attachment figures can interpret an infant's cues properly and respond in an appropriate, balanced, positive way, the child develops a secure attachment which will allow them to lead a positive, independent life.

What is secure attachment used for in daily life?

As infants, staying attached to our mothers allows us to survive. We are so underdeveloped when we are born that we can't fend for ourselves. What would happen to us if no one took care of us? In order to develop we need to eat, drink, keep safe and clean and receive plenty of stimulation. Infants display attachment behavior to ensure all their needs are met by their main caregiver; proximity maintenance, a secure base from which to explore the world and a haven where they can seek comfort and protection.

From a neurobiologial perspective, the brain gives top priority to information relating to safety and danger. From the day they are born, infants are equipped with genetically coded programming that provides them with the tools necessary to attach themselves to the person who will help them survive.

Originally, it was thought that this emotional bonding was only created with one specific, emotionally significant person who was not interchangeable. This view is outdated now that we know that children can establish attachment bonds with different figures who have carried out the parenting role appropriately. This knowledge brings a whole new dimension to relational growth: the infant can benefit from being under the watchful gaze of different people who are keen to support her emotional development.

How does attachment help us in terms of our personal development?

Attachment helps us to build a picture of ourselves (who we are) and of our relationships with others too (what to expect and how to react to others). This means that, to a large extent, the way attachment is programmed with our main caregivers will shape our life in the future; making us very self-confident or, conversely, extremely insecure.

Similarly, it will also affect the way we relate to others throughout our life. By this we mean that the type of attachment you had with your parents has great bearing on how you choose your partners; how you face critical situations; the dangers you pick up on and how you react to them; and of course, your attitude to, and style of, parenting. An adult who has been programmed with secure attachment will be able to establish symmetrical relationships because they are self-sufficent (self-assured and capable of managing their emotions), and can achieve intimacy (trust the other person both cognitively and emotionally and self-regulate via this relationship).

However, remember that all the relationships and experiences we have during our life can help our initial attachment style to evolve into what is known as «earned secure attachment». So, whilst it is important to be aware of the significance of bonding and attachment in the early years, we must ensure we maintain a spirit of personal growth and care that opens the possibility of healing relational wounds and moving forward towards greater well-being over the course of our lifetime.

These final chapters look at how attachment has proven to be a key ingredient in brain development, and how it affects all aspects of life. So, when did the experts start to take this on board?

The first author to realize the importance of attachment was John Bowlby in the 1950s. His theoretical construct is one of the most robust in terms of social-emotional development. Subsequently, other authors such as Mary Ainsworth or Mary Main, among others, have expanded on his findings and come up with more complex models that provide more answers. If you would like to examine their findings more closely you will find specific references at the end of this chapter.

How can you create a secure base?

By being sensitive, predictable and consistent in your responses; by empathizing; paying attention to your baby's cues; responding promptly to her needs; by being emotionally available; and, of course, by making her feel good about herself.

Before we elaborate on how a secure base for attachment is built, it is worth taking a moment to reflect on this healing mantra: «Everything we did was out of our deep love for our child. We did things the best we could bearing in mind our personal circumstances and experiences». This is important because, from now until the end of the book, we offer guidelines on how to provide a secure, controlled, consistent environment. Perhaps when we reflect on how we have faced the challenges of parenting up to now, we may have some doubts about the decisions we made or the attitudes we adopted. Be kind to yourselves because the one thing we do know about families is that everything we do is out of love. We mobilize every possible personal resource available, bravely facing the challenges with total commitment. Bear in mind too that this book is not about how to raise the perfect child. It is about how you can best support your child's development based on your own personal circumstances. Remember, development is a lifelong process. You are reading this book so you must believe this too. There is still a great deal you can do; your positive, healing «superpowers» are just as valid now as they ever were.

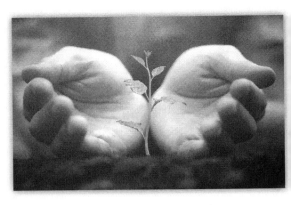

Maternal sensitivity (empathy, availability, acceptance, the ability to provide an in-tune response...) seems to be one of the most reliable predictors of secure attachment. If you are emotionally available for your baby and respond to her behavior in a predictable, warm way, looking out for her well-being and containing her emotional states, before long she will begin to trust your response and her behavior will become more predictable (which will definitely make parenting easier!).

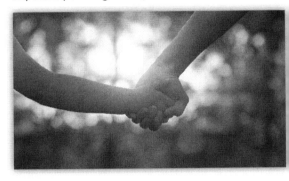

A sensitive, predictable and consistent presence fosters secure attachment.

- Empathy means (rationally) understanding and being (emotionally) attuned to what the child feels in each situation. You need to spend time with her, get to know her; learn how to recognize her special cues in order to figure out how she feels and what she needs. You also need to use a lot of common sense. How would you feel if a bunch of strange ladies stroked your cheeks and talked to you in high-pitched voices, taking turns to hold you, endlessly passing you round and round from one to another? Uncomfortable, maybe? Like you wanted to run away, perhaps? Your baby can't run. Get her out of there. When you feel it's ok for someone to hold her, hold her yourself for a couple of minutes between each stranger (or strangers!). If she cries in their arms, don't hesitate, remove her. It's a sure fire sign that she is uneasy and needs to feel safe again. She is activating the attachment system.

- Responsiveness is the ability to respond (tune in) in a timely, effective and appropriate way to the child's needs. This isn't always easy, especially at the beginning. It doesn't matter so much if you get it right the first time (or the third time). What's important is that she notices you are taking care of her, responding to her need.

- Similarly, it is very important to provide the maximum emotional availability possible. That is to say, the ability to offer your child the security of your presence or assistance (both physical and emotional) in any situation she may need it. By offering your baby predictable responses, you are helping her to control herself and remain calm. If she learns that she will get a proper response, she will display less anxiety when she calls for you.

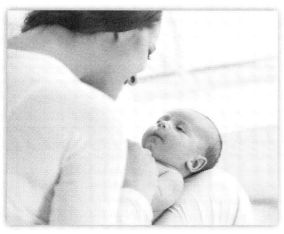

Spend time with your baby. Place her on your knees in front of you so that your faces are close together and your hands are free to caress and engage with her. These moments promote mutual awareness and create attunement.

- To be able to do this, it's just as important to look after your own needs as it is your baby's. Self-care is essential; you can only tune in to your baby if you are feeling good about yourself. Make it a personal project to equip yourself with emotional management tools (including therapy where necessary); make sure to surround yourself with a good social network (friends and family) and use it; lean on your partner if you have one; share experiences with other moms and dads; let off steam; pick up ideas; have fun, dance, laugh.

Don't forget about yourself.

You can only offer emotional nourishment to others if you are sufficiently self-nourished yourself.

- On the other hand, consistency in the way you interact with your baby is good for her mental health. Always say what you want to say, do what you said you were going to do and express your feelings openly. Even when she is an infant, if you sometimes react one way in front of her and at other times in a completely different way, she won't know what to expect. She will feel she is navigating a minefield and this will lead her to be more intent on reorganizing your behavior to gain a little security, than anything else. If, on the other hand, you offer a consistent, predictable response, she will soon learn what your reaction is and how to engage your help whenever it is needed. She will learn to trust what you say and the emotions she perceives in others and will be able to develop more and better by maximizing the full potential of her temperament and the experiences that lie ahead.

- Finally, how much time do we spend observing and showcasing the special qualities children have? Do we accept them for who they are? A very valuable strategy in life is to validate your child's feelings: send her positive messages about herself; show how much you appreciate her through words, gestures and looks; always offer her emotional support. Take a positive approach to parenting and enjoy every moment. By showing her the joy of relationships, you are conveying strength and serenity and teaching her how to find happiness in the simplest things in life.

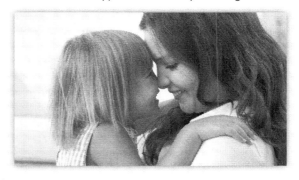

How to recognize different attachment styles

What happens when there is no secure base? As well as secure attachment, which is the most desirable, there are other attachment styles that most of us use too. All these styles form part of a multidimensional continuum and show the strategies an individual puts in place to seek security in situations they perceive as threatening. For this reason, only some people have extreme (pathological) styles and the rest are distributed somewhere along the continuum. Sometimes they mix their own different styles of strategies (depending on the occasion or the moment), or adopt a style that is most identifiable with a specific strategy: and whilst this doesn't mean their positions are immobile, it does make them predictable.

Attachment behavior is adaptable and functional: it developed as the best way to find the resources needed for protection and survival.

Remember this attachment behavior is adaptable and functional; it developed as the best way to find the resources needed for protection and survival. This is precisely why you should stop and ask yourself what factors could have caused this behavior in your child and set the ball rolling if we want things to change. Remember, it's never too late to repair your relationship and the dynamics between you.

How can we recognize the type of attachment we have and the style of bonding we are offering our children?

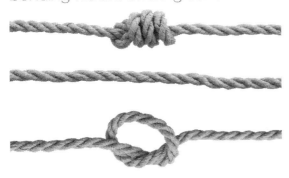

Infants who develop a **SECURE ATTACHMENT** style, clearly perceive that their attachment figures care for them in a sensitive, consistent way. They feel safe in their presence and regulate their well-being via the emotional tuning that exists between them, characterized by calm, intimate, complicit interactions.

These children's primary attachment figures are responsive and available to satisfy their demands. They respond in a timely, effective and consistent way. They know how to interpret the infant's cues correctly and show warmth towards them. Their mere presence is soothing. In other words, your baby may seem slightly anxious or distressed in your absence, but, as soon as you return, she recovers immediately because she trusts you. She has learned that you provide a secure base for her when she is upset because you have been there for her and calmed her down before.

During the Preschool years and once she is over the age of two, a secure attachment child will be confident and will express her emotion honestly. She will turn to you when she is upset because she feels she can access your care freely. She won't sense too many dangers and will know how to correctly interpret the emotional and cognitive cues she receives from others. In other words, the world will seem like a safe place. Also, because she will hardly need to dedicate resources to triggering attachment behavior in her parents and will explore her environment from a secure base, she will make swift headway in her studies and psychosocial and motor development.

This behavior will continue for years. Then when she reaches adolescence (with all the frantic neurogical development it entails), she will have the chance to learn from her experiences and, therefore, reassess her mental models and improve her overall functioning.

This type of caregiver makes plans with their children and these plans consider the needs of the whole family. They listen carefully to their thoughts and feelings and are understanding yet containing (supporting them with their emotions and helping to channel them).

INSECURE-AVOIDANT ATTACHMENT refers to those relationships in which there is emotional distance, detachment, strict boundaries and even rejection. So, what leads loving parents to behave this way? Their own personal attachment wounds. Parents of infants with avoidant attachment have had difficult, possibly traumatic experiences during their childhood and have still not healed their emotional wounds. It's likely they experienced an avoidant (distancing) attachment style in their infancy, one in which their emotions were invisible, so they were unable to learn how to manage them. Perhaps they are scared at having to manage the intense emotions and demands of children who depend on them, when they are barely able to support themselves.

When their attachment figures are absent, infants are quite independent and show little «separation anxiety» (crying, distress, etc.) and clear disinterest in them when they return. Even if the adult tries to get close to them, the infants end up rejecting this contact in their own way. They have learned not to trust the availability of this figure and the separation triggers major activation of their nervous system: they become scared, even if they don't show it. This is why, even if these children usually appear confident about separations, we must ask ourselves if they really are okay.

This type of attachment figure feels swamped and overwhelmed. Their relationship style is based more on action than emotion and they have difficulty tuning in to their children's needs and emotional states. All their energy goes into managing their emotions and attempting to control them, so they feel unable to deal with another person's emotions as well. Not even their own children's.

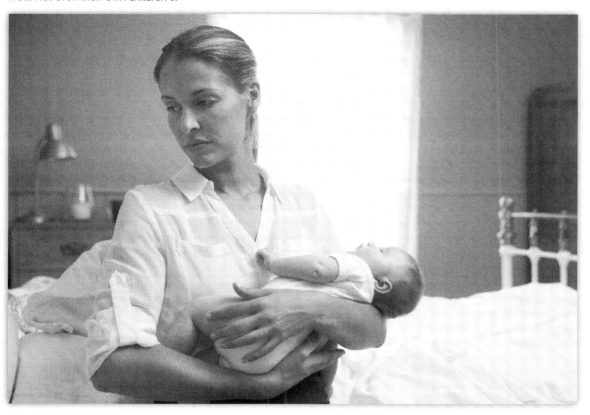

Some research indicates that depression makes it difficult for mothers to be in tune with their children because they can't be emotionally available for them. A psychotherapist can help you to feel better about yourself and improve the attachment with your baby.

In these situations the adult will display avoidance behavior, coldness or even rejection. His body will stiffen, and he will find physical and emotional contact with his child uncomfortable. He will probably punish them and scold them excessively, adhering more to rules than feelings. The infant or child feels this rejection and realizes that when she expresses her needs, her parents are so overwhelmed that they steer clear of her.

As the main objective is to keep them close, these children learn not to show intense emotions, to become «invisible». If they express themselves, their parents are overwhelmed. If their parents are overwhelmed, they withdraw and that is even scarier and harder to deal with. So, they disconnect from their own needs and attempt to self-regulate. They prefer to go to their room when they are sad or angry instead of turning to their parents for comfort. They don't turn to them when they're going through a tough time either.

At Preschool they learn to be obliging and independent and in extreme cases they even feel responsible for their parents' emotions: if they can just manage to keep their «stress» to acceptable levels, everything will be ok.

When the child shows few signs of emotion or affection, her caregivers will be more available and seem more prepared to offer close, intimate contact. However, as soon as the child starts to trust them and expresses herself, the caregiver quickly becomes overhelmed again, withdrawing and rejecting her.

Since emotions are scary and unreliable, they avoid them and hence lose the ability to recognize their feelings and the depth necessary to experience and manage them. They focus on a visible show of positive emotion and on developing their cognitive side to the fullest (their studies, verbal expression...) which are the areas they obtain the most attention and recognition from their parents. They are increasingly demanding of themselves to the point of extreme perfectionism yet they ignore the emotional information. They are always very aware of their parents' mood and skilled at only showing them things they will find pleasing. They truly become the «caregivers of the caregivers». When their parents reject them or are cold towards them, these children feel ashamed. This feeling will accompany them for a long time though they will try to disguise it with academic triumphs and excessive self-sufficiency.

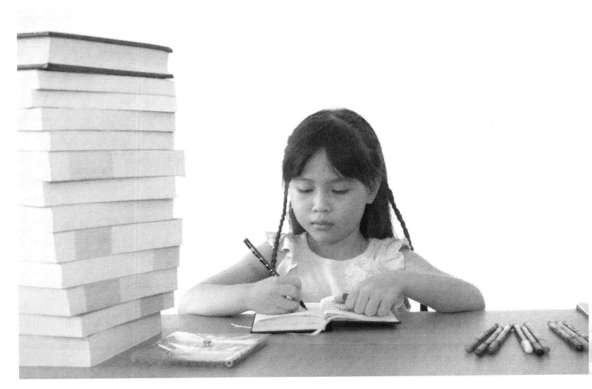

They give the appearance of being very independent and self-sufficient in a bid to avoid overwhelming their attachment figures. They may seek recognition from them through academic success.

When they reach adolescence, they have great difficulty socializing and connecting with others. Their attempts at affectionate exchanges are abrupt, brief and out of context and intimacy makes them feel uncomfortable.

Conversely, parents who over-stimulate their babies or are very intrusive can also create this type of attachment because there is emotional disconnection here too. Needs are neither understood nor met, hence why it is so important for adults to develop the ability to manage their emotions. It helps them to be more available and responsive to their baby so they can offer the right amount of stimulation or quiet time as required.

An infant with an **ANXIOUS-AMBIVALENT ATTACHMENT** style has separation anxiety and doesn't calm down when the attachment figure returns. She is left feeling extremely concerned when the adult departs and stops exploring her environment. She doesn't feel sure that her attachment figure will return or that when they do, they will calm her down.

She is incapable of feeling safe in an unpredictable environment and fears emotional abandonment. The infant's distress may manifest as irritability, or may make her clingy, or reject contact altogether. In other words, she will have ambivalent responses to ambivalent care.

This type of attachment figure is characterized by a high level of emotional expressivity (including sadness, anger and feeling overwhelmed), by only being available at certain times and by not responding in a consistent way to their children's demands. They were probably brought up in an inconsistent setting too and are now being held hostage by their own emotions which dominate their mental state. They may even explicitly blame the children for feeling overwhelmed. These are very worried, anxious individuals who, because they have failed to acquire the right emotional tools, are still suffering and trying to resolve their own difficult experiences.

Probably, the times they attend to their children and the times they don't makes some kind of sense to these adults, but not to the infants or small children in their care. They need a consistent framework to feel safe and secure.

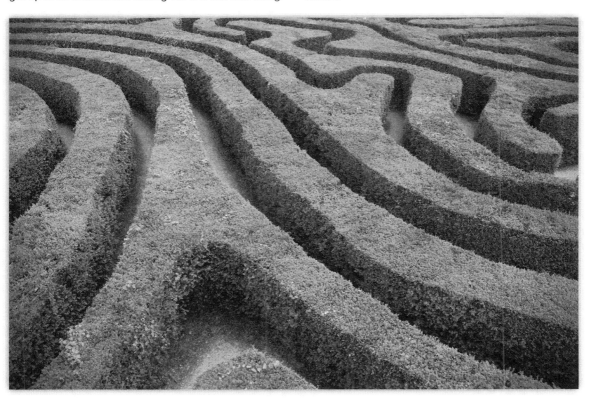

Children with anxious-ambivalent attachment feel very confused about what to expect from their attachment figure because their responses are confusing and unpredictable.

These children are unable to predict what is going to happen and develop deep-seated feelings of anger, fear and uncertainty. As young as 9 months they are capable of identifying the figure whose inconsistency causes these emotions in them and of reacting towards them with intense anger and, at the same time, a deep-rooted fear of abandonment. They suffer separation anxiety, are more fearful of exploring the world, and lack confidence and feel insecure in relationships, despite a strong desire for intimacy and contact.

To engage their parents and keep them at arms length, they use a complex system of highly-charged emotional expression. These expressions will vary as their brain matures but will be firmly focused on seeking the security of the (ideal) emotional connection. Anger is a good method for attracting attention, although it can have its dangers depending on the caregiver's response. It takes a great emotional toll on these children to set up and maintain a system that makes them feel safe because they were unable to develop reliable cognitive scaffolding. This highly-charged, emotionally demanding environment undermines the cognitive development and functioning of school-age children, as well as their exploratory behavior. It also increases the likelihood of learning disabilities, attention deficit and information processing deficits which can be (erroneously) diagnosed as behavioral disorders and/or hyperactivity. These children may develop dependent behavior and feel they are responsible for looking after other people's emotions, even those of adults.

The **DISORGANIZED/DISORIENTED ATTACHMENT** style is seen most often in childhoods where there was neglect or abuse of some kind. But it is not limited to these extreme situations: when one of the main attachment figures has undergone a traumatic experience or loss and their grief is unresolved, they show a high level of psycho-physiological activation in situations that evoke memories of the traumatic event. This means they can't be supporting, soothing figures for their children and in fact, are possibly quite the opposite. They are trapped in their own experiences and disconnected from the child's emotions at that instant in time.

Children with disorganized attachment are insecure, terrified, «emotionally blocked» and their behavior is disorganized and confusing. Their programming was traumatic and now their affective and behavioral strategies have collapsed. They don't know how to get people to attend to their as yet unmet needs. They haven't been «seen» either physically or emotionally so it is very difficult for them to build up a picture of who they are and how to cope.

On the one hand they are very dependent on their role model, and on the other they are filled with fear at this individual's reactions because their behavior is scary, threatening or incoherent (they are detached from the infant's needs or cues). These children find themselves faced with the constant dilemma of getting closer to seek comfort and safety or withdrawing to protect themselves. In order to «survive» they have to cling to the person who hurts them. Disorganized attachment is associated with emotional disorders and severe psychopathology. In other words, abuse and neglect have serious consequences in the long-term.

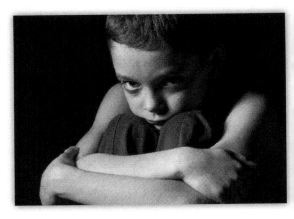

There is a great deal psycotherapy can do to heal the attachment wounds in children with disorganized attachment: by offering them a positive, consistent, protective presence; by restoring their trust in relationships. This is where other role models who are able to respond as attachment figures become especially important by allowing them to feel secure and wholeheartedly trust the relationship as a safe place where they feel seen and well-loved.

These children experience a high degree of muscle tension and learning disabilities (because they didn't develop properly). They play fight, hit objects and provoke their classmates; the only way they know how to connect with others is through negative emotions. They usually challenge their caregivers and teachers by needing and demanding constant attention. They don't know how to regulate interpersonal relationships, or their own emotions and there are flaws in their cognitive and affective ability to interpret relationships. They suffer because they know it is something they don't do well, but they don't know how to improve. Very often the symptoms are so confusing and diverse that it is difficult to distinguish from other diagnostic conditions such as ADHD or behavioral disorders, even for the professionals.

It's never too late to heal these attachment wounds, including seeking help through counseling. The role of the caregiver is to help the infant's brain to develop (broadly speaking, through affection and stimulation), by supporting their children in a manner appropriate to each developmental stage. So, why not join me in the next chapter to discover what opportunities are on offer at each stage, right from the start?

SUMMARY

Attachment behavior is the behavior your baby develops in order to trigger your care behavior when she needs to feel safe and protected. This relationship begins from the moment she is born.

Everybody develops «attachment» towards their main caregivers. The key lies in the quality:

- With secure attachment, the key is consistency, emotional availability, being responsive to her needs, showing predictable positive responses and empathy. She feels safe because she clearly realizes there is someone in her world keeping her safe, responding to her needs and that, therefore, she has nothing to be afraid of. She can explore, learn and experiment.

- With insecure-avoidant attachment the consistent response is emotional distance and even rejection of the child's demands. A pattern of emotional detachment is established because the attachment figures do not have the necessary resources to tune in to the child's emotions and they feel overwhelmed. Hence the child learns to control his parents' proximity by hiding her own emotions to avoid overwhelming them and gain greater access to them.

- With anxious ambivalent attachment the response is inconsistent: sometimes it is sensitive and supportive and other times it's not. Faced with the impossible task of predicting the attachment figure's response, the child simultaneously feels intense desire and fear of both proximity and distance in relationships. They switch between highly charged emotional behavior and «disarming» behavior which halts their parents' intense emotions. Their quest for attachment security drains them of the emotional energy to progress in other areas such as learning, for example.

- With disorganized/disoriented attachment, attachment bonding is a traumatic process because the person who should provide security, is a source of intense fear. The attachment system cannot be organized effectively, and this affects the development of the child's identity.

- It is possible to develop an earned secure attachment. Even if our childhood was complicated, the experiences we have throughout life can modulate and restore our ability to feel safe in relationships and in ourselves.

- It's never too late to heal attachment wounds and reshape relational dynamics. A psychotherapist trained in family therapy and attachment will be able to guide you through this process.

What can you do?
HELPFUL PRACTICAL ADVICE

- Create a calm, consistent space where you can attend to her and connecting emotionally with her needs and you will be directly contributing to healthy development on all levels.

- In order to provide a framework within which she can feel safe, secure and cared-for, you need to familiarize yourself with the needs infants have for stimulation and attention at each stage of their development. Nurture emotional tuning with her by connecting through your gaze and touch; observe her reactions and adjust your behavior accordingly to cater for her rythms.

- It is only natural there will be flaws in this tuning process (upsets, misunderstandings between you, confusion). You don't need to be perfect, the most important thing is you can fix the bond between you by showing her affection, proximity and availability; containing and regulating her distress with calm, comforting words. It's a bit like when someone loses their step when dancing with a partner: watch what they do to recover and dance in unison again.

- It is possible to provide a secure base; the key thing is to «be there». Pay close attention to her needs, emotions and rhythms (and your own!). Try to remain calm so you can interpret her cues. Transmit a sense of availability and predictable presence through your responses and give her emotional support throughout her development.

BIBLIOGRAPHY

«From a neurobiological point of view, attachment behavior is based on the premise that learned motivation exists, that it is genetically coded and allows the infant to create a bond with a specific figure to provide him with a secure base from which to explore the outside world»:

Kaplan H, Sadock B. Textbook of Psychiatry. Reactive attachment disorder of infancy and early childhood. Cap. 44 LWW. 10th ed.; 2005.

«Originally, it was thought that this emotional bonding was only created with one specific, emotionally significant person who was not interchangeable, although some recent research shows that children are capable of establishing attachment bonds with different figures»:

Oliva Delgado, A. Estado actual de la Teoría del Apego. Revista de Psiquiatría y Psicología del Niño y el Adolescente. 2004;4(1):65-81.

«The Attachment theory, which stems from research started by Bowlby in the 1950s, is one of the most robust theoretical constructs in terms of social-emotional development»:

Bowlby J. Vínculos afectivos: formación, desarrollo y pérdida. [Edición renovada, 2014]. Madrid: Ediciones Morata; 1986.

Bowlby J. El apego y la pérdida (volúmenes I y II). Paidós Ibérica; 1993.

Bowlby J. Una base segura. Aplicaciones clínicas de una teoría del apego. Barcelona: Ed. Paidós; 1989.

«Mary Ainsworth (1952) describes three attachment styles: secure attachment, insecure-avoidant attachment and anxious-ambivalent attachment. Subsequently a fourth style was added called disorganized attachment»:

Ainsworth MD. Patterns of attachment behavior shown by the infant in interaction with his mother. Merrill-Palmer Quarterly of Behavior and Development. 1964;10:51-8.

Ainsworth MD, Bell SM. Attachment, exploration, and separation: Illustrated by the behavior of one-year-old in a strange situation. Child Development. 1970;41:49-67.

Main M., Morgan H. Discovery of a new insecure-disorganized/disoriented attachment patern. En: Brazelton TB, Yogman M, eds. Affective Development in Infancy. Norwood, NJ: Ablex; 1986. p. 95-114.

«We know that neuroendocrine changes occur that favor bonding and that attachment behavior has a direct impact on an infant's neural development». If you would like to learn more about the neurological basis of attachment and the emotional factors affecting brain development:

Aguado R. El vínculo como potenciador de la activación de las redes neuronales. xxiv Reunión de la AEP (Asociación Española de Psicodrama). Bilbao; 2009.

Schore AN. Affect regulation and the origin of the self: The neurobiology of emotional development. Routledge; 2015.

Vargas A, Chaskel R. Neurobiología del apego. Avances en psiquiatría biológica. 2007;8:43-56.

Regarding the effects of attachment disorders throughout life: insecure attachment established in childhood acts as a vulnerability factor for future emotional disorders and disorganized attachment as a causal factor of a potentially severe psychopathology.

Cortina M, Liotti G. Attachment is about safety and protection, intersubjectivity is about sharing and social understanding: The relationships between attachment and intersubjectivity. Psychoanalytic Psychology. 2010;27(4):410.

Holmes J. Teoría del apego y psicoterapia. En busca de la base segura. Bilbao: Desclée de Brouwer;2009.

Johnson SC, DweckCS, Chen FS, Stern HL, Ok SJ, Barth M. At the intersection of social and cognitive development: Internal working models of attachment in infancy. Cognitive Science. 2010;34(5):807-25.

Lecannelier F, Ascanio L, Flores F, Hoffmann M. Apego y psicopatología: una revisión actualizada sobre los modelos etiológicos parentales del apego desorganizado. Terapia psicológica. 2011;29(1):107-16.

Liotti G. Disorganized/disoriented attachment in the etiology of the dissociative disorders. Dissociation: Progress in the Dissociative Disorders. 1992;5(4):196-204.

Mansukhani A. Dependencias interpersonales: las vinculaciones patológicas. Conceptualización, diagnóstico y tratamiento. Actualizaciones en sexología clínica y educativa. Huelva: Servicio de Publicaciones de la Universidad de Huelva; 2013.

Siegel DJ. La mente en desarrollo. Cómo interactúan las relaciones y el cerebro para modelar nuestro ser. Madrid: Desclée de Brower; 2007

Chapter 13

Creating invisible bonds
How to bond effectively from the start

Jara Acín y Rivera

Healthy bonding starts right from the beginning. However, the beginning doesn't refer to the birth, rather the prenatal stage, or even way before that! The relationship between the two of you can be nurtured at each stage, becoming richer and more complex along the way.

Prenatal stage: expectations, awareness and self-reparation

Bonding begins well before birth and is heavily influenced by the mother's attitude and expectations about the imminent arrival of her baby. This is why it is so important to allay any fears and insecurities that might interfere with the happy event and redirect the mother's energy towards the search for answers and self-reparation.

During pregnancy we find a special mental state called psychic transparency (Bydlowski) where there is a state of greater susceptibility and unconscious aspects are more accessible to our conscious part which helps us to revisit our own early attachment experiences. Previously unresolved conflicts such as awareness of neglect, abandonment, the absence of attachment figures, or previous pregnancy losses, can resurface. The resulting sadness, fear and stress will have an impact on the bond we are creating with our baby as well as on his physiological development in this prenatal stage.

On the other hand, if you stroke your belly, talk to your baby, communicate with him in a mindful way, etc. you are strengthening this bond and laying the foundations for a secure, attuned relationship in the future.

This is an excellent moment for undergoing psychotherapy as it stirs memories that require re-visiting to achieve better emotional bonding with your newborn. It's worth looking after yourself, taking stock and finding inner balance.

Pregnancy is a very intense life experience because it forces you to think about yourself: previously unresolved psychological problems may resurface in the process.

Previous pregnancy losses can condition your expectations and stress levels during pregnancy. It is vital you have processed this grief properly in order to face another pregnancy with renewed confidence and hope. In the next chapter we will explore more fully what can be a devastating process.

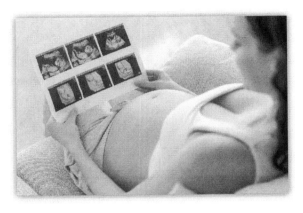

This mental process prior to pregnancy has a preparatory function to ensure proper mother–infant bonding. Fathers can build a clearer picture of their baby too thanks to increasingly sophisticated ultrasound techniques, helping them to feel more attuned to their future child.

From a practical perspective, shops, friends and family will all tell you what you must have ready for when your baby arrives: a crib, changing table, stroller and a whole host of other gadgets. But, has anyone warned you about the need to prepare yourself emotionally for his arrival? Getting the baby's room ready will help you to realize some of the changes that are about to take place in your family – but not the most important ones. This is why there is no better way of spending time during your pregnancy than dedicating it to this all-important emotional preparation: reading, talking with others, asking questions, looking inside yourself and re-adjusting your mindset as necessary.

During pregnancy the perception you have of your baby will go through different phases. According to Winnicott, in the final months you build a more realistic, differentiated perception of your baby.

Did you know that in the final trimester of pregnancy, your baby can hear sounds from the outside? This means he can recognize your voice and those of the people close to you. What goes on around you during pregnancy is important.

Everything that happens in the first few moments after birth will be permanently stored in his brain. Ideally, as soon as infants are born, they should be united with their mother and enjoy skin-to-skin contact and the intimacy of that first shared connection.

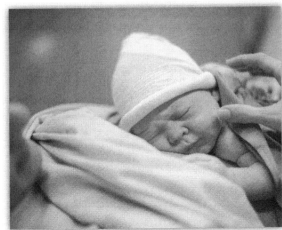

This is why the bond between infants who are born very prematurely (with a birthweight less than 3 pounds 3 ounces) and their mothers is affected right from the start as the «psycho-biological nesting» process is interrupted. In the next chapter there is a section on the constraints and opportunities found in this scenario.

Perinatal: hormones and falling in love

The way we experience labor is also conditioned by how we prepare beforehand, the expectations we have, how we were accompanied during the process, but above all by our hormones. Primarily oxytocin, which triggers the necessary uterine contractions for the baby to be born; facilitates milk letdown; promotes a calm, serene emotional state; helps regulate stress; has relationship enhancing effects; increases eye contact and general well-being. The infant receives oxytocin from the mother during labor and again through her milk when he breastfeeds.

As well as oxytocin, vasopressin, prolactin, cortisol and other catecholamines also play a role in the process by modulating the behavior of both mother and infant. It has been noted that, not only does the attachment relationship between mother and infant have a direct impact on the infant's neurodevelopment, but it also produces neuroendocrine changes in the mother.

As we saw in the first chapter, labor can be experienced differently to the birth itself. Yet, at the same time, during that shared moment there is a special mother-infant connection -a natural, neurochemical connection that is almost magical.

Thanks to this neurochemistry, what happens in those first few moments will be indelibly stored in the infant's memory. This is the start of the attachment process. The purpose of these chemical changes in both brains is to help them meet each other and to make this encounter subconsciously enjoyable. According to Ibone Olza, the oxytocin and endorphins that flood the mother's brain help her to «fall in love» with her baby. In other words, she has a feeling of profound love and well-being when she meets her baby for the first time. The infant's brain will clearly perceive this, and he will feel the same complete satisfaction just as profoundly.

In those first few moments the infant is capable of moving towards his mother using his sense of smell, allowing him to locate her nipple and begin breast feeding on his own. At this point and against this background of love and well-being (bonding), it is likely mother and infant gaze at each other for the first time, assisted by the high levels of oxytocin in both of them. This starts to generate new neural connections in their brains. After about an hour, the infant enters a sleep cycle and his brain consolidates everything he has learned as he sleeps; he can only maintain a feeling of security when he is close to his mother and able to smell her.

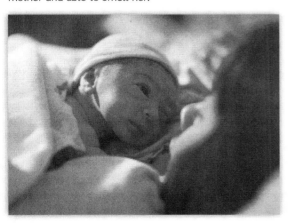

This first gaze represents a milestone in their bonding process and is the result of the neurohormonal communication between them.

Research into the long-term impact of skin-to-skin contact in the first two hours of life (known as the sensitive period) found that when this contact took place, there was a better mother-infant relationship by the age of one (greater attunement, reciprocity and complicity), than when they were separated during that period.

This close relationship between them is maintained for the next few weeks and the mother continues to have a regulating effect on the infant's basic functions (breathing, heart rate...) through skin-to-skin contact and breastfeeding. Almost as if he was still in her womb!

So, as you can see, this moment is vitally important for the mother-infant bond to get off to a good start and nature prepares us very thoroughly for it. This is why any external elements that interfere at this stage will have a direct impact on his development.

It is such a delicate moment that certain techniques and instructions, but above all, the chemical substances that are sometimes administered, can alter the natural neurochemical conditions and interrupt the natural flow of the process. In this sense, induced labor and scheduled C-sections (if the labor process hasn't started spontaneously beforehand), present a totally different neurohormonal scenario to that found when these interventions take place during the final stage of labor. Along the same lines, there are also differences when the mother and infant are separated at birth or when the baby is formula-fed, as we saw earlier.

Not only does separation at birth hamper emotional bonding and breastfeeding, but it also makes it difficult for the infant's stress levels to return to normal: a few hours later the level of stress hormones in their blood can be twice that of infants who had skin-to-skin contact!

This situation can affect an infant's neurodevelopment. However, there are plenty of things you can do afterwards to reduce his initial stress levels and offset the interruption to your bonding process. In Chapter 14 we give you some specific ideas to try out. Whatever happens, it's never too late to build or repair your bond!

Postnatal: touching and gazing at each other

Maternal bonding behavior in the immediate postnatal period plays an essential, decisive role in regulating the infant's heart rate, breathing and general endocrine status and we know that oxytocin is a key player in this process.

The three areas of the neonate's brain essential for developing attachment at this early stage are: the olfactory bulb, locus coeruleus and the amygdala. Simply put, the sucking action liberates oxytocin which flows to the baby through the mother's milk. He then experiences physiological changes of peace, calm and pleasure (it acts like a natural anti-anxiety medication); his quality of sleep improves; he has a lower stress response and a greater desire for social interaction. This is how he is conditioned to associate the maternal smell with a sense of peace and safety.

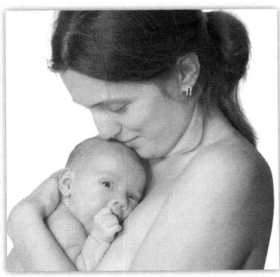

The mother provides physiological regulation for her baby through skin-to-skin contact and he is conditioned to associate the maternal smell with a sense of peace and safety.

In addition to the three brain areas described in research on the neurobiology of attachment, I would venture to add that skin is the fourth pillar upon which bonding is built. As we saw in previous chapters, touch is a key tool not just for an infant's neurological development, but also for developing his sense of Self: when an infant feels touched, he feels appreciated, cared for, wanted, loved. He senses his presence is felt. This is why it is so important to give him skin-to-skin contact, physically touch him and find ways of soothing him that are not merely associated with sucking but also with coordinated movement between you and caresses, for example.

How do you achieve that physical bond?

Breastfeeding and breast milk itself both have important functions. Don't turn them into a pacifier!

As we already know, breastfeeding has many functions: as well as being nutritious, regulating the nervous system and enhancing the infant's immune system, it has a calming and bonding effect. It also develops the baby's face, restores the shape of his skull and prepares him for speech in the future, etc. For all these things to happen, you must be fully in the moment with your baby whenever he breastfeeds: look into each other's eyes, don't let anything distract you and stroke his hands to stimulate suction (the Babkin reflex we saw earlier in the book).

This is a once-in-a-lifetime moment in terms of attachment and neurodevelopment. Make the most of it!

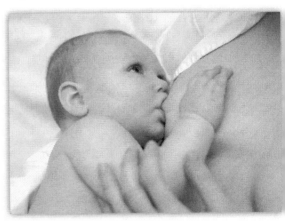

Breastfeeding is not just nutritious, but it also has a calming, bonding effect. Other ways you can promote a sense of calm and encourage bonding include providing skin-to-skin contact, speaking to your baby using a soothing, affectionate tone and prosody, rocking him gently in your arms...

What are the risks of putting him indiscriminately to your breast each time he complains? Have you ever wondered why children and adults who suffer from anxiety tend to have habits that involve their mouths? They suck their thumb, bite their lip, eat, drink or smoke too much, chew their hair, clothes or pens. Breastfeeding programs the brain. We need to find other ways of calming him down when it's not time to eat.

So, how do you bond when breastfeeding isn't an option? There are lots of reasons why you may not be able to breastfeed and in this case there are things you can do to compensate, for example: give your baby extra skin-to-skin time; hold him in your arms each time you bottlefeed him (the two most emotionally significant people in the infant's life should do this), paying the same care and attention you would if you were breastfeeding; find a private space that allows close communication with caresses and the right kind of stimulation.

What's the father's role in all of this?

Some authors have begun to include fathers as very significant figures in the infant's life since, nowadays, they tend to develop a close relationship with their children from the outset.

Historically the roles of both sexes were more conditioned by biological and cultural functions: the mother nurtures, protects and soothes..., the father plays games with varying levels of risk and sets the boundaries. Cultural changes mean that this pattern of parental roles is becoming more balanced and duties are shared in a more natural, sensible way. These days, fathers are involved in every aspect of parenting, not just the fun side and they play important roles as attachment figures.

Starting with the pregnancy, fathers can support the mother's emotional states, communicate with the fetus by talking to it and stroking the mother's belly. When the baby is born this voice and rhythm will be familiar to him. During breastfeeding, fathers can take part in feeding, stimulation and bonding from day one. Men don't experience the same hormonal tsunami as a pregnant woman does but they can bond in an intuitive, mindful way through their skin, their smell and their voice.

From a more emotional perspective, one of the most useful roles fathers have fulfilled has been to broaden the horizons of the mother-infant relationship, expanding its world, bringing new, valuable energy to it. Similarly, by playing with his children, stimulating their movement and even including a certain amount of risk (chasing them, tickling them and lifting them off the floor, etc.), he is making a significant contribution to his offspring's neurodevelopment.

It is unhealthy and limiting to stick to our traditional roles. It means we have no respect for ourselves and we are not giving parenting our best shot. What impact do you think the traditional male upbringing has had on the paternal role in society? Don't show your emotions or feelings of any kind, don't touch – it has clearly hampered bonding between fathers and their children. Everyone has the right to express their emotions, to kiss, show tenderness, etc.

If we overcome these cultural barriers we can develop more fully as people, as well as enjoying truer, healthier, more constructive two-way bonding.

Everyone has their own «superpowers», regardless of gender. This concept is already evident in other areas of life so why don't we apply it to parenting?

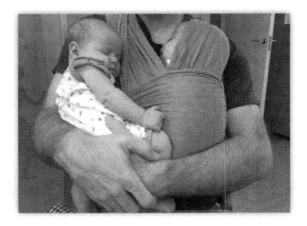

If we actively participate in all aspects of parenting, we will bond better and more deeply from the start.

Consider yourself for a moment. When you were little, or even today, who do you turn to when you are sad and need comforting? Who do you call to share your latest success, your mom, your dad, someone else? Does it follow the expected pattern? Maybe it does, maybe it doesn't. This shows that, even at a time when there was less equality than there is nowadays, your father possibly knew how to tune in to you and comfort you. Because he had the ability and knew how to connect with you. Your mother set the boundaries and implemented the consequences because she could, and because powerful energy came naturally to her.

Perhaps the person you have chosen is someone other than your mother or father. Sometimes we find significant emotional role models outside the nuclear family. This is because they are close to you, present and available for you.

So, it doesn't matter if you create a traditional family, one with two members of the same sex, a single parent family or any other kind of family unit. Parenting should make the most of all the resources the entire tribe has to offer so that each person contributes whatever they can, and the end result enhances the infant's life.

Is it possible to parent with secure attachment and limits at the same time?

We have seen how important it is to respond promptly when they are babies and small children. Later when he asks you for other things, you will have learned how to tell if he has a real need (pain, fear, etc.) and therefore still requires a prompt response, or, if on the other hand, it's just something he wants (to stay in the bathtub playing with his toys forever, for example). In this case our response will be less urgent and our approach kind but firm. Staying very calm you say: «Honey, I know you want to, but right now, you can't» whilst, slowly but firmly, lifting him out of the bathtub.

It is very beneficial for them to have a certain amount of initiative when it comes to choosing what they want to do and how to do it. They can choose: what they want to play with; which of the two snacks on offer they want today; which story they want you to read to them; which park they want to go to; which T-shirt they prefer. All of this is ok as long as we use our common sense and take their age and circumstances into account. Some things are negotiable, others aren't.

A parenting style that includes reasonable limits makes children feel more secure, more contained and less anxious both now and in the future.

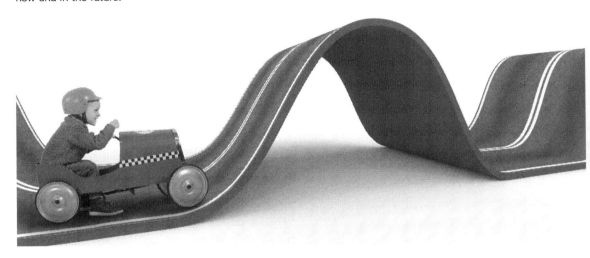

The presence of limits and a certain dose of frustration in conjunction with emotional support and the right resources, helps children face future challenges in a confident, decisive manner.

Children whose caregivers don't set limits because they wish to protect them from the negative emotions caused by the word «no», grow into insecure adults who are less able to empathize and have low negative emotion tolerance because they haven't had the chance to experience it. Their brain hasn't been programmed to accept or resolve the situation and move on. You won't be able to shield them from these negative emotions throughout their life and when they appear, as they will, they won't know how to handle them and will be left feeling confused, paralyzed and deeply troubled, without knowing how to return to normal.

The aim is for them to become more independent and capable of self-regulating. Until such time we need to guide them, teach them and be familiar with their needs and possibilities so that we respond in the right way.

Tackling parenting myths

Historically a lot of childhood behavior has been labeled «attention-seeking». That's exactly what it is.They are attracting your attention.

The question is, are we getting the message? Do we really understand what the child needs? Is what the child wants different to what they need? The little girl who cries and screams when things don't go her way is really drawing attention to the fact that she needs someone to teach her how to manage her frustration. The little boy who becomes so distressed when faced with a new situation might be asking someone to help him feel calm and safe again so he can go and explore.

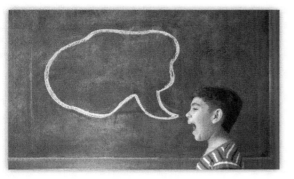

Do we really understand what they are asking for?

Frustration is necessary in parenting. They won't be traumatized, quite the opposite. It's essential to teach them how to live in a frustrating world because things won't always go their way and you must prepare them for that as best you can. Say no to them, allow them to be frustrated, and then stick by their side to show them how to modulate and regulate this emotion.

In this sense, anger is one of the strategies most widely deployed by children. The scene they create will differ depending on their age: tantrums, door-slamming, threats...: all of them aimed at drawing attention to their lack of control. You need to see through this kind of behavior and respond accurately to what they really need. The higher their level of anger, the lower their ability to cope with handling other emotions such as vulnerability, sadness and fear.

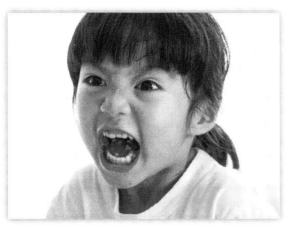

The strength of their anger is an indication of how intensely difficult they find it to manage their underlying sadness, vulnerability or fear.

Families often feel hijacked by the threat of their child's terrible rage. As we have seen, this emotional expression is a desperate attempt to get a consistent, organized response to his plea for help. He has learned that anger is a trigger and gets a response from you. In other words, it is prompted out of necessity within this relational exchange that you are party to and therefore partly responsible for. Whilst this may sound like bad news, in fact being aware that you are part of the problem opens the door for you to become part of the solution. Luckily there is a lot you can do to take back control and restore your family's well-being. In systems such as the family, when one element changes, the general dynamics change. So, bearing in mind that your brain is fully developed, it seems clear you have to make the first move. If you seem more consistent and sensitive and give logical, proportionate, coherent, responses, his brain will finally sense there is a secure framework and these intense, emotional outbursts that everyone finds so unpleasant will cease to be necessary.

Other things we are used to hearing about infants and toddlers include phrases such as «he does it to annoy me», «he seems to know which buttons to push». It is important to know that the areas of the brain that enable us to develop a strategy for doing something just «to annoy», don't develop until several years later. Also, in addition to requiring advanced brain connections, it also requires the will to annoy.

Therefore, babies don't actually mean «to annoy» you. They are merely trying to attract attention to what they consider pressing needs that are causing them some level of discomfort, which they believe you should soothe. Yes, he probably has got you «wrapped around his little finger». That's his job: to trigger you to respond to his needs, because he needs you.

«If you're always holding him, he'll never want you to put him down». By this stage in the book you are already aware just how important skin-to-skin contact and carrying your baby are for neurodevelopment and bonding. When he's ready to leave the nest and fly away, nothing will stop him. Not even you!

«Leave him to cry it out so he learns to self-soothe». No, please don't! When an infant cries, he needs something. If he stops crying, it's because he's realized you are not going to provide it. He has stopped trying to trigger a response from you. He's given up. Beyond that, in extreme cases, some studies suggest that the increase in cortisol (the stress hormone) that occurs when he asks for help and doesn't get it, may damage his neurodevelopment. You can find more details of these studies in the bibliography. The emotional dysregulation produced is so intense that it has a negative impact on healthy neural development, making it difficult for the individual to self-regulate later. When a baby is silent after a prolonged bout of intense crying it is because his autonomic nervous system is experiencing hypoarousal due to the fact that his level of physiological arousal has exceeded its window of tolerance (for more information see: Porges' Polivagal Theory).

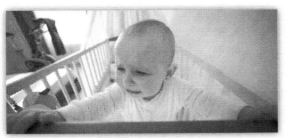

Leaving him to cry it out will only make him feel abandoned, that he can't rely on you, and may even cause such a high level of arousal that it exceeds his window of tolerance. He may be in discomfort or frightened but at least he can cry near to you and this is a lot more comforting for him.

Do you want him to stop counting on you? In the future he will try to satisfy his needs on his own (he won't tell you his problems, he will «keep it all inside», preferring to come up with his own poor solution rather than asking for help...), but he won't be ready. There must be «co-regulation» (emotional calmness, containment and management) from the outset: children need someone to help them gradually «self-regulate» one step at a time. It's a vertical relationship where you have all the tools and they barely have any. Now your job is to give him these tools. When some day in the future, after years of helping him deal with his emotions, you see he can manage them on his own, you'll know you did well. Nice job!

Last but not least, everyone thinks they are qualified to give an opinion about the best way to raise other people's babies. Your baby. Remember, every family is free to decide what they are willing and able to do in terms of parenting. It is essential you feel comfortable and in tune with what you do. It makes no sense to follow a course of action you are uncomfortable with because it will make bonding and connecting with your baby more difficult. Read about it, ask questions, make mistakes, try out strategies..., but above all else, do some soul-searching and trust yourself. You are the best possible mom or dad for your baby.

How pediatric physiotherapy can help your child to remain calm

The brain is our most undifferentiated organ at birth and both our early experiences and our genes, will mastermind the way the neurons interconnect. This will shape the specialized circuits involved in mental processes, regulation, memory, emotions, etc. The main structures are formed during our early years and grow stronger over our lifetime.

At the beginning the brain is very plastic and malleable so these early experiences are crucial for neurological development. Did you know that when we suffer a traumatic experience during childhood, the lessons we learned during this stage of maturation will probably be blocked? Or that if we suffered sustained stress in our first years of life, our levels of stress hormones will remain high for a long time, possibly even throughout our life? This is because emotional experiences have a real physiological impact on the way our brain develops. We are not just referring to traumatic experiences here either, even those we have in everyday life have an impact. Not just during our development either, in the prenatal stage too.

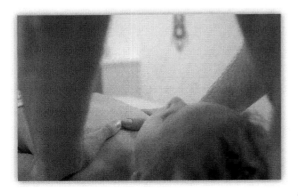

Body-mind psychotherapy (such as EMDRor Sensorimotor), is not alone in helping to regulate responses to trauma and stress. Pediatric physiotherapy (especially PIMT), can also be very effective when treatment is combined with a psychotherapist. This is done using skin and breathing techniques and targeted exercises. There is incredible potential in the collaboration between psychology and physiotherapy.

We find that by applying the model put forward by several authors («bottom-up» processing and regulation proposed by Van derKolk, amongst others), in our approach to treating trauma, pediatric physiotherapy can also help to readjust a child's self-regulation system from the bottom-up when treatment is combined with a psychotherapist specializing in the treatment of trauma.

Newborns come with «hidden» equipment for self-regulation (for organizing sleep-wake cycles, heart rate, breathing and digestion). Subsequently, as the brain matures and with the mediation of the attachment process, emotions and how they affect relationships, become more important. At this point, regulation is determined by social interactions. His caregivers are the ones who will help him self-regulate.

Not only do his role models affect his core functions through these interactions, they also affect his mental states, and this has a direct impact on his way of feeling and thinking. The basic objective during his maturation and development is for the child to be able to self-regulate at the end of this interim support stage. As we saw earlier, this is achieved by modeling (learning by observing a model, i.e. you!) and also by providing him with specific tools adapted to each of the challenges he will face in his development.

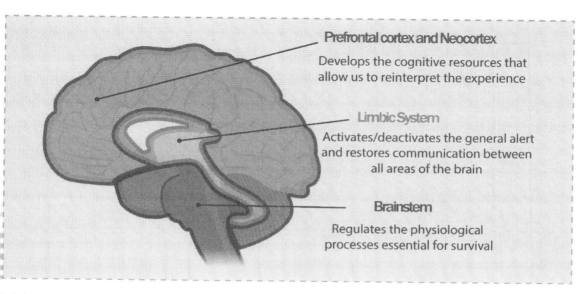

Prefrontal cortex and Neocortex
Develops the cognitive resources that allow us to reinterpret the experience

Limbic System
Activates/deactivates the general alert and restores communication between all areas of the brain

Brainstem
Regulates the physiological processes essential for survival

This is why it is essential he develops the capacity to regulate the activation produced by his emotions. Many psychological and psychiatric disorders are the result of this lack of self-regulation. Acute anxiety, anger and fear are at the root of childhood (and adult) problems such as: panic attacks, obsessive compulsive disorders, violent outbursts, self-harming, depression, etc. Returning to a regulated state involves recovering stability in several areas of the brain; from the lower brain (the brainstem that restores the most basic, physical calm), to the intermediate brain (limbic system: deactivates general state of alarm and restores communication between all areas of the brain) and the higher brain (incorporates new cognitive resources that allow us to approach the experience in a different way and understand that we are no longer in danger).

The therapeutic approach must be multidisciplinary to ensure it is coordinated at all these levels. The measures aimed at restoring calm to more vital parameters (breathing and heart rate) are very valuable from a psychological perspective, because experiencing moments of calm and well-being, moments of regulated functioning, creates an imprint on his brain dynamics, a new «neural pathway» that he can use from now on. This becomes apparent in his everyday life as it opens up new ways he can relate to himself (experiences in his own body) and the world (he will be able to experience the world in a more receptive, less invasive and disturbing way). Each time he uses this new pathway it will become more preferential. This will enable him to reduce the general state of alarm and make use of all the available tools: those that were already there but were inaccessible due to dysregulation, and the new ones that have been incorporated thanks to psychotherapy). In this sense, our experience of joint collaboration on regulation in children is quite revealing in that it achieves better results by acting at the different level involved.

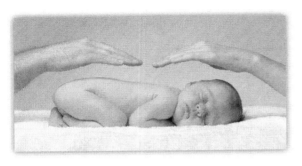

You can calm your baby

Now you have even more reasons to learn to self-regulate and teach your children how to do it through healthy bonding. A calm brain that no longer needs to waste energy on the superhuman effort of being permanently in a state of alarm, on surviving, is ready to grow, interact with others and learn.

This is just one of the beats to the new dance we are choreographing between pediatric developmental physiotherapy and perinatal and infant psychology. But this is only the beginning; there's still a whole lot more music left to dance to.

SUMMARY

Healthy bonding starts at the very beginning, even before the prenatal stage. The relationship between the two of you will grow in wealth and complexity as you continue to nurture it at each stage.

Bonding is heavily influenced by the mother's attitude and expectations about the imminent arrival of her baby. This is why it is so important to allay any fears and insecurities and address any issues of previous pregnancy losses that might interfere with the happy event, re-directing her energy towards the search for answers and self-reparation.

The way we experience labor is also conditioned by how we prepare beforehand, the expectations we have, how we were accompanied during the process, but above all by our hormones. Primarily oxytocin which; triggers the uterine contractions required for the baby to be born; causes milk letdown; promotes a calm, serene emotional state; helps regulate stress; has relationship enhancing effects; increases eye contact and general well-being.

Thanks to this neurochemistry, what happens in those first few moments will remain indelibly stored in the infant's memory. This is the start of the attachment process.

When skin-to-skin contact is made possible in the first two hours of life (known as the sensitive period) we find that there is a better mother-infant relationship by the age of one (greater attunement, reciprocity and complicity). Not only does separation at birth hamper the development of an emotional bond and breastfeeding, but it also makes it difficult for the baby's stress levels to return to normal.

Maternal bonding behavior in the immediate postnatal period plays an essential, decisive role in regulating the baby's physiological functions and oxytocin is a key player in this process.

Skin is the fourth pillar upon which bonding is built. Touch is a key tool not just for a baby's neurological development but also for developing his sense of Self: when an infant feels touched, he feels appreciated, cared for, wanted, loved. He senses his presence is felt. This is why it is so important to give him skin-to-skin contact, physically touch him and find ways of soothing him that are not merely associated with sucking but also with coordinated movement between you and caresses for example.

Cultural changes mean that the pattern of parental roles is becoming more balanced and duties are shared in a more natural, sensible way. These days, fathers are involved in every aspect of parenting, not just the fun ones and they have important roles as attachment figures.

In the case of intense, unattended crying, the increase in cortisol (the stress hormone) that occurs when he asks for help and doesn't receive it, can damage his neurodevelopment. The emotional dysregulation produced is so intense that it has a negative impact on healthy neural development, making it difficult for him to self-regulate later.

Newborns come with «hidden» equipment for self-regulation. Subsequently, as the brain matures and through the process of attachment, emotions and how they affect relationships, become more important. At this point, regulation is determined by social interactions. His caregivers are the ones who will help him self-regulate.

What can you do?
HELPFUL PRACTICAL ADVICE

- Make the most of the waiting process to prepare yourself emotionally. Give priority to people and spaces that help you stay calm, positive and balanced; surround yourself with a good support network that gives you the right kind of advice and knows how to assist you through the whole process. Revisit your fears and any unresolved emotional or relationship issues. This will better prepare you for the arrival of your new baby.

- Keep stress in check during pregnancy and after the birth. You can only transmit a feeling of security to him if you are calm yourself. Postnatal support groups and psychotherapists can provide you with the necessary tools to ensure you remain emotionally available and aligned with your core values when giving care and attention to your baby.

- The labor-birth moment is unique and life-changing. Trust yourself, stay attuned to what your bodymind is telling you and entrust yourself to experts who respect your wishes.

- If the opportunity of skin-to-skin contact is offered to you in those first few moments after the birth, don't turn it down and keep your baby close to you for as long as possible.

- When this isn't an option you can still enhance bonding with your baby through touch, gentle movement, affectionate gazes and loving, soothing words, to name just a few. Remember, attachment is built and reinforced when you are available to provide safety and well-being when he needs you. There will be plenty of disconnections throughout your lives, but the most important thing is to get back in step with each other.

- The first hour after the birth is a unique time. Where possible, allow your baby to go at his own pace so that important events occur naturally, i.e. let him crawl up your body to reach your breast and start sucking in a natural way: let him sleep afterwards so that he starts to regulate his sleep-wake cycles: let him to start to recognize your smell as a sign he is in a safe place...

- In the weeks and months that follow, stay tuned to his cycles and synchronize with them. Nourish this communication through loving touch. Spend time caressing him and stimulating his senses with your smell, words or songs, movement as you rock him in your arms and visual contact as you interact with each other...

- The paternal figure can do all of these things too, actively enhancing the father-infant bond from birth and breaking with stereotypes and social conventions. Having several attachment figures actively involved is extremely beneficial for children in terms of their emotional life and overall neurodevelopment. It offers them the chance to enjoy a wide range of relational styles and to become more confident and stimulated thanks to the personal traits each individual brings to the relationship.

- If your child is no longer a baby and you feel that some areas haven't been programmed satisfactorily or haven't developed properly, or maybe you want to improve family dynamics, then working with a psychotherapist can help you achieve these goals. It is possible to change the dynamics, reprogram what has been learned, develop whatever didn't develop properly at the time and repair any significant attachment ruptures that may have occurred along the way. It can be done.

BIBLIOGRAPHY

PRENATAL STAGE:

«Pregnancy is a period of crisis that turns our sense of identity upside down and reactivates previous unresolved psychological processes»:

Bibring GL, Valenstein AF. Psychological aspects of pregnancy. Clinical Obstetrics and Gynecology. 1976;19:357-71.

Bydlowski M. Le regard intérieur de la femme enceinte, transparence psychique et représentation de l'objet interne. Devenir. 2001;13(2):41-52.

«In the final months a more realistic, differentiated perception of the infant develops and very early interaction begins»:

AmmanitiM. Maternal representations during pregnancy and early mother-infant interactions. Infant Mental HealthJournal. 1991;12:246-55.

Gómez Masera R, Alonso Martín P, Rivera Pavón I. Relación materno fetal y establecimiento del apego durante la etapa de gestación. International Journal of Development and Educational Psychology. INFAD Revista de Psicología. 2011;1(1):425-34.

Hepper PG. Fetal memory: does it exist? What does it do? ActaPaediatr. 1996;85(s416):16-20.

Winnicott D. Escritos de pediatría y psicoanálisis. Barcelona: Laia; 1979.

«Bonding between very premature babies and their mothers is affected from the outset as the "psycho-biological nesting" process is interrupted»:

> Jofré R, Enríquez D. Nivel de estrés de las madres con recién nacidos hospitalizados en la UCI en Hospital Guillermo Grant. Ciencia y Enfermería. 2002;8:31-6.

> Ruiz AL, Ceriani Cernadas JM, Cravedi V, Rodríguez D. Estrés y depresión en madres de prematuros: un programa de intervención. Archivos argentinos de pediatría. 2005;103(1):36-45.

PERINATAL STAGE:

«Attachment is a neurohormonal process that bonds mothers and infants»:

> Olza-Fernández I, Gabriel MA, Gil-Sánchez A, García-Segura LM, Arévalo MA. Neuroendocrinology of childbirth and mother-child attachment: The basis of an etiopathogenic model of perinatal neurobiological disorders. Frontiers in neuroendocrinology. 2014;35(4):459-72.

POSTNATAL STAGE:

«Research into the long-term impact of skin-to-skin contact in the first two hours of life (known as the sensitive period) found that when this contact took place, there was a better mother-infant relationship by the age of one (greater attunement, reciprocity and complicity), than when they were separated during that period».

> Hales DJ, Lozoff B, Sosa R, Kennell JH. Defining the limits of the maternal sensitive period. Developmental Medicine & Child Neurology. 1977;19(4):454-61.

> Moore ER, Anderson GC, Bergman N, Dowswell T. Early skin-to-skin contact for mothers and their healthy newborn infants. Cochrane Database Syst Rev. 2012;5(3):CD003519.

«The three areas of the newborn's brain that are essential for developing attachment are the olfactory bulb, locus coeruleus and the amygdala»:

> Vargas A, Chaskel R. Neurobiología del apego. Avances en psiquiatría biológica. 2007;8:43-56.

Paternal-infant bonding: «Some authors have begun to include fathers as very significant figures in the infant's life since, nowadays, they tend to develop a close relationship with their children from the outset»:

> Aguado R. El vínculo como potenciador de la activación de las redes neuronales. xxiv Reunión de la AEP (Asociación Española de Psicodrama). Bilbao; 2009.

> Eimil B, Palacios I. El estrés materno en la organización del vínculo madre-bebé prematuro de bajo peso maternal (Stress in theOrganization of the Mother). Clínica. 2013;4(2):171-83.

Hernández-Martínez C, Canals Sans J, Fernández-Ballart J. Parent's perceptions of their neonates and their relation to infant development. Child: Care, health and development. 2011;37(4):484-92.

To learn more about how early bonding develops:

Brazelton TB, Cramer BG. La relación más temprana. Padres, bebés y el drama del apego inicial. Barcelona: Paidós; 1990.

Winnicott D. Desarrollo emocional primitivo. En: Escritos de pediatría y psicoanálisis. Barcelona: Laia, 1945. p.104-219.

Winnicott D. Preocupación maternal primaria. En: Escritos de pediatría y psicoanálisis. Barcelona: Espasa Libros; 2012.

Tackling parenting myths: resources for parenting based on a constructive, respectful relationship:

Faber A, Mazlish E. Cómo hablar para que los niños escuchen y cómo escuchar para que los niños hablen. 38.ªed. México D. F.: Diana; 2009.

Faber A, Mazlish E. Cómo hablar para que los adolescentes le escuchen y cómo escuchar para que los adolescentes le hablen. Medici; 1997.

Nelsen J. Positive discipline: The classic guide to helping children develop self-discipline, responsibility, cooperation, and problem-solving skills. Ballantine Books; 2011.

Siegel DJ. Tormenta cerebral: el poder y el propósito del cerebro adolescente. Alba Editorial; 2014.

Siegel DJ. El cerebro del niño. Alba Editorial; 2016.

For more on psycho-physiological regulation:

Van der Kolk BA. El cuerpo lleva la cuenta: cerebro, mente y cuerpo en la superación del trauma. Editorial Eleftheria; 2016.

PorgesSW. La Teoría Polivagal. Fundamentos neurofisiológicos de las emociones, el apego, la comunicación y la autorregulación. [Traducción de Miriam Ramos Morrison; Revisión de Anabel González.] Ediciones Pléyades; 2017.

Chapter 14

When life isn't always a bed of roses

Finding support when the going gets tough

Jara Acín y Rivera

Life doesn't always go according to plan and sometimes puts us to the test. Babies arrives early, or not at all; they are born on the other side of the world; they behave unexpectedly or experience situations that are hard to come to terms with. As a result, we adults have feelings that are both overwhelming and confusing and, at times, we may feel incompetent, incapable, miserable even. It is important that we can feel competent and capable again and that we have the right support, because, far from being unusual, the situations described here are very common place, although it may not always seem so. The world is full of people who have experienced emotional upheavals/turmoil at some point or other in their lives, or have been diagnosed with a learning disability, or whose parents couldn't care for and protect them, or simply didn't know how to do so.

We want to dedicate this chapter to all those people whose lives have been no bed of roses. Because the most valuable human asset is to be different, and what may seem like a weakness to us now, may turn out to be something extraordinary in the future. Because we learn from every experience in our lives. Because, although it may be hard to grasp, all human behavior has a survival function. Because our brain is always keen to grow and heal and it is never too late to correct it and ourselves too. Because anything is possible when we have a strong, positive outlook. This chapter is dedicated to all those individuals who always strive to push ahead in life, despite all the difficulties they face.

Surviving is success in itself.

When they arrive ahead of schedule

After a baby is born, the parent's role is to help her self-regulate physiologically and emotionally. Physiological regulation is achieved through pathways that operate deep in the brainstem and involves achieving balance in functions as vital as the infant's heart rate, breathing, digestion or introducing sleep-wake cycles. All of these promote a state of emotional calm.

So, what can you do to accompany your baby in this crucial mission? You can engage with her through emotional and physiological stimulation; gaze at her, caress her, rock her in your arms, talk to her in a soothing, loving way. In other words, tune into her.

In the case of very premature babies (a birthweight of less than 3 lbs) the difficulty lies, amongst other things, in the baby's immaturity because she cannot receive or respond appropriately to any stimulation from you. On top of this, you must deal with limited or non-existent physical access to her while she is in the incubator, and cope with your emotions about the uncertainty surrounding her progress, as well as experiencing anxiety, distress, guilt or grief.

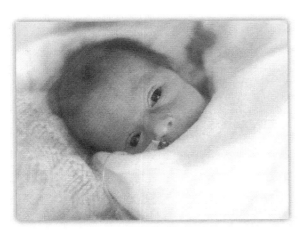

By engaging calmly and responsively with your baby you are helping her self-regulate and establish a secure attachment. She will identify you as role models for her safety and well-being.

If you have been in this situation, you know only too well just how stressful it is when your baby is hospitalized. Not just because it's a sign that «something is wrong» (your alarm bell goes off), but also because it means the natural thread of the mother-infant relationship is severed. This break in the continuity of your relationship causes emotional upset for both of you.

The effect of skin-to-skin contact is evident in those first few hours, and just as important as the mother-infant neurohormonal connection and the modulating role of oxytocinin the perception of well-being that we discussed earlier. The infant's system both expects and needs this contact to provide a sense of well-being and if it doesn't materialize, she will have to rapidly adapt to the environment around her which, in the absence of her mother, will seem hostile. In previous chapters we saw how skin-to-skin contact reduces the levels of cortisol required during labor and how it continues to do so for the next few weeks, months even. Without this contact, not only do the levels not decrease, they increase, and become toxic for the newborn's nervous system, causing a hormonal, metabolic and cognitive dysregulation that can last a long time.

In this respect, we have long known that the first year of life is a window of opportunity for many things; one of which is the chance to reduce your baby's cortisol level, something that will prove extraordinarily beneficial for her.

It's very likely you are extremely worried about your baby's immediate future, particularly as her vital functions may sometimes be hooked up to myriad wires and tubes.

Did you know that your care directly helps reduce the levels of «stress hormone» in your baby? Make sure the time you spend with her is positive and relaxing, so this shared moment of calm resets her system.

The image is so shocking and far removed from the one of tender, well-being you dreamed of, that it could cause a lifelong psychological impact. In this sense, the need to deal with the real risks that accompany every step of her progress will test your ability to make swift decisions and develop infinite patience and calm.

On the other hand, she is so fragile and vulnerable because of her immaturity that, in extreme cases, she will only be able to respond to one sense at a time. This will probably increase your stress as the exchanges between you are upsetting, out of synch and confusing for both of you.

In this emotionally demanding context, the coping mechanism your brain triggers will be directly related to the way your response to danger is programmed. As you know, this is something that has been forming since your early infancy. You may feel defeated, blocked or even practically frozen to the spot (like a deer caught in the headlights). You may also feel very anxious (hyperactive), your mind may be racing and your core body functions impaired (tachycardia, insomnia, panic attacks...), as you try to fight the danger «like a wounded lion» by triggering all systems, albeit in a futile, chaotic way.

Your system is reacting as well as it can to a critical situation. It is crucial you are informed honestly about the process so that you can begin to accept the reality of the situation.

It's possible that this deep shock is too much for you to bear. It may even lead to post-traumatic stress disorder where you are constantly hypervigilant even after the danger has passed: as though you were still in that moment, re-living it in vivid detail and reacting equally intensely. You can increase your capacity for self-regulation with the help of a sensorimotor psychotherapist to ensure this overwhelming experience doesn't trigger your own learned survival responses that might get in the way of your ability to soothe your baby and bond with her.

If you felt overwhelmed by the experience, it is likely this will condition the way you relate to your baby throughout her lifetime; maybe you will be excessively over-protective or suffer separation anxiety when you're not with her.

Although it is difficult to imagine you will ever feel normal again while we are still suffering the consequences of this traumatic episode, an EMDR therapist can help you get back to your old self in just a few sessions. Ensuring your own well-being is the best way of ensuring your baby's. There is a lot you can do to help her!

Similarly, your baby may show signs of stress (of being overwhelmed), such as trembling, restlessness, crying, changes in breathing..., in response to your actions. She may also «freeze» (remain still, tense) and although she may appear to be calm, she isn't at all! She is very scared and confused, just like you. Naturally this increases your worry and confusion too because the fact that your baby has a very disorganized neurological pattern, means that her behaviour is often incomprehensible. Therefore, the more organized, coherent and serene your responses are, the easier it will be for the two of you to get closer.

The loss of this natural reciprocity in the interactions between you, of learning from one another through skin contact, prevents an interactive regulating response from occurring. In other words, it severely hampers the tuning and synchronization so essential for creating a bond during this stage.

The loss of this natural reciprocity in your interactions, of learning from one another through skin contact, prevents an interactive regulating response.

In such a delicate situation, it is essential parents receive counseling and that other basic support networks are mobilized too. Support groups as well as family and friends can provide emotional support and help you through the most critical moments. Additionally, it is paramount that your baby receives specialized attention both from midwives and developmental physiotherapists, so that a daily early stimulation program can be set up to guide and optimize her progress. It is vital you keep a positive mindset so you can celebrate each breakthrough and make the most of your time together. Surround yourself by people who will help you to believe that everything is going to be just fine! The greatest stories always begin with the biggest challenges.

Further down the road, your baby will also require attention and her traumatic experience will need to be addressed. Did you know that somatosensory memory develops in the womb? Or that in psychotherapy we often work on pre-verbal traumatic experiences such as difficult births or incubator stays? There is a lot we can do to help all of you!

Learning how to relate to such a fragile infant, how to hold her and care for her, requires a great deal of emotional preparedness and resilience. The objective is to approach each encounter with a deep sense of calm and availibility so that your time together is constructive and positive for both of you. There is evidence that the early mother-infant relationship is one of the key factors in maximizing or minimizing the potentially adverse effects of premature birth. In the previous chapters we discussed the neurobiological benefits of skin-to-skin contact, including stabilizing the infant's vital signs and improving the development of her immune system. Now we see the parallel role it plays in emotional «attunement».

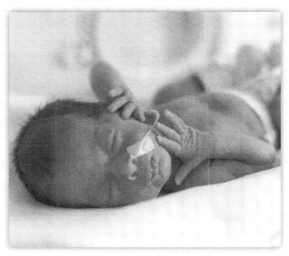

The objective is to approach each encounter with a deep sense of calm and availability so that your time together is constructive and positive for both of you.

So, we know that making the most of each encounter with your baby to share skin-to-skin time (kangaroo care) and engaging with her in a calm, loving way will help her overall development and preserve the bond between you. This bond will develop more fully later. Each encounter is soothing, stimulating and constructive and, in the background, it is programming a synchronized, connected relationship between the two of you that forms the basis for well-being. Just hearing your voice, sensing your smell, your skin, contributes to her vitality.

When the going gets tough – challenging births

In the previous chapter we looked at the complicated neurohormonal, physiological and emotional processes that steer the labor-birthing process. But what happens when there are complications? Many of you will have experienced births that, whilst not ultimately requiring a cesarean, were tremendously difficult, and many births where the babies needed a strong will to survive. There may have been fetal distress, the baby got stuck or suffered bone deformity during the struggle to be born. Occasionally, after these births we may find the newborn has physical injuries such as plagiocephaly, congenital torticollis, hypoxia or dural tension.

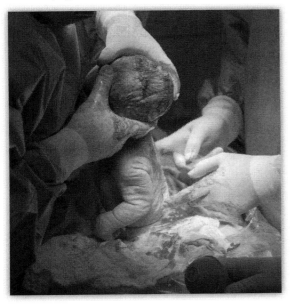

These physical injuries cause the infant great discomfort that translates into restlessness, crying, difficulties feeding or sleeping and makes her less available for positive, enjoyable bonding with you. It is also more than likely you will have exhausted every strategy you know, as well as all your positive energy, attempting to soothe her and calm her down. I never cease to be amazed by the sheer effort and creativity of the moms and dads who visit my consulting room when they explain the lengths they go to to comfort their babies.

In the context of this new sense of well-being you are both experiencing, there is potentially a two-way relationship based on enjoyment and calmness, a mutual contentedness.

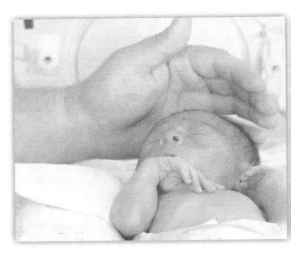

Following a complicated labor-birth it is essential the baby has a check-up with a specialist physiotherapist who can provide precise information about what is wrong with her and what can be done about it. Quite often, a few sessions (or even just one!) are enough for the infant to find relief. In the context of this new sense of well-being you are both experiencing, there is potentially a two-way relationship based on enjoyment and calmness, a mutual contentedness. When she stops feeling pain and sensing she is in danger, her brain is better prepared for stronger bonding.

When there was a previous pregnancy loss

Bonding commences even before the prenatal stage. So, what happens if you have suffered a previous pregnancy loss? How do you know when the time is right to try again?

It doesn't matter when the loss occurred. It doesn't matter if nobody else knew you were pregnant. It doesn't matter if it only lasted a few weeks. It doesn't matter if people say, «you were barely pregnant» or «you'll soon fall pregnant again». It was your baby, your child, and when you lose them, you must acknowledge your loss and grant it the importance it deserves.

The grieving process is very important: a life that was growing inside you is no longer there. You are a mother who has lost her child.

It is very likely that some people won't see it the same way. However, it is important you validate your own experience, your own emotions, so that you can start to process your loss. I suggest you don't push yourself into rapidly appearing back to normal if you're not: or jump straight into trying again without taking your time to close the previous process. Showing how you really feel helps to keep you balanced and integrated and enables others to gauge your emotions and offer better support. It's an opportunity to strengthen the bonds with the people who care about you.

Not only is the loss itself hard, but so too are the physical and even surgical processes involved. It is not a mere formality, it is a farewell, but it is rarely viewed this way.

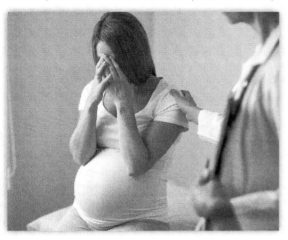

It is important to make pregnancy loss visible as real grief that takes time to process.

The deep sense of emptiness, the pain, the loss, the feeling of something missing, all take time to integrate. A lot longer than the time we are allowed and the time we afford ourselves.

This is why you need to connect with yourself and with your emotions; face your sadness, cry, get angry, complain and talk with whoever you can: whoever understands you. It is important to process your grief and there is no better way of doing it than in good company. Did you know that tears have healing powers that reduce the levels of cortisol and increase the levels of endorphins? And that when we cry with someone, we dare to face our pain more deeply than when we are alone with no-one else to support us. It is far more healing to cry on someone else's shoulder.

Invent your own ritual, find the right words and a good moment to say goodbye. Give her a name, the one you dreamed about and tell her she will always have a place in your family. If this wound doesn't heal properly, you will never be able to bond completely freely with the children you may have in the future. This is something you should do when you are ready, when both of you are ready. Don't rush into it as a way of escaping. You cannot replace someone you have lost. You will only be ready to receive when your heart is free from the pain of loss.

If you wish to try again, change absolutely everything. Choose another name, a new color, a different way of doing things. A new cycle begins when the old one ends, not before. Get help if you need it. There are therapists who know how to support you through this all-important grief process that is so profound, yet, at the same time, so invisible.

When our child is born halfway around the world

There are myriad paths to adoption: infertility, families with no wish to have biological children, new family structures (single-parent, LGBT parents, for example).

In all these cases there is a lengthy process prior to meeting your child: a detailed assessment, an unpredictable waiting time, uncertainty and a lack of control. Perhaps even grief for the biological children you couldn't have...

In this last case it is very important to have grieved properly over your infertility. If you don't embrace the fact that you can't have children, you are not really giving up on having a biological child and he or she will remain idealized in your mind as a benchmark against which to compare your future children. The best starting point for quality bonding with your child, is to be able to approach the encounter with your mind free of ideals and full of curiosity about getting to know them.

A key fact about bonding in cases of adoption is that, for the adoption to take place, the child must previously have been abandoned. This is a fact. There can be several reasons for this but, for the child, the reality is the same: they have experienced at least one interrupted bond.

In cases where very young infants of the same ethnicity are adopted, there is a temptation to hide the fact they are adopted. The opposite is true when their skin color is different, or they were older when they arrived: it goes without saying that they know they are adopted and, therefore, the subject isn't often broached. In both cases it is the parents' fear that blocks this conversation. Their fear may have to do with facing their grief over infertility;

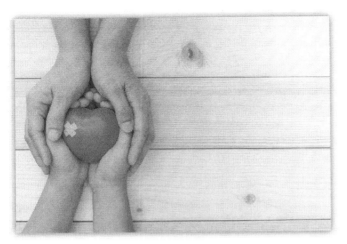

or questions about the child's past (previous experiences and genetic inheritance); or their birth parents, or perhaps the idea they may want to meet them in the future. It is crucial you work on these fears because your child is capable of processing and confronting their situation, but only with your support and control. You need to be able to talk about the adoption, not just name it.

Usually there is little information about their history. If they ask, it's a good idea to give them the information you have but make sure you choose the right way and time so that they can take it on board. It will boost their confidence in you. If, on the other hand, you hide information from them or they discover they were adopted through other channels, this breach of trust could damage their bond with you. In addition, depending on their age, they might think that you are hiding the truth because there is something wrong and this could trigger a more intense process of guilt and shame. You need to accompany them in this process of accepting and coping with their pain, with trust, affection and the security of knowing that, although they were abandoned, they are worthy of love.

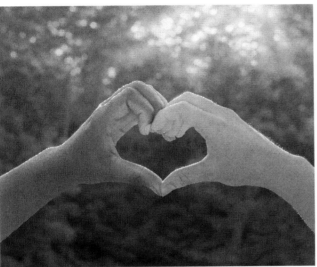

Two fundamental ideas must support the relationship between you: That they are worthy of being loved and that you will not abandon them.

The bond with a biological infant starts in pregnancy. The real bond with an adopted infant is built gradually through contact, daily experiences and signs of trust you share once you are together.

The amount of time and the relational circumstances surrounding the child from the time they are born to the time they come home with you is crucial. Perhaps they were in an orphanage and were the caregiver's favorite, so she always carried them around and responded lovingly and reliably to their demands. Or perhaps they were in several foster homes and experienced successive interrupted bonds. This information will enable you to better interpret their behavior with you. A child who has been neglected or abused or who has lived with several different families will take longer to trust their new parents.

The circumstances surrounding the abandonment will have had a direct effect on their neurodevelopment.

212

In the same way, the circumstances surrounding the abandonment will have had a direct effect on their neurodevelopment. If they have not been caressed or hugged, not only will they not have felt loved, but they will not have received adequate stimulation either. It is highly likely that they are still somewhat dysfunctional from a psychological or physiological perspective, (they sleep badly, are tense and nervous...), their primitive reflexes are still present, and they haven't completed motor development stages satisfactorily, all of which hinders optimal brain development. A lack of adequate nutrition and stimulation (physical and emotional), mean their weight and development are commonly below the norm for their age. This is a sure sign they need specialist attention to set their bodies on the right track. The lack of stimulation results in psychomotor awkwardness, learning disabilities, hyperactive behaviour, attention deficit or behavioral difficulties, or hormonal or immune system disorders. Did you know that adopted children are more likely to go through the hormonal changes of the teen years earlier?

Children who have syndromes caused by exposure to toxins during pregnancy, such as fetal alcoholism, are special cases. The degree to which they are affected determines the severity of the symptoms which can range from behavioral disorders to severe failings in prefrontal lobe development. These cases require global care from a multidisciplinary team (neuropsychology, family counseling, developmental physiotherapy, speech therapy, special education, occupational therapy, etc.) that can cater for the needs of the child and their family and accompany their progress.

We have already seen in previous chapters how the right stimulation, movement affective ties, develop the brain. Adopted children require extra help and you can provide it by enlisting the help of a developmental physiotherapist and a psychotherapist specializing in attachment. Accompanying your child as they progress along this path is good for the well-being of the whole family because they feel more capable and you are making a real contribution to their optimal development.

The right stimulation, movement and affective ties develop the brain. Adopted children require extra help.

Early experiences of emotional deprivation, or even being deprived of nutrition, space etc., will have left an imprint on their brain. They will probably overreact to some stimuli (the shower, cold, wind, certain sounds or smells). Their brain has undergone extremely unpleasant or threatening experiences in the past that they may not be able to explain in words and, as we will see later in this chapter, will require re-programming with a safe experience.

Naturally, in these cases it is more important than ever to show consistent, dependable sensitivity and availability. It is normal for children to verify this by putting you to the test. The underlying questions always relate to their wound, and this is something they will attempt to figure out as they go through the different stages of maturation: «Are you going to stay? Will you always love me? Can I trust you? Is there something wrong with me? Am I the type that gets abandoned?». They need answers: explicit and implicit answers. They need to feel that you will love them whatever they do; that you are not going to abandon them; that they are cherished for who they are; that they are «lovable», and your love is solid. Their doubts can take the form of intense separation anxiety, dependency, clinginess, or conversely, behaviour that is oppositional, challenging and even aggressive. It's nothing personal. Or maybe it is. The very fact that they are working through their unease with you means you have become their attachment figure. That's great news!

Are you going to stay? Can I trust you? Is there something wrong with me? Am I the type that gets abandoned?

Very often they have their own doubts about why they were abandoned (sometimes they romanticize about it because they are still not ready to face reality), or what their birth parents look like (they have no idea what they're going to look like when they grow up!). Later on, they may even want to visit their country of birth or get in touch with their biological relatives. All these processes are aimed at building a solid identity and finding out who they are. Their brain wants to heal the wound. They often feel different, inadequate or even ashamed. You must address these feelings by creating opportunities where they feel they can talk about their emotions and by providing an appropriate response each time. You must work hard at making them feel they fit in, that they are accepted, appreciated, seen, listened to and that they belong.

You must work hard at making them feel they fit in, that they are accepted, appreciated, seen, listened to and that they belong.

Something that can help them build a full picture of who they are is to create a story that includes all the key moments in their life: from the day they were born (or even before if possible). Tell them how a baby grows inside a birth mother, what their birth might have been like, who looked after them and where they were until they met you (if you can show them photos, all the better!). Tell them what the process was like for you (full of longing to be together); what the journey was like; the first time you set eyes on each other; how you felt and how they reacted; the homecoming; how the rest of the family welcomed them; the progress they have made... You can turn it into a story and read it each time they ask. Later, they can read it for themselves. It is important to be aware of your own emotions as you write: if it makes you feel upset or overwhelmed, you need to work through this before continuing with their story. It will only be healing for them if you are feeling stable and emotionally available to accompany them through the process.

Raising a child with an attachment wound and a lack of early stimulation is a delicate task that requires commitment, consistency, sensitivity and at the same time, terrific strength. It turns the experience of being a mom or dad into an unparalleled opportunity for personal growth.

When there is nowhere to hide

As we saw in the previous chapter, the attachment system is activated in stressful situations when we fear our attachment figure might leave us, or when we feel there's a threat: when we sense danger, the nervous system becomes dysregulated and we do everything we can to return to a calm, balanced state. We do this by activating protection and proximity behavior in our attachment figure: to protect us and calm us down. So, what happens when the person harming us is the person we are attached to? This is the case of children who suffer abuse in the family environment.

The attachment mechanism («if I am close to him or her, I will be protected, calm, safe»), overrules the survival-defense mechanism («if something hurts me, I move away from it»). This is precisely why abusive relationships are perpetuated. A paradoxical bond is established whereby: the more fear I feel, the greater the need to feel close to that figure; the nearer I am to them, the greater the danger I am in. It is impossible for them to develop a coherent, orderly mindset against this backdrop.

The attachment response system overrules the survival-defense response system. This is precisely why abusive relationships are perpetua-

ted. A paradoxical bond is established whereby: the more fear I feel, the greater the need to feel close to that figure; the nearer I am to them, the greater the danger I am in.

Personality development is deeply affected in these ongoing situations. They feel guilt, profound sadness, anger..., and these emotions are programming a future style of relating full of suffering and emotional detachment from themselves and others, in a bid to numb the pain.

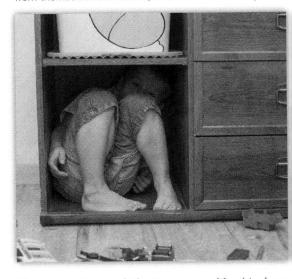

There is nowhere to hide. Experiences like this shape a future full of a fear of close relationships, aggressiveness and supressed guilt.

In the future, these children will probably feel very scared, terrified even, when a relationship becomes too intense or intimate and, without realizing it, they will trigger their defense response to get away from this person who might potentially be harmful. In order to stay alive, they have had to be very vigilant. Consequently, their brain has been programmed with «modified» criteria (although at the time they were adaptive) which dictates where and when danger may appear. They become hypervigilant.

As we know, this defense response can appear in the form of fight or flight, and whether behavior is expressed in one way or another varies depending on the maturity of the brain, the lived experiences and perceived support from others. However, when these experiences of danger have been present every day since early childhood, the danger response system is programmed in the pre-cortex. Consequently, even if you are an adult at the time, if you perceive the current situation as a severe threat, you will be unable to access the cognitive or emotional resources you may have acquired in earlier phases. At that crucial time in the early years of your life, a response system was programmed that will be activated today

In the early years of life, a response system to situations perceived as threatening was programmed. Today it will be activated.

These early experiences of exposure to systematic risk have a physiological effect on the architecture of our brain. Subsequently, this will be reflected in the way we process information, how our memory works, which stimuli we respond to and if we are able to interact with others (and how we interact), and learn. Hence, development is traumatic as the damaging consequences of these experiences continue to be present much later and interfere with our personal life and relationships.

However, the brain always finds a way to organize itself, to adjust and survive. In order to do this, it sets all the available defense mechanisms in motion, even if they are primitive and inefficient. They are the only ones it has. When fight or flight are, literally, out of the question, one of these mechanisms may be dissociation (emotional detachment to avoid pain and negative emotions and sensations in the mind and body). It is a way of encapsulating the pain so that you can move on. At times it is the best way. This strategy may be used in both childhood and adulthood whenever the lived emotional experience exceeds our ability to integrate it into the continuum of life.

When an emotion is dissociated it isn't stored with all our other memories, so it may seem as though it never happened. Our brain activates this mechanism to allow us to survive situations that, otherwise, would be unbearable. «That never happened».

Our brain activates mechanisms which allow us to survive situations that, otherwise, would be unbearable.

The problem is that it is an emergency tool and it has limited effectiveness. It doesn't solve the problem: it just

puts it away so it can be processed later. Encapsulating the trauma doesn't make it disappear. So, the effect of these experiences, the images of those memories or the physical sensations associated with them, can suddenly appear at any point in your life. This can have a dramatic impact on you and reveal information about yourself that you had completely «forgotten». At times you will doubt the veracity of these memories («I've just remembered something, but I'm not sure if it really happened or not. I find it hard to believe that could really have happened to me»).

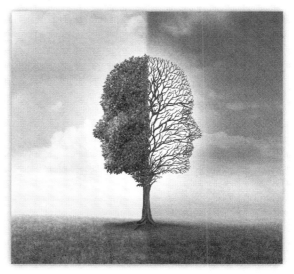

If this has happened to you, or if it is happening to you now as you read this book, it is crucial you contact a trauma therapist. If your brain is starting to open that box it is because it is ready to face whatever is stored in there, even if it will require a lot of help to do so.

Your brain wants to solve this, reorganize itself and move on. Without counselling you won't be able to muster the resources you were missing at the time and will have to fight with the same weapons and lose again. A psychologist with training in this field can help you reprogram what you have learned and provide you with new tools so that, little by little (and accompanied this time), you can integrate the experience as just another part of your life. A terrifying one admittedly, but one you survived.

Did you know that a team comprising a psychologist and physiotherapist specializing in trauma can treat children and adults to help them regain a state of calm? They do this by working together to reduce their «neuroception» of danger: when you feel threatened your brain triggers an alert system that activates your whole body. When you can't defend yourself or run away, your system collapses either due to over-activation or by default. Both responses

The only way to reprogram the brain to recover a state of calm and sense of security is through mind-body counseling.

are immobilizing. Consequently, the only way to reprogram your brain to regain a state of calm and sense of security is by working on both your mind and your body. On the one hand, this is achieved by providing calming experiences through your body: and, on the other, by helping to correctly mobilize the defense responses that were blocked when faced with the impossibility of responding.

Children with childhood attachment trauma, who have an attachment wound, are at a higher risk of suffering other traumas during their lifetime and are poorer at resolving them. They are more at risk of suffering psychological disorders (obsessive-compulsive disorder, eating or personality disorders, dissociation, phobias...) and other difficulties. They are vulnerable people. On the other hand, people who enjoyed secure attachment in their childhood can clearly identify what is healthy and what is harmful and know when to get away quickly.

Violent, abusive people choose people at risk. Therefore, establishing secure attachment in childhood is a form of protection against abuse and other dangerous situations.

Did you know studies show there is abnormal cortical development in boys who suffer childhood sexual or physical abuse? Or that girls who suffer postraumatic stress disorder due to serious childhood sexual abuse have reduced gray matter in some areas of the brain?

Abuse clearly affects brain development. We also know that the combination of a healthy, positive upbringing, proper nutrition and EMDR counseling to repair emotional damage, can be effective and help children to flourish and catch up at an incredible rate. It's never too late to start the healing process.

Children with childhood attachment trauma are at a higher risk of suffering other traumas during their lifetime. On the other hand, people who enjoyed secure attachment in their childhood can clearly identify what is healthy and what is harmful and know when to get away quickly.

When we are hijacked by anger

Does your child have extreme tantrums? Does she throw things on the floor or break them in a fit of rage? Does she «punish» you when you don't do what she wants? Does she attack you verbally or physically?

Displays of anger in children are an extreme attempt to activate the attachment system in their caregivers. It appears in early childhood and is an extreme expression of the ambivalent attachment style. Their goal is to control the relationship with the attachment figure; sometimes they hurt them and at other times they get closer to them in order to bond. This is why they alternate between angry and disarming behavior that placates their caregivers. They set the pace of a relationship which, while containing a lot of negative emotion, does at least guarantee them your full attention.

This is their way of being in control. They feel they can't concede control to adults because they behave inconsistently and incoherently towards them. How do you feel when you don't know what is going on? In danger, scared?Their aggressive behavior is a way of managing their fear. The more scared they are and the more in-

secure they feel, the worse they behave. They feel the attachment figure is the one causing this anxiety, which is why they usually attack this important figure the most, the very one they want the most availability and security from.

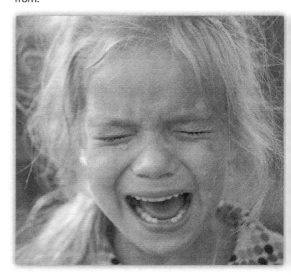

Aggressive behavior and expressions of intense anger are her way of managing her fear. She is experiencing emotional overload.

As their brain matures, their tactics become more sophisticated, though not necessarily more efficient. Interestingly, around the age of two or three, children fine-tune their ability to «dominate» their caregivers using these strategies (sometimes causing the latter to erupt) and this coincides with an increase in their motor skills (so they can run away if the going gets tough). In other words, they create danger for themselves and assume the consequences through this behavior.

Therefore, it is more effective to work on making them feel safe and secure again, than trying to control their angry, aggressive behavior directly. This behavior is their way of coping with the situation, their defense mechanism. However, it is not an effective way of achieving the care they need. In this sense, intervention must be at a systemic, family level so that the adults can examine and fix the inconsistencies in their care and learn about new resources; and the children can bond with their parents (who are now emotionally available and consistent) so they have the chance to trust them and hand back control.

Only then, with the help of specialized family counseling, will the wound be able to heal, and their behavior cease to be so disruptive or even dangerous for them. Procedures aimed at eliminating the tantrums and fits of rage in a purely behavioral way (for example, «extinction»), have a very limited effect. It is possible, (though unlikely) that they may reduce the crises, but they don't repair anything. A brain with disorganized attachment will turn to these responses when it feels in danger because that's what it is programmed to do. Of course, the problem won't have been «extinguished», but it will have left a child who is asking for a coherent framework where her brain can mature, with no way of expressing her emotions. Hence, she will experience defenselessness. How are you supposed to feel when all your tools are taken away, however inappropriate they may be? Probably even more defenseless. They are your tools and they are the only ones you have.

When traumas go unnoticed

t is possible for a «traumatic» experience to leave a lasting impression, although not all cases are that serious. So, what is trauma exactly? Is it some terrible thing that happens to other families?

Generally speaking, trauma is a complex, global neuroendocrine response to an experience that exceeds our resources.

From a more psychological perspective, trauma is seen as an emotional wound; the consequences of an experience we have been unable to integrate emotionally. It may be something small, almost invisible, which is why the cause of our unease so often goes unnoticed. Our ability to integrate this experience into the fabric of our life depends on several factors: your age at the time (the brain is constantly evolving so the exact same experience may be fun for a teenager but intolerable for a 5 year old child); the cognitive and emotional resources you had at the time of the event; the skill of the adults around you in making sense of the experience; experience; the context; the gravity of the repercussions (if there is physical as well as emotional suffering, for example)... These circumstances amongst others, can mean the difference between moving forward with your life or, getting trapped by the experience.

Did you know that some people are particularly vulnerable to trauma?

Did you know that some people are particularly vulnerable to trauma? As we have seen, early experiences can link to chronic disorders in brain functioning, lowering its sensitivity threshold to emotionally charged situations. The range of strategic responses is reduced. The brain may be especially alert to certain stimuli (according to what was dangerous in the past) or, conversely, may have learned to ignore the warning signs of danger in order to maintain the relationship with our attachment figures.

On the one hand, our brain «protects» us from a negative image of our parents; yet, on the other, it learns to ignore information that would be relevant for avoiding dangerous situations in the future.

However, an accumulation of stressful experiences in a short period of time can exhaust the adaptation resources of both children and adults. In this sense, when parents are experiencing grief, stress, depression, etc., they have fewer resources available to contain their children and help them to integrate difficult experiences.

So, which experiences can be potentially «traumatic»? The list is varied and, in some cases, quite surprising: falls and all kinds of accidents; experiencing «suffocation» (choking, being winded by a fall); getting momentarily lost on the street or in a shopping mall; serious illnesses; dental and surgical procedures (intravenous lines, invasive exploratory examinations, repeated injections or stitches); prolonged immobilization (casts, orthopedic corsets…); sentimental losses (death of a loved one or even a pet); separation and divorce; moving house; bullying; witnessing a violent attack (in the home, on the street, in video games or movies); sudden, loud noises as an infant, and other stressors such as extreme temperatures; going without food for a long time, and a long list of etc. Not forgetting of course, kidnappings, sexual abuse and aggressions, natural disasters, terrorist attacks, wars and displacement.

Any one of us can be exposed to circumstances that can, potentially, lead to a sudden shift in our well-being.

Any one of us, i.e. any «normal» person leading a «normal» life, can be exposed to circumstances that can, potentially, lead to a sudden shift in our well-being. In many cases, these situations are bound to happen sooner or later: children fall, break bones and need casts and stitches; they choke on something or they get lost. You must be ready to see them for what they are: normal life situations and opportunities for growth.

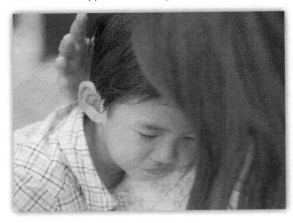

Situations that adults get over easily, can cause children great distress.

Therefore, you must equip yourself with all the right tools: cultivate your own resources for handling critical situations. Children rely on you to identify their emotions, to put them into words and offload their negative feelings. They are emotionally fused with you: if they fall and see a look of terror on your face, their fear will multiply, not just because of their own discomfort, but because they sense that the person who should keep them safe is unable to cope and, therefore, can't help them. Adults must always be on their guard. That isn't to say that you shouldn't show your fear or helplessness (you should!), but do it with other adults, never in front of the children.

If they fall and see a look of terror on your face, their fear will multiply, not just because of their own discomfort, but because they sense that the person who should keep them safe is unable to cope and, therefore, can't help them.

So, you have two jobs to do: First, increase your resource responses and second, activate your adult support network. By doing so you will be able to meet your child's needs at that moment in time, (providing her with safety and calm, helping her to recover her well-being and acquire resources for next time). This will strengthen your position as a role model and improve the bond between you.

She will know that you are responsive and available, capable of containing her and helping her move forward. What more can you ask for!

It is essential you recognize the core indicators of childhood trauma in order to tell if you should seek help for your child. How do I know if my child has fully got over that situation or if she has got stuck? The symptoms of childhood trauma can be disguised or confusing. Some are ostensibly non-specific and may be common to other conditions (neurodevelopmental problems or issues associated with early-life abandonment, for example). Hence why it is so important to choose the right professional who can distinguish between them and work as part of a team.

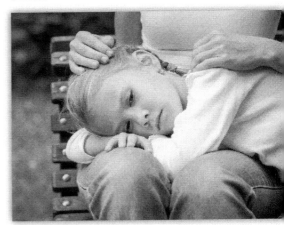

The symptoms of childhood trauma can be disguised or confusing. Some are ostensibly non-specific and may be common to other conditions (neurodevelopmental problems or issues associated with early-life abandonment, for example).

Reactions to a threatening situation can be divided into two groups: active defense responses (fight, flight or attachment cry) and passive defense responses (freezing and submission). Your brain quickly analyzes which is the best option of all those available to you at the time, taking into account the circumstances surrounding the threat and your real possibilities at that moment, and chooses the one that offers the best guarantees of survival. This happens in milliseconds and sets in motion different neural circuits of response in the autonomic nervous system (ANS).

When our experiences are so overwhelming that they can't be integrated as just another episode in the fabric of our life, our response mechanisms remain activated It is exactly the same for infants, children and adults. So, what symptoms might your child have in that situation? In infants and young children, a submissive response may take the form of lethargy; distancing themselves from people; refusing to play; excessive shyness; sadness; loss of enjoyment in previously rewarding activities; loss of muscle tone; a slowdown of breathing and heart rate or modified body posture (drooped shoulders and arms, a hunched back...). When the response is one of hyperactivation they may: be very distressed; cry inconsolably; have tantrums they didn't previously have; be hypervigilant and alert; be short-tempered and irritable; reject any changes (even small changes of plan!); get very anxious and be unable to return to a relaxed state; suffer chronic muscle tension in their shoulders and back; experience disorders affecting the digestive system and gut or skin disorders.

Moreover, all these vague symptoms can appear unexpectedly and, as far as the adults are concerned, not seem directly related to what is going on at the time. Their nervous system is trapped in this state of hypo- or hyperactivation and needs help to return to a balanced, secure state.

In this sense, we know that the alarm in our brain activates our entire body. However, little children have difficulty expressing physical discomfort. Infants will appear agitated or, conversely, immobile. In later stages, we see gastrointestinal problems, headaches, very rapid shallow breathing and even problems related to food (the may reject certain textures and types of food, or develop a fear of swallowing, for example). When they are trapped in a traumatic experience, it's as though the threat were still present, resulting in chronic stress for their body. They need to switch off the alarm in their brain in order to rest. Therefore, it is good to remind them they are here in the present where the danger has passed, and they can feel safe again.

When our experiences are so overwhelming that they can't be integrated as just another episode in the fabric of our life, our response mechanisms remain activated

When they are trapped in a traumatic experience, it's as though the threat were still present, resulting in chronic stress. They need to switch off the alarm in their brain in order to rest.

They often show signs of re-living the event (when playing or sleeping). Their brain is trying to process what happened. You can see this in repetitive games where they act out the event in some way or, at least the most shocking part of it, the way they experienced it. Keep an eye on them, let them play and with support, little by little they will start to introduce more comforting, reassuring elements and different endings to the story. If not, you need to consult a psychotherapist.

They may also revert to more childish behavior from stages they have already successfully completed (for example wetting themselves or using baby-talk again). All these are signs they are crying out for love and safety, hugs, warmth and relaxing games for as long as it takes. No two children will react in the same way to the same experience and they will require different amounts of time to get over it. One way of staying quietly connected and accepting of them is to respect this time.

Sometimes trauma symptoms are mistakenly diagnosed as attention deficit, behavioral disorders or hyperactivity.

In later stages children also display blocking or hyperactivation, although the way it is expressed may differ slightly: difficulty paying attention and «daydreaming», (sometimes mistakenly diagnosed as ADHD or behavioral disorders!); decreased academic performance; irritability; increased fears and aggressive behavior such as hitting things or even people, (they often pick a fight as a way of mobilizing the physical energy that was blocked during the event). When the alarm goes off, the body generates a lot of energy to be able to escape or fight. When this isn't possible, this energy is trapped inside the body, causing discomfort and even pain.

This energy must be released in a controlled way. Many children will be able to process what happened adequately if they are allowed to, and it is chaneled correctly.

They also have stomachaches and headaches (with no physical cause), as well as many of the potential signs of trauma in younger children. In addition, we usually see feelings of helplessness and hopelessness because they are now capable of reasoning about the consequences of what happened. There are times they feel they influence everything going on around them, that they are the centre of the universe. So, you often find them lost in thought, pondering what they could have done differently and feeling guilty.

The symptoms in adolescents are more like those of adults.

This aspect is exacerbated in adolescents who are capable of more sophisticated thinking. Their symptoms are more like those of adults. Their brain creates flashbacks of the traumatic event and, to avoid the negative feelings this causes, they avoid all the situations, places, people, smells... that might remind them of the experience. If their memories are very intense and they don't handle them adequately, or, conversely, encapsulate them, they may try to desensitize themselves through drugs, alcohol and other kinds of risky behavior. On the one hand, this type of behavior acts as an «anesthetic» (when they are highly activated and upset). On the other, it can be a way of feeling alive again after «freezing» with fear (self-harming, etc.). You need to be particularly mindful to symptoms of numbness in parts of their body, or an increase in their pain threshold (they say they don't feel anything, that nothing hurts them). These are signs they are having great difficulty assimilating the traumatic experience.

In cases where there is no natural, forward progression and the symptoms persist, a psychotherapist is a must.

In cases where there is no natural, forward progression and the symptoms persist, a psychotherapist who can help to find a solution is a must. In the same way you would take them to hospital if a wound wouldn't stop bleeding or their temperature wouldn't come down. As their caregiver you may not have all the necessary tools to help them fix the situation, but your role is essential.

However, your role isn't to apply techniques for overcoming post-traumatic stress. Your role is to notice when something is wrong, let them know you are keeping an eye on them and that you will do whatever it takes to stop them suffering. Always in their own time and at their own pace. This healing, in the moment, attitude will help to restore their confidence that things will be okay again because they are safe and secure with you.

When fitting in is a challenge

Our expectations are a product of our education, culture, experience, the time and place we live in, but also of our personal limitations! For this reason, we often find that our children don't live up to these expectations. Do they move about a lot, not pay attention or behave as expected? Perhaps they don't learn at the same speed as the rest?

Sometimes, our children don't live up to expectations.

A diagnosis of ADHD (Attention Deficit Hyperactivity Disorder), or conduct disorder, or other similar terms that are so common place these days, do nothing but label people and limit their perspective as well as that of those around them. These labels describe what is absent, not what is present, and can be even more limiting if the clinical approach is one-dimensional. If the framework of understanding is narrow, we only see part of the picture. If we get to see the whole picture, we will have a deeper appreciation of the possibilities that present themsleves and will be able to offer a more accurate picture of what is going on.

In the chapter on learning disabilities we raised awareness of the risks of diagnostic labels and the need for a holistic map of the child that considers their limitations but also their potential. If we take normality to be a continuum, we see that the extremes do not have to be limiting. They simply inform us about each person's individual characteristics.

During childhood, having diffuse awareness, or attention deficit is likely to be a problem at school. Attending to several stimuli at the same time, being impulsive.

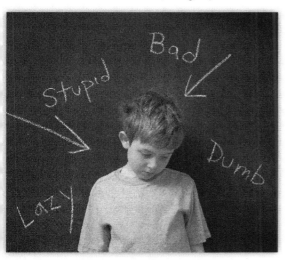

However, if you were asked to select a creative director, the manager of a large company, a mediator, a fireman, the person in charge of managing a crisis... would you prefer a person capable of generating ideas, of reacting quickly, etc., or someone who is very intellectual?

The fact is that all strengths are valuable. Probably not all the time and not in every context, but we should value them because they play an essential role in the overall dynamics. Every brain is different, this is the richness of humans. Were you aware that Steve Jobs had an ADHD diagnosis? So too do chef Jamie Oliver, the amazing Bill Gates, Will Smith and Michael Phelps? Did you know that singer Tony Bennett and author Agatha Christie were both dyslexic? Do they seem like successful people to you? How about Leonardo da Vinci, Albert Einstein...? All these people were able to find their place, use their strengths and stand out.

Every brain is different, this is the richness of humans.

So, how does a child with these characteristics become a happy, fulfilled adult? Through the acceptance and approval they receive from their role models. From you. That's all. That's what they tell us.

Your child's identity starts to take shape through the way you look at her, right from infancy: what you can see and appreciate in her, what you tell her about herself through your comments and gestures... This is how you can showcase her strengths, give her hope that her time will come, accompany her along the way and provide options. Alternatively, you can convey the idea that she is inadequate, inferior, stupid. It's up to you to make her feel good about herself!

Your child's identity starts to take shape through the way you look at her, right from infancy: what you can see and appreciate in her, what you tell her about herself through your comments and gestures...

Quite often we are most demanding with the children who are most like us. Did you know there is a strong genetic component to some learning disabilities? Sometimes we see ourselves clearly reflected in them, at others, we do it subconsciously. We connect with the experiences we had in our childhood and sometimes react as though we were re-living them now. This complicates the adult-child relationship because we are functioning on an emotional rather than a rational level. Hence, it's likely that if you are the parent of children with attention deficit, who also had problems concentrating at school themselves, you are more demanding and less understanding now. Or perhaps the reverse is true, you shun the help that is available now because «I experienced that too and got through it without help and it's made me a stronger adult. It's not such a big deal, there's nothing wrong with her».

It's a good idea to check if your expectations have more to do with your own limitations than her potential. Ditch the past and look afresh; appreciate her for who she is and be thankful. Because the best way to grow is to feel seen and accepted for who we really are.

We tend to be more demanding with the children who are most like us.

Have you stopped to think what she is telling you with this hyperactivity? It may be functional behavior (that is, it has a function, serves a purpose and achieves its aim). Possibly to mobilize you. Maybe she has an ambivalent attachment pattern and tries to attract your attention through disruptive behavior. She may do this with her teacher too and annoy her classmates by interrupting. If she doesn't get what she needs (containment, coherence), her behavior will probably continue to escalate until she has real behavioral problems. Maybe she has a disorganized attachment pattern and is incapable of self-regulating because her attachment figures are also scared and disoriented.

Does she have a problem paying attention? While her head seems to be in the clouds, she could be focusing all her attention on emotional aspects, for example. She is focusing very intensely, just not on what she's been asked to do.

These circumstances among others, together with those directly related to neurodevelopment can create difficulties learning at school. There needs to be a global assessment of the situation to explore all the possible causes and find integrated solutions that can really make a difference. It's likely a team will be required, comprising a family and child psychologist, a developmental physiotherapist, a speech therapist and other professionals who can draw a clear, global roadmap.

But the diagnosis doesn't matter. They're only words. Find reliable professionals to guide you and, meanwhile, take a moment each day to observe her progress in relation to her potential in context. Be her secure role model. Help her grow. Consider what motivates her. Not just what she's good at but what she likes. If something excites her, she will spend endless time and energy on it. Appreciate her ability, effort, motivation and achievements. And tell her. Create opportunities to talk about how she feels about it and welcome her emotions. Talk to her about how you felt at her age and offer her what you learned about how to handle it. By doing this, not only will you be strengthening her self-concept, but also the bond between you which is what is so often at stake.

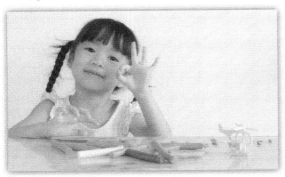

Be her secure role model. Help her grow. Appreciate her ability, effort, motivation and achievements. And tell her.

SUMMARY

In premature babies, bonding can be created through responsive synchronization with their rhythms; through your touch, where possible; your gaze; your voice, which should be softer than ever...

The level of calm and self-regulation with which you approach her as parents, will have a direct effect on her well-being and development. If you are in-tune with yourselves, you will be open to noticing what she feels and converying to her that you will be a source of calm, safety and love for her.

Following a difficult labor-birth, it is essential any negative feelings that may have arisen in the mother (pain, suffering, worry) are worked on, and that the infant has a physiotherapy examination to help restore her physical well-being and increase her physiological regulation. Subsequently, joint mother-infant perinatal therapy will be able to restore the interrupted tuning between the two.

When there have been previous pregnancy losses it is vital to complete the grieving process before trying again. Give yourself as much time as you need and get all the help you need to get you through it. This way you will be ready to welcome a new parenting adventure when the time is right.

Adopted children have lived through an initial situation of abandonment that has left a significant emotional imprint on their internal regulation system. It is possible that their prior experiences have impacted their nervous system in other ways too, so a specialized psychological examination is needed in order to be able to accompany them in the development process if necessary. As you build a bond with your child, you must include the repair of this initial interrupted bond in a conscious, directed way. It is a path of constant growth along which every interaction between you weaves a safety net of love.

When the family environment is confusing, stressful or threatening in some way, a child's brain develops in a particular way, and the attachment system that determines how we will relate to ourselves and others in the future is clearly affected. If possible, individual or family therapy is needed in these cases to heal emotional wounds, provide the child with regulation tools, and to restructure or reprogram the bonding patterns that will accompany them throughout the rest of their life.

In the case of conduct disorders, extreme irritability, persistent anger or angry outbursts, these are emotional difficulties that require your external regulation. The way to tackle these situations is to adopt a two-pillared approach; this involves having a clear vision of what is behind the behavior and acquiring the parenting strategies to provide them with whatever they need to feel good about themselves again.

The way children respond to traumatic experiences that exceed their capacity to cope and overwhelm them emotionally, can vary greatly and include lethargy or, conversely, hyperactivity. They may also present difficulties with attention, irritability, immune system disorders, unremitting physical pain, etc. Therefore, it is essential you consult a specialist psychotherapist if you notice changes in your child following a shocking or painful experience, or the loss of a significant person in their life. The therapist will be able to activate all the physiological, emotional and cognitive resources to enable them to calm down in readiness for the therapeutic work of integrating the experience into the fabric of their life in an adaptive way. Experiences that are not processed leave a neuro-biological imprint on the brain so there is a strong case for consulting an expert.

In the case of learning disabilities, attention deficit, symptoms of hyperactivity, it is possible to help a child manage their neurodevelopmental deficiences through combined treatment. It is important to take care of their self-esteem by highlighting the skills they excel at and creating opportunities for them to feel appreciated and valuable. A diagnosis does not define who a person is or what they are like, it merely provides information about how they function in certain areas at a specific moment in time. A human being is constantly evolving, especially when they are accompanied by professionals in their learning process. Development knows no bounds and you must restore this potential for change in your child through the way you see them.

What can you do?

HELPFUL PRACTICAL ADVICE

- If you have experienced pregnancy losses, take your time and air your feelings. Share them, make them visible and give the process the importance it deserves. When you are ready, hold a meaningful memorial or farewell ceremony. If you feel that you are not progressing through your grief, you need to see a grief counselor who will accompany you through all the stages so that you can return to your usual self.

- If you want to increase your self-regulation resources, try practising yoga or mindfulness or any other activity you feel «re-situates» you and makes you feel calm again. Even plain old walking helps build better connections between the two brain hemispheres, making it easier to process whatever we are dealing with. There are some very simple things that can help you to feel balanced and stay within your window of tolerance.

- Focus on the support you receive from loved ones and share your experiences with them. Surround yourself with positive people who are glad to be alive and who will help you to savor every single moment. Be less self-demanding and keep an eye on your responses. If you stop for a second to observe how you feel, your gut feeling will tell you what you need to feel even better. You should listen to your gut feelings.

- In those cases where there were problems in the early stages (difficult births, separation due to hospitalization, prematurity, adoption...), the professionals best qualified to help you and your baby are psychotherapists specializing in EMDR or Sensorimotor psychotherapists with a family-centered approach.

- In the case of adoption, it is more important than ever to reinforce the consistency, availability and predictability of your responses because, not only do you need to build an attachment relationship, you also need to repair a missing relationship too. When looking for a professional, it is essential they have intensive training in family and attachment therapy and, more specifically in early-life abandonment related trauma treatment.

- If some of your lived experiences still have a big impact on you now and affect the way you live, or if they continue to act as strong trigger whenever you recall them..., it's important you know that they will also be affecting the way you bond. In these cases, the DMS recommends EMDR therapy as the most efficient (fast and effective) way of working on postraumatic stress and dissociation, as well as experiences that may have become «stuck» in your memory. Sensorimotor therapy can help you to work on the trauma through the body. You can find the therapist best suited to your needs at: http://emdr-es.orgl/web-2-0-directory and https://www.sensorimotorpsychotherapy.org

- In the case of learning disabilities, don't accept a one-dimensional diagnosis: look for a team of professionals who work in an integrated way, who communicate with each other and with the school, and involve you in the process. The team should include an educational psychologist, a speech therapist, a developmental physiotherapist, an optometrist and a clinical psychologist. This team will offer you myriad options and accompany you on the path to your child's growth and development.

- Don't forget that, sometimes, the symptoms children display can be confusing, (for example, excessive moment could be a sign of significant emotion dysregulation that would be aggravated by certain drugs). If you only have one view of the case, it can lead to a very limited range of options. Having a professional trained in a broad range of child development on board, can provide cross-cutting responses resulting in more accurate solutions and the possibility of tapping in to help from any other professionals he or she deem necessary.

BIBLIOGRAPHY

When they arrive ahead of schedule:

To learn more about the effects of maternal deprivation due to hospitalization and about the benefits of skin-to-skin contact:

Brazelton TB. *Niños prematuros. En: BrazeltonTB. Momentos clave en la vida de tu hijo. Barcelona: Plaza y Janés; 2001.*

Bergman N, Bergman J. *Kangaroo mother care. Kangaroo Mother Care Promotions; 2005.*

De Bellis M, Keshavan M, Clarck D, Casey B, Giedd J, Boring A, et al. *Developmental traumatology. Part II: Brain Development. Biological Psychiatry. 1999;45:1271-84.*

Hernández-Martínez C, Canals Sans J, Fernández-Ballart J. *Parents' perceptions of their neonates and their relation to infant development. Child: care, health and development. 2011;37(4):484-92.*

Neu M, Robinson J, Schmiege SJ. *Influence of holding practice on pre-term infant development. MCN. The American journal of maternal child nursing. 2013;38(3):136.*

Rutter M. *Maternal deprivation reassessed. Short-term effects of «maternal deprivation». Cap. 3 (29-52). Harmondsworth, Middlesex, Inglaterra: Penguin Books; 1972.*

Wijnroks L. *Maternal recollected anxiety and mother infant interaction in preterm infants. Infant Mental Health Journal. 1999;20(4):393-409.*

When our child is born halfway round the world:

Limiñana AMR, Bueno AB. *La construcción del vínculo afectivo en la adopción: La teoría del apego como marco de referencia en la intervención post-adoptiva. International Journal of Developmental and Educational Psychology: INFAD. Revista de Psicología. 2011;1(1):333-40.*

Montano, G. *Alteraciones del apego en adopciones tardías. Sus consecuencias y posibles abordajes terapéuticos. Revista de psicoterapia psicoanalítica. 2011;12(4):29-41.*

Ricart Carratalà E. *Factores de buen pronóstico en la adopción: cómo valorarlos. Temas de Psicoanálisis. 2014 Jul;8.*

Román M, Palacios J. *Separación, pérdida y nuevas vinculaciones: el apego en la adopción. Acción Psicológica. 2011;8(2).*

Rosas M, Gallardo I, Angulo P. Factores que influyen en el apego y la adaptación de los niños adoptados. Revista de Psicología. 2000;9(1):145.

Sánchez EL. Una aproximación a la adopción desde la teoría del apego. Informació psicològica.2015;82:14-20.

When there is nowhere to hide:

Ballester CG, Mañes RJM, Llario MDG. Desorganización del apego y el trastorno traumático del desarrollo (TTD). International Journal of Developmental and Educational Psychology. Revista INFAD de Psicología. 2016;3(1):375-84.

Farina B, Liotti G. Dimensione dissociativa e trauma dello sviluppo. Cognitivismo clinico. 2011;8(1):3-17.

Hesse E, Main M. Second-generation effects of unresolved trauma in non maltreating parents: Dissociated, frightened and threatening parental behavior. Psychoanalytic Inquiry. 1999;19(4):481-540.

Lecannelier F, Ascanio L, Flores F, Hoffmann M. Apego y psicopatología: una revisión actualizada sobre los modelos etiológicos parentales del apego desorganizado. Terapia psicológica. 2011;29(1):107-16.

Liotti G. Disorganized attachment in the etiology of the dissociative disorders. Dissociation. 1992;5(4):196-204.

Liotti G, Farina B. Sviluppi traumatici: eziopatogenesi, clinica e terapia della dimensione dissociativa. R. Cortina Ed.; 2011.

Main, M, Hesse E. Parents' unresolved traumatic experiences are related to infant disorganized attachment status: Is frightened and/or frightening parental behavior the linking mechanism? En: Greenberg M, Cicchetti D, Cummings M, eds. Attachment in the Preschool Years. Chicago: University of Chicago Press; 1990. p. 161-84.

Main M, Solomon J. Procedures for identifying infants as disorganized/disoriented during the Ainsworth Strange Situation. Attachment in the Preschool Years. En: Greenberg M, Cicchetti D, Cummings M, eds. Attachment in the Preschool Years. Chicago: University of Chicago Press; 1990. p. 121-60.

Morris-Smith J, Silvestre M. EMDR para la próxima generación. EMDR Biblioteca; 2017.

Teicher MH, Andersen SL, Polcari A, Anderson CM, Navalta CP. Developmental neurobiology of childhood stress and trauma. Psychiatr Clin North Am. 2002;25:397-426.

Teicher MH, Samson JA, Polcari A, McGreenery CE. Sticks stones and hurtful words: relative effects of various forms of childhood maltreatment. American Journal Psychiatry.2006;163:993-1000.

When we are hijacked by anger:

Crittenden PM. Apego y psicopatología. Nuevas implicaciones clínicas de la teoría del apego.Valencia: Promolibro; 2002.

Siegel DJ. La mente en desarrollo. Madrid: Desclée de Brower; 2007.

When traumas go unnoticed:

To find out more about how trauma affects us:

Levine PA, Kline M. El trauma visto por los niños. Editorial Eleftheria; 2016.

Odgen P, Fisher J. Sensoriomotor Psychotherapy: Interventions for Trauma and Attachment [Trad. cast.: Psicoterapia sensoriomotriz: Intervenciones para el trauma y el apego. Bilbao: Desclée de Brouwer, 2016]. Nueva York: Norton.

Ogden P, Minton K, Pain C. El trauma y el cuerpo. Un modelo sensorio-motor de psicoterapia. Desclée de Brouwer; 2009.

Porges SW. The Polyvagal Theory. Madrid: Pléyades; 2017.

Porges SW. Neuroception: A subconscious system for detecting threats and safety. Zero to Three Journal. 2004 8 May;24(5):19-24.

Salvador M. El trauma psicológico: un proceso neurofisiológico con consecuencias psicológicas. Revista de psicoterapia. 2009;20(80):5-16.

Shore, AN. Affect dysregulation and disorders of the self: The neurobiology as emotional development. Hillsdale, NJ: Lawrence Erlbaum Associates; 1994.

Van der Kolk BA, Pelcovitz D, Roth S, Mandel FS, McFarlane A, Herman JL. Dissociation, somatization, and affect dysregulation: The complexity of adaptation to trauma. American Journal of Psychiatry. 1996;153:83-93.

Van der Kolk, BA. El cuerpo lleva la cuenta. Cerebro, mente y cuerpo en la superación del trauma. Editorial Eleftheria; 2014.

Acknowledgements

Thank you Jara, for accepting the invitation to take on this project that was custom-made for us. Your view of children and your deep understanding of their struggles in life has, gently but surely, shaped mine too.

. . . .

Thank you Lucila for having faith in this project from the moment we put pen to paper. Your guts and zeal to produce this book from scratch, were invaluable.

Thank you Noa and Dana, for the adventure of being your dad and the wonderful daily challenge that represents; for everything I learn about myself, my strengths and my weaknesses; for the way you confront me with the fragility of life and, at the same time, its incredible force. For the pure joy of living.

Thanks Iryna, for making my path smoother in life, for filling my gaze with flowers and my existence with the fresh aroma of newly cut grass.

Thanks Gema, for the true meaning of unconditional.

Huge thanks to all of you, health professionals, psychologists, teachers, moms and dads, everyone who read the draft, for your encouragement, ideas, wishes, editing, hopes and love for this project.

Iñaki Pastor Pons

I want to thank Iñaki, my comrade in arms in inspirational projects, for giving me this extraordinary opportunity to convey our shared practice of whole-hearted commitment to helping children and supporting their families.

. . . .

My mother and father, for having the courage to overcome every parenting challenge they faced and continue developing as role models, fostering my curiosity and desire for permanent growth, teaching me to commit myself and to continue to seek a more conscious presence in the world.

My sister Rebeca, for her valor and clarity that are like a beacon in every project I undertake.

My grandma Pilar, for being a source of unconditional love.

Teresa, for her dependability. For being my safe place where I can work on all things great and small in life.

Mercedes, whose outlook on life is a constant source of growth and support.

Bruno, Blanca, Marco, Lorién and Daniel, whose very existence fills my life with joy.

And Robert, for the simple, resolute way he navigates the world that has helped me to grow beyond anything I ever thought posible, keeping my feet on the ground yet, at the same time, allowing me to fly.

Because emotional role models hold together the jigsaw puzzle that is the ground beneath our feet.

They are all pieces of my jigsaw.

Jara Acín y Rivera

How can I find pediatric physiotherapists who specialize in development?

Physiotherapists trained in Pediatric Integrative Manual Therapy (PIMT) have a good understanding of the model of infant and child development you have seen in this book. They have the skill to treat dysfunctions in the spine or skull and also to reprogram and reeducate the nervous system to improve its function.

You will find a list of PIMT physiotherapists in different countries on the following website: **www.tmpi-pimt.com**

These professionals can help you and your child with different health problems, whether they are caused by pain (eg headaches, neck pain or colic in babies, etc.), neuro-orthopedic problems (eg plagiocephaly), morphological changes to the feet or back, etc.) or by mild to moderate developmental problems (eg. learning, attention, or coordination issues, etc.).

For cases involving neurological damage or respiratory physiotherapy, you can turn to the professional body or association of physiotherapists or kinesiologists in your area or country, where no doubt they will be able to inform you of the specialists with the appropriate professional training. In Spain there is a Spanish Society of Pediatric Physiotherapy (SEFIP) which brings together physiotherapists involved in the field of pediatrics and associated health professions: **www.sefip.org**.

How do I find psychotherapists who specialize in attachment and trauma?

In order to work on bonding and attachment it is essential to have an overview of the dynamics between the family members. Therefore, it is important you contact a child and adolescent psychotherapist trained in family intervention (preferably one who specializes in systemic family intervention). They will work on the relationships between you and involve you in the process, mobilizing the resources of each family member to achieve the balance necessary for well-being.

For traumatic situations, the WHO recommends EMDR therapy as the most efficient (effective and timely) way of managing post-traumatic stress and dissociation, as well as experiences that have become "stuck" in the memory. You can find more information on the website **emdr-es.org**.To find the practitioner best suited to your needs, go to: **http://emdr-es.org/web-2-0-directory/**.

You will find professionals who specialize in children and adolescents, and attachment and grief, among others, in the EMDR Association.

This is the link for the EMDR Iberoamérica (in Spanish and Portuguese):

http://www.emdriberoamerica.org/

The link for the rest of the world is: **http://www.emdria.org/**

Sensorimotor therapy will help you use your body to work through trauma and address your bonding history. You can find a therapist here:

https://www.sensorimotorpsychotherapy.org

ADHD: Attention Deficit Hyperactivity Disorder.

Amygdala: a structure in the brain that forms part of the limbic system and processes all aspects of our emotional responses.

Attachment trauma: this term refers to situations in which the traumatic experience occurs in an individual's relationships with their attachment figures.

Autonomic nervous system: this is the part of the nervous system that regulates and coordinates many unconscious and automatic bodily functions such as: organ function, respiratory rate, the secretion of several hormones and stress adaptation. It is divided into two branches: sympathetic and parasympathetic, which have antagonistic effects that achieve a functional balance.

Brainstem: is the largest communication highway between the forebrain, the spinal cord and the peripheral nerves. It also controls several functions such as breathing and regulating heart rate.

Central nervous system: a biological structure present in individuals of the animal kingdom that includes the brain and spinal cord. It is organized into levels, each of which is controlled by those above it. It is a very complex system responsible for perceiving stimuli from the outside world, processing information and transmitting impulses to nerves and muscles.

Cortex: a coating on the surface of the cerebral hemispheres composed of gray matter. The most evolved part of the brain, it is highly developed in humans.

Cortisol: hormone produced by the adrenal gland, which is released as a response to stress, triggering the body's response to perceived threats.

Embryo: is the initial stage in the development of a living being while it is in the egg or mother's uterus.

EMDR: the English abbreviation of Eye Movement Desensitization and Reprocessing. It is a psychotherapeutic approach based on neurobiology. See more on emdr-es.org.

Epigenetics: refers to the study of factors which play a very important role in modern genetics by interacting with the genes, although, strictly speaking, they are not considered to be components of classical genetics.

Dissociation: the brain's reaction to an extremely traumatic experience, whether a big emotional impact or a situation in which there is a constant threat or emotional neglect.

Genetics: the field of biology that studies genes and the mechanisms that regulate the transmission of hereditary traits.

Immune system: responsible for protecting the body against external biological agents and for repairing damaged tissues.

Locus coeruleus: the region of the brainstem involved in the response to threatening situations that cause stress and panic.

Mesencephalon: is the upper structure of the brainstem, also known as the mid-brain.

Methylphenidate: is the active ingredient of the psychostimulant drug approved for treating Attention Deficit Hyperactivity Disorder.

Motor: refers to motion or movement.

Motor system: made up of the organs, brain areas and nerves responsible for preparing, organizing and executing movement.

Myelination: is the process of forming a myelin sheath around a nerve. This substance protects and improves nerve conduction.

Nociception: is the perception of damage that travels from the body to the brain through specialized nerve pathways.

Occupational Therapist: a health professional who promotes health and well-being in children and adults through holistic approaches to functional rehabilitation.

Olfactory bulb: a structure in the brain involved in the sense of smell that helps to manage the information obtained through this sense.

Perinatal: refers to the period around childbirth.

PIMT: Pediatric Integrative Manual Therapy: a field of physiotherapy that involves assessing and treating muscle, bone and joint dysfunctions in infants and children in the framework of sensorimotor development. Find out more at www.tmpi-pimt.com.

Postnatal: refers to the period after childbirth.

Prenatal: refers to the period before childbirth.

Primitive reflexes: automatic stereotypic movements present in the fetus before birth that are needed in the early months of life for survival and for maturation of the nervous system.

Proprioception: is the sense that informs the body of the position and tension of the muscles and the location of the bones.

Psychophysiological regulation: the process of re-establishing the balance and correct functioning of the autonomic nervous system which restores physical and emotional well-being.

PTSD (Post-traumatic Stress Disorder): is a range of specific symptoms found in people who have seen or been directly involved in, an extremely traumatic event which caused them to experience reactions of intense fear, helplessness or horror. The symptoms can be grouped into several areas including avoidance, persistent negative alterations in cognition and mood swings, as well as enhanced psychophysiological activation.

Sensory system: consists of organs, brain areas and nerves that are responsible for detecting and processing information from the environment or the body itself.

Speech therapist: professional who deals with the prevention, evaluation and intervention of human communication disorders.

Stabilization reflexes: automatisms responsible for stabilizing the gaze when the head moves.

Thalamus: nervous structure located within the brain responsible for receiving sensory information from the body and relaying it to the nerve centers in charge of processing it.

Trauma: experiencing a threatening situation we cannot escape from or effectively neutralize because it excedes our capacity for emotional management. Trauma triggers (psychological and physical) defense mechanisms.

Vestibular system: consists of organs, brain areas and nerves responsible for sensing movement and positioning of the head.

Printed in Great Britain
by Amazon